'This timely collection by leading experts will be an excellent resource for academics and practitioners alike as the need to agree on criteria for establishing good healthcare becomes ever more urgent. Highly recommended'.
– **Graham Scambler**, *Emeritus Professor of Sociology, University College London*

'At a time when national health services across Europe are facing huge pressures, there is an urgent need for a book which maps their changing features and considers how they can be sustained. This excellent edited collection provides a detailed understanding of these issues and the key actors involved and offers some proposals for their future directions'.
– **Jon Gabe**, *Emeritus Professor, Royal Holloway University London*

'[This] is an example of solid scholarship, an excellent, illuminating and much-needed book that students of comparative welfare, policymakers, health professionals and concerned citizens cannot afford to miss'.
– **Alberto Martinelli**, *Emeritus Professor, University of Milan*

National Health Services of Western Europe

This book draws on research within neo-Weberian and neo-institutionalist perspectives to critically analyse National Health Services (NHSs) in Western Europe. Exploring the challenges posed by neo-liberal policies, it also looks at the impact of the role of the state, the medical profession, the public and the medical–industrial complex in their development.

Bringing together a top-line range of expert international contributors, this book includes national studies from three European macro-regions: Britain, Scandinavia and the Mediterranean. In the first part, the NHSs of each country considered are examined historically and in a contemporary context in face of emerging challenges – from cost containment to governance. The second part looks across the macro-regions at the influence of the main actors involved in their evolution and sustainability. Comparing and contrasting the NHSs of Western Europe, the book ends with a discussion of future directions.

This book makes a vital contribution at the time when health services globally have been under great pressure in the wake of the COVID-19 pandemic. It is written for academics and advanced students of healthcare, management, public policy, social policy and sociology – in addition to health professionals and policymakers.

Guido Giarelli is Professor of Sociology at the Magna Græcia University of Catanzaro, Italy.

Mike Saks is Emeritus Professor at the University of Suffolk, UK, where he was previously Research Professor in Health Policy.

Routledge Studies in Health and Social Welfare

The Ethics of Care
Moral Knowledge, Communication and the Art of Caregiving
Edited by Alan Blum and Stuart Murray

Diverse Perspectives on Aging in a Changing World
Edited by Gillian Joseph

**Globalization and the Health of Indigenous Peoples:
From Colonization to Self-Rule**
Ahsan Ullah

Participation in Health and Welfare Services
Professional Concepts and Lived Experience
Edited by Arne Henning Eide, Staffan Josephsson, Kjersti Vik

Governance Ethics in Healthcare Organizations
Gerard Magill and Lawrence Prybil

Transforming Healthcare with Qualitative Research
Edited by Frances Rapport and Jeffrey Braithwaite

Peer Research in Health and Social Development
International Perspectives on Participatory Research
Edited by Stephen Bell, Peter Aggleton and Ally Gibson

National Health Services of Western Europe
Challenges, Reforms and Future Perspectives
Edited by Guido Giarelli and Mike Saks

For more information about this series, please visit: https://www.routledge.com/Routledge-Studies-in-Health-and-Social-Welfare/book-series/RSHSW

National Health Services of Western Europe

Challenges, Reforms and Future Perspectives

**Edited by Guido Giarelli
and Mike Saks**

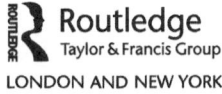

Routledge
Taylor & Francis Group

LONDON AND NEW YORK

Cover image: Getty Images

First published 2024
by Routledge
4 Park Square, Milton Park, Abingdon, Oxon OX14 4RN

and by Routledge
605 Third Avenue, New York, NY 10158

Routledge is an imprint of the Taylor & Francis Group, an informa business

British Library Cataloguing-in-Publication Data
A catalogue record for this book is available from the British Library

ISBN: 978-0-367-68959-9 (hbk)
ISBN: 978-1-032-53572-2 (pbk)
ISBN: 978-1-003-13979-9 (ebk)

DOI: 10.4324/9781003139799

Typeset in Sabon
by Apex CoVantage, LLC

Contents

The Mediterranean macro-region

The editors

Guido Giarelli is Professor of Sociology at the University Magna Græcia of Catanzaro in Italy, where he teaches sociology, sociology of health and medicine, social and health policies and the sociology of globalisation. He obtained his PhD degree at University College London in the United Kingdom (UK) and was Director of the Centro di Ricerca Interdipartimentale sui Sistemi sanitari e le Politiche di welfare in Italy. He was Founder and first President of the Società Italiana di Sociologia della Salute; Secretary and then member and Coordinator of the Board of the Section of Sociologia della salute e della medicina of the Associazione Italiana di Sociologia; member of the Board and then elected President of the European Society for Health and Medical Sociology; member of the Board and then Vice President of the International Sociological Association (ISA) Research Committee on the Sociology of Health; and he is currently Coordinator of the Board of the Research Network on the Sociology of Health and Medicine of the European Sociological Association. His main research interests are in the sociology of health and medicine, comparative health systems, self-help and civil society in healthcare reforms, non-conventional medicines and integrated medicine, illness narratives, person-centred medicine, and ageing and life course. Drawing on his knowledge of such areas, he has given presentations in many countries and published widely in many books and articles. Internationally in the course of his career, he has been Research Associate at the Institute of African Studies of the University of Nairobi, Adjunct Associate Professor at the School of Health Sciences of the Oakland University of Rochester in Michigan, Visiting Scholar at the New York Academy of Medicine and the Harvard Medical School in Boston in the United States (US), Visiting Professor at the University of Oviedo in Spain, the Escola de Saúde Pública do Ceará di Fortaleza in Brazil, the Centre for Sociological Theory and Research on Health Division and Population Health at University College London, the University of Coimbra and the University of Lisbon in Portugal, and at the Panteion University of Social and Political Sciences of Athens and the Miguel Hernandez University of Alicante in Spain.

Mike Saks is Emeritus Professor at the University of Suffolk and Visiting Professor at the University of Lincoln and the University of Westminster in the

UK and the University of Toronto, Canada. He was previously Visiting Chair at the University of Essex, Plymouth Marjon University and the Royal Veterinary College, University of London, in the UK. He received his PhD degree in sociology at the London School of Economics, where he also taught, and is Fellow of the Institute of Directors, the Institute of Knowledge Exchange, the Research Council for Complementary Medicine and the Royal Society of Arts. He was Provost and Chief Executive at University Campus Suffolk (UCS), Deputy Vice Chancellor at the University of Lincoln and Dean of Faculty of Health and Community Studies at De Montfort University – after contributing extensively to the Schools of Business, Law, Public Administration and Social Sciences there. He was until recently a Board member at Rose Bruford College of Theatre and Performance in London – having earlier served on the Executive at the University of Essex and University of East Anglia, which owned UCS. Professor Saks has published extensively in this context on health, professions, regulation and research methods. Aside from many keynote presentations at international conferences – a number of which he has co-organised – he has produced many journal articles/chapters, as well as over 20 edited and single-authored books with top publishers. His work spans the social sciences, from politics and social policy to his base discipline of sociology. He has won a number of national excellence awards in his university career and has a strong enterprise profile as highlighted by his membership of the Innovation Council, along with the chief executives of multinational corporations. He has also been a chair/member of many National Health Service committees at all levels – covering fields from the changing healthcare workforce to research and development. He was a member of, and academic adviser to, the National Institute of Health Research (NIHR) Research for Patient Benefit Committee and Suffolk NHS Primary Care Trust in the UK. He has formally advised the UK Departments of Health and professional bodies, including the General Medical Council and most recently the Royal College of Podiatry. In addition, he has been Chair of the UK Human Tissue Bank, the Research Council for Complementary Medicine and the British Acupuncture Accreditation Board. Internationally, he has participated in funded research on areas from the changing attitudes of physicians with the Russian Academy of Sciences in Moscow to care in the community with the University of Toronto. In 2013, he was Co-Chair and Speaker at the International Humanitarian Conference in Azerbaijan, with 14 Nobel Prize winners and eight heads of state, and gave the annual Distinguished Professor lecture at Arizona State University in the US. In 2014, he advised the Canadian government on health policy, receiving the Best Brains Exchange Award from Health Canada/Canadian Institutes of Health Research. In 2015, he was invited to the University of California in the US to discuss with its leaders health and educational governance. In 2016, he was a visitor to Wuhan University sponsored by the Chinese government. In 2017, he was appointed to the Advisory Council of the School of Creative Arts in Accra in Ghana. In 2018, he became Honorary Senior Adviser on Leadership to the United Nations (UN) and Co-Founder of the UN-endorsed Institute for Responsible Leadership, which he currently chairs. He was a previous President of the ISA Research Committee on Professional Groups, and is the current Vice President of the ISA Research Committee on the Sociology of Health – and a Board member of several top international journals, including serving as Associate Editor of the *Journal of Professions and Organization*. He is presently an appointed member on the World Health Organization Technical Expert Group on global health practitioner regulation.

Contributors

Joana Almeida is Senior Lecturer in applied social sciences (health and social care) in the School of Applied Social Sciences in the Faculty of Health and Social Sciences at the University of Bedfordshire in the UK.

Rob Baggott was until recently Professor of Public Policy and Director of the Health Policy Research Unit at De Montfort University in the UK.

Paula Blomqvist is Associate Professor in the Department of Government at Uppsala University in Sweden.

Mike Dent is Emeritus Professor in the School of Justice, Security and Sustainability at Staffordshire University in the UK.

Sigita Doblytė is Assistant Professor in the Department of Sociology at the University of Oviedo in Spain.

Charalambos Economou is Professor of Sociology and Health Policy in the Department of Sociology at the Panteion University of Social and Political Sciences in Greece.

Guido Giarelli is Professor of Sociology at the University Magna Græcia of Catanzaro in Italy.

Ana M. Guillén is Professor in the Department of Sociology at the University of Oviedo in Spain.

David Hughes is Emeritus Professor in the Faculty of Medicine, Health and Life Sciences at Swansea University in the UK.

Jon Magnussen is Professor of Health Economics in the Department of Public Health and General Practice at the Norwegian University of Science and Technology in Norway.

Pål E. Martinussen is Professor of Political Science in the Department of Sociology and Political Science at the Norwegian University of Science and Technology in Norway.

Mike Saks is Emeritus Professor at the University of Suffolk in the UK and Visiting Professor at the University of Lincoln and the University of Westminster in the UK and the University of Toronto in Canada.

Mauro Serapioni is Senior Researcher and Professor in the doctoral programme on 'Democracy in the Twenty-First Century' at the Centre for Social Studies in the Faculty of Economics at the University of Coimbra in Portugal.

Giovanna Vicarelli was Professor in the Department of Economics and Social Sciences at the University Polytechnic of Marche in Italy.

Karsten Vrangbæk is Professor of Health Policy in the Faculty of Health and Medical Sciences at the University of Copenhagen in Denmark.

Ulrika Winblad is Professor of Health Services Research in the Department of Public Health and Caring Sciences at Uppsala University in Sweden.

Introduction

The National Health Services of Western Europe: a historical-comparative perspective

Guido Giarelli and Mike Saks

What is a National Health Service? Typologies of healthcare systems

It is not very well known that in 1938, during the first Labour government of New Zealand – the independence of which had recently been granted by the United Kingdom (UK) – the Parliament approved a greatly expanded Social Security Act, including tax-funded healthcare provision covering the total population. According to Roemer (1991:206):

> [T]his was the first country with a free-market economy to do so. (Britain and the Scandinavian countries made coverage universal later, and the Soviet Union – with universal entitlement to health services in the 1920s – did not have a free-market economy).

However, as a result of opposition from the medical profession, the provisions of the Act were not implemented until 1941, and the scope of the services provided under the New Zealand Health Service was not comprehensive at the outset. In fact, in the words of Goodyear-Smith and Ashton (2019:432), despite the vision of the government

> for New Zealanders to have universally available access to a comprehensive range of health services provided free of charge . . . the medical profession strongly resisted the government's proposal to pay for general practice (GP) services via capitation funding.

This led to

> a compromise in which the government subsidy was paid on a fee-for-service basis, and GPs could charge co-payments over and above the government subsidy. The result was fully funded public hospitals operating alongside privately owned GPs with partial public funding.

Notwithstanding such partial implementation in New Zealand, the three fundamental pillars on which a National Health Service (NHS) in a country

DOI: 10.4324/9781003139799-1

with a free-market economy is based were planted: universal coverage regardless of income, funding from tax revenue and a comprehensive range of public health services provided free of charge at the point of delivery to all. And these pillars on which this book is based in a Western European context are the same as those we find in the establishment of the NHS in the UK in 1948. This was part of the new welfare state (Titmuss, 1958) centred on social citizenship entitlements that the Labour Government introduced for the first time in the West in a social security system based on the collectivisation of the risks of individual life (Marshall, 1950).

The apparent paradox of a state-run healthcare system in the home country of liberalism and a liberal state, where a minimal state-supported health system of workhouse hospitals for the poor and a national insurance system for workers previously existed, can be seen in pragmatic terms as related to the favourable context for radical change. The first aspect of this was the epidemiological pressure of World War II, with large-scale civilian casualties and returning wounded or disabled soldiers, and the new therapeutic potential offered by the incipient pharmacological revolution with the discovery of antibiotics and sulphonamides which were unaffordable for most people. Although there are deeper theoretical debates about the reasons for the gestation of the NHS (see Saks, 2015b), it was felt that a flat-rate universal contribution could be exchanged for a flat-rate universal benefit run by the state, as suggested in the Beveridge Report (Abel-Smith, 1992) – even though, as Blank and Burau (2007:44) note, 'the NHS did not resolve the tension between laissez-faire liberalism and collectivism and instead a generous entitlement philosophy has coexisted with rationed service provision'. In fact, since its inception and at least until the 1990s, the NHS suffered from chronic underfunding because 'there was a lack of political will to commit the resources necessary to meet Bevan's remit for the service' (Gabe, 1997:6) despite the naïve assumption that it would lead to a reduction in healthcare costs as diseases were cleared up and demand was reduced (Berridge, Webster and Walt, 1993).

However, the four principles on which the NHS was grounded – collectivism, comprehensiveness, equality and universalism (Allsop, 1995) – together outlined a new model of a healthcare system based on the direct responsibility of the state for the health of its citizens in a market economy. This was an alternative model to both the traditional Continental Europe Bismarckian system of social health insurance and the private fee-for-service model in the United States (US). It was also different from the model developed in the post-revolutionary former Soviet Union since the 1920s, where the state had large-scale control of the healthcare system (Saks, 2018). These international differences offered the basis for the development of the categorisation used here to compare various healthcare systems in the relatively new field of interdisciplinary comparative analysis.

If 'classification is integral to comparison' (Freeman and Frisina, 2010:101), a short history of the classification of the healthcare systems can help us to better understand the common defining characteristics of the NHSs compared with other healthcare systems of the world. In fact, 'the emergence of a standard or "normal" classificatory scheme' (Freeman and Frisina, 2010:104) can be identified in comparative studies of healthcare systems. The problem we wish to tackle is whether this standard classification still has a heuristic value: in other words, whether it continues to usefully highlight by mutually exclusive and exhaustive categories the fundamental features of the cluster of different healthcare systems considered in this volume.

The genesis of such classificatory schemes started with Anderson (1963), who attempted to single out significant criteria or dimensions by which to compare the healthcare systems of the US, the UK and Sweden. He identified them as different arrangements for the funding and delivery of healthcare, on which there was a continuum of cases from the private to the state rather than categorical distinctions between types. Subsequently, one of the earliest typologies was proposed by Terris (1978), who identified 'the three world systems of medical care' on the basis of the nature of the economic system, clustering together very different systems in the same category: *public assistance* in the pre-capitalist societies of Asia, Africa and Latin America; *health insurance* in the capitalist societies of Europe, Northern America, Israel, Japan, Australia and New Zealand; and *NHS* in the socialist societies of Eastern Europe, China and some other Asian countries, and Cuba. A more elaborated and influential typology was developed by Field (1973, 1980) based on analysing the concept of healthcare as a national social good, the status of physicians, the role of professional associations, the ownership of health facilities and the terms of payment for treatment. On these criteria, he identified five types of systems: *anomic* or *private* (Western countries and Russia in the nineteenth century); *pluralistic* (US in the twentieth century); *insurance/social security* (Continental Europe, Scandinavia, Canada and Japan); *NHS* (UK); and *socialised* (Soviet Union). Field was thus the first to identify a specific 'national health service' type in Western countries. He was also one of the first scholars – albeit contentiously (Saks, 2015b) – to assert a 'theory of convergence' by arguing that the five forms represented a progression, since all systems were moving towards the last type.

The classificatory scheme was canonised in its final form in a landmark study by the Organization for Economic Cooperation and Development (OECD) (1987), which also defined a policy agenda on the basis of three dimensions: funding, coverage and ownership. This trichotomous classification of healthcare systems has become a paradigmatic reference point for subsequent studies: a *private insurance* model based on private insurance financing, private insurance coverage and healthcare provision in private ownerships; a *social insurance* model based on funding by social insurance contributions, almost universal coverage by social insurances, and healthcare provision by both private and public ownership; and a *NHS* model based on funding out of general taxes, universal coverage based on citizenship and provision of healthcare in public ownership. In the following years, various scholars consolidated this classification. Giaimo and Manow (1999), for example, adopted the influential typology elaborated by Esping-Andersen (1990) on 'welfare regimes', focused on system-specific modes of financing, provision and access to healthcare in three prototypical countries by distinguishing *state-led* systems in the UK, *corporate-governed* systems in Germany, and *market-driven* systems in the US. In turn, Tuohy (1999) focused on mechanisms of social control ruling the decision-making processes in healthcare in three countries, identifying them in the *hierarchy* in the NHS in the UK, in the *collegiality* in the Canadian Medicare system, and in the *market* in the US private insurance system. This is a similar tripartite classification to that elaborated by Rico, Saltman and Boerma (2003), who distinguished three types of coordination and control of healthcare by using the terms *hierarchy*, *networks* and *market*.

However, Mechanic and Rochefort (1996) criticised some limitations and weaknesses of this standard classification, claiming that there was no accepted authoritative taxonomy of healthcare systems. Apart from the inappropriate use of the term 'taxonomy' instead of 'typology',[1] there are undoubtedly some interesting issues that the classification raises. One of them is to what extent the classification of healthcare systems should correspond to the more general classification of welfare states, since

> health care is a big component of welfare provision, it is striking that many of the major contributions that have in recent years shaped debates about the welfare states . . . have had health policy at the corner of their eye rather than in the centre of their vision.
>
> (Moran, 2000:136)

In this vein, Wendt, Frisina and Rothgang (2009) argue that Esping-Andersen's welfare typology is largely inapplicable for at least two reasons. First, his typology of welfare regimes – *social democratic*, *conservative-corporatist* and *liberal* – is based on dimensions of 'decommodification' and 'destratification'[2] which do not establish an adequate basis for differentiating the key features of healthcare systems. This is in spite of attempts by contributors like Bambra (2005) to adapt Esping-Andersen's concept of decommodification to healthcare systems. Second, in countries like the UK, the type of overall welfare regime can significantly differ from specific sectors of welfare like healthcare.

If a different and specific typology for healthcare systems is needed, this means that we should perhaps not pay too much attention to the social and institutional frameworks in which they are embedded. However, the 'typology developed by the OECD is a descriptive categorisation of how health care is organised in different countries and reflects its specific origins in applied policy analysis' (Blank and Burau, 2007:65), largely influenced by economists and focused on the internal functioning of healthcare rather than its context. This is the reason why Moran (1999, 2000) focused on the institutional embeddedness of healthcare and revising the typology of healthcare systems by shifting the level of analysis from its internal organisation to its governance. For this purpose, he introduced the concept of 'healthcare state', consisting of the institutions governing the consumption, provision and production of healthcare. The government of consumption is concerned with the mechanisms by which patients have access to healthcare and is collectively organised and financed by the state: commercial insurance markets in the US, earned insurance entitlements in the Bismarckian system and social citizenship in the Beveridge model. The institution governing the provision of healthcare includes the mechanisms for regulating hospitals and doctors. In both cases, according to Moran (2000:143), there is a significant differentiation *within* the same categories of consumption government – for example:

> 'national health service' systems include those where the central state owns much of the 'means of production' (the United Kingdom); ownership is public but often decentralised (some Scandinavian systems); and a formally 'nationalised' hospital system in practice coexists with a large institutional private sector (Greece, Portugal).

Likewise,

> variations in the government of professional providers map poorly onto consumption categories. Take 'national health service' systems again: they coincide with some Scandinavian systems where doctors are in the main salaried public servants; with the UK system where the key primary deliverer, the general practitioner, has been a self-employed contractor but one with little freedom to generate discretionary income; and the Mediterranean arrangements in which there is an extensive private practice by medical professionals allowing the generation of significant discretionary income.

Finally, the government of the production of healthcare focuses on mechanisms regulating medical innovations and technology. Here there is a remarkable uniformity by contrast with consumption and provision, given the key role played by private corporations and their relative autonomy from public decision-making by the state, resulting in a form of polyarchy.

The four 'families' of 'healthcare states' Moran (2000) constructed on the basis of the above criteria represent one of the most interesting attempts to rethink the canonic classification scheme: in the *entrenched command and control* family (the UK and Scandinavia), the state plays a key role in all three governing arenas, whereas in the *corporatist* family (Germany), consumption is dominated by public law bodies (statutory insurance funds), provision by public law associations of doctors and hospitals, with some limited constraints on medical innovation due to the marginal role of the state limited to setting the regulatory frameworks; and in the *supply* family (the US and Switzerland), private insurances dominate consumption, private hospitals and doctors dominate provision, and there are no public constraints on medical innovation. Moran (2000:154) also add a fourth family of *insecure command and control* states (Portugal, Spain, Italy and Greece) as a sort of sub-type of the first family of most recent creation during the late 1970s and the early 1980s, as

> in none has command and control been able to entrench itself in the manner of the north European systems. In all the insecure systems, despite the existence of a formal apparatus of citizenship entitlements, the reality is far from one of universal coverage.

The two factors identified by Moran as at the origin of the 'insecure' character of these states were the scarce administrative rationality of their bureaucracies due in part to corruption, and the later period of development of their national health systems compared with the Northern European countries, when the 'Golden Age' of the welfare state had come to an end and a new political climate had begun to assert itself.

Neo-liberal reforms from the 1980s

Since the 1980s, a series of challenges significantly affected Western industrialised countries changing the previous optimistic scenario based on the model of indefinite development of the post-war era. First and foremost, the economic recession that followed the oil price shocks of the 1970s marked the end of the continuous economic growth that had characterised all Western capitalist economies in the previous 30 years. The reduced availability of economic resources resulting from declining gross domestic product also inevitably affected healthcare systems, creating enormous pressures for greater efficiency and costs containment in a period of so-called 'medical inflation'. Second, advances in longevity in these countries coupled with the reduction of birth rates resulted in increasingly ageing demographic structure. As Mechanic and Rochefort (1996:245) point out, 'as people live longer they have more chronic disease and disabilities. Ageing is associated with greater need across the entire spectrum of health services, but especially for long-term care of both institutional and noninstitutional form'. Changing demography therefore brought a third important challenge, namely a new pattern of disease characterised by the 'epidemiological transition' (Omran, 1971), involving the declining relevance of infectious diseases (even though they continued to resurge periodically) compared with the growing prevalence of chronic degenerative conditions and behavioural disorders resulting in increasing disabilities and dependency (Wilkinson, 1994).

These changes in disease patterns in turn modified traditional cultural conceptions of illness and health, altering patients' expectations; since 'illness less often threatens life itself, but more often endangers the ability of persons to perform their usual activities and achieve a desired quality of life' (Mechanic and Rochefort, 1996:248), a series of personal and social conditions (such as impairment, disabilities, infertility, distress, personal maladjustments and eating disorders) became medicalised, raising public expectations and demands for biomedical knowledge and technology. Realisation of the limits of such biomedical knowledge and technologies in healing these chronic degenerative conditions produced a social climate of mistrust towards science and its applications (Ehrenreich, 1978). The fourth challenge of medicalisation and pharmaceuticalisation of life and society (Conrad, 2007; Gabe, 2016), supported by the mass media and advertising campaigns of 'Big Pharma' and the health technology and medical aids industry, thus generated a cultural crisis given biomedicine's inability to meet the growing and unrealistic expectations of the public.

In addition to resulting in the sort of 'medical nemesis' to which Illich (1976) attributed 'iatrogenesis' (doctor-induced disease and suffering), this crisis generated a fifth challenge to biomedicine: the resurgence of unconventional medicines after nearly a century of almost undisputed monopoly on Western healthcare systems by biomedicine (Saks, 2003, 2015a). The unmet demands of the public by biomedicine turned to once marginalised heterodox forms of medicine such as herbalism and homeopathy in the search for more humanised therapeutic relationships and in-depth communication. This questioned the 'social contract' between state, society and biomedicine (Pescosolido and Kronenfeld, 1995) forged nearly a century before, that granted the latter control of Western healthcare systems in exchange for its effectiveness in healing diseases. The end of this exclusive legitimation opened an 'uncertain era' of a possible return to medical pluralism (Cant and Sharma, 1999) that intersected with the incipient crisis of the welfare state as it had emerged during the post-war years (Moran, 1988).

Precisely because the welfare state represented the social and institutional frameworks in which Western healthcare systems were embedded, the crisis could not but affect healthcare systems as well – and this was more so in the case of the NHSs, in which the state played a dominant role. Putting it simply, 'if the essence of the welfare state is government-protected minimum standards of income, nutrition, health, housing, and education assured to every citizen' (Wilensky, 1975:1), then the crisis of the welfare state can be synthesised as a triple crisis of the capacity of the state to raise resources, of its capacity to transform these resources into service and of a model of social citizenship. Therefore, by the 1980s, 'this model of institutionalized, bureaucratic provision and social rights' was radically questioned by the new 'political rhetoric of deregulation, privatization, the efficiency of the "free market" and rolling back the frontiers of the state' (Kennet, 2004:1).

How did this new neo-liberal rhetoric translate into healthcare systems and NHSs in particular? If we use the British NHS as the most famous case, we can summarise neo-liberal reform policies in four words: marketisation, managerialism, empowerment of the consumer and welfare pluralism (Gabe, 1997). In 1990, the Thatcher Conservative Government introduced an 'internal market' system by splitting the NHS into providers (hospitals, community health services and general practitioners) and purchasers (district health authorities and GP fundholders) of health services on the assumption that competition among providers could minimise the price of their services to remain competitive, even with greater private sector efficiency (Enthoven, 1993). The opportunity offered to providers to become self-governing trusts to enjoy more financial freedom and greater autonomy therefore moved in the same direction as the marketisation of the NHS. However, an actual internal market was never established because of its impracticability in the health context, meaning that the changed structure of the NHS has been defined as a 'quasi-market' (Hughes, 1991; Le Grand and Bartlett, 1993).

The marketisation process was coupled with the managerialisation of governance of the NHS to support the application of private sector business principles to the public sector as a way to control expenditure, the so-called 'New Public Management' (Pettigrew, Ferlie and McKee, 2009). The introduction of general managers in place of teams composed of representatives of doctors, nurses and administrative staff significantly altered the balance of power in favour of managers at the expense of doctors and their clinical freedom, even though the latter were able to master the new managerial techniques and, in some cases, become managers themselves (Elston, 1991). The legitimation of the managerialisation process was mainly based on an emphasis on the empowerment of patients and public renamed as 'consumers'; the management-led consumerist approach was officially aimed at fostering freedom of choice through the market through market research into consumer preferences. Actually, behind this rhetoric of empowerment in this 'supermarket approach', as Gabe (1997:33) notes, 'the consumer is confined to purchasing what appears on the shelf or complaining when a product is faulty, and has no direct voice in determining what appears on the shelf in the first place', while citizen's rights are reduced to consumer rights without real participation in decision-making processes. This was evident in the White Paper *Working for Patients* produced by the Conservative government of 1989, in which the role of the Community Health Councils in contributing to local health policies was significantly reduced 'by withdrawing their right to nominate representatives to attend meetings of the board governing Health Authorities' (Gabe, 1997:33).

The neo-liberal reforms of the 1980s and 1990s also shifted the balance between public and private health services in favour of greater private sector funding and delivery in line with the New Right policy loathing of the public monopoly of services. Controls on private hospital development were relaxed, consultants' contracts in the NHS were modified to foster private practice, private health insurance was made more attractive, health authorities were directed to contract out patient care to the private sector as a way of reducing NHS waiting lists and pay-bed provision was expanded in both public and private sectors. This imbalance of the NHS in favour of the private sector could have also favoured the integration of unconventional medicines into the system, creating greater welfare pluralism, but in practice, it simply meant in many cases 'the shift to a new public/private mix of services, a mixed economy of health care. . . . As such it arguably represents an attempt to "privatize from within"' (Gabe, 1997:43).

Since the 1980s, these neo-liberal reform policies spread throughout various Western healthcare systems like a virus (Maynard, 2005:S255), well beyond the NHSs, with different degrees, ways of implementation and outcomes. A key purpose of this book is to document such variability with specific reference to the European systems which adopted a NHS type of healthcare, namely the Scandinavian countries after World War II and some Mediterranean ones during the 1970s and 1980s. These policies were also adopted in the Bismarckian systems based on social health insurance in Continental Europe (Germany, Austria, France, Belgium, Luxembourg, and, to a lesser extent, The Netherlands and Switzerland). An interesting question is whether they have followed the same model of reform. According to Hassenteufel and Palier (2007:586), the answer is negative:

> At a first glance structural changes introduced by the reforms adopted in the last decade seem to follow similar patterns to national health service. But a closer look underlines their links with the specific problems we have underlined previously. These changes also led to specific health insurance system trajectories: the silent privatisation of healthcare coverage, the limits imposed on financing by social contributions, the lack of regulation of the health care supply.

The 'specific problems' of the Bismarckian health insurance systems, according to the two authors, derive from their institutional organisation based on sickness funds or mutual insurance societies; compared with the NHSs, they allow for more 'patient choice, comfort and often quality of care to guaranteed, but most often at the cost of high health spending, and occasionally, inequality of access to health care' (Hassenteufel and Palier, 2007:576).

Given their institutional settings of healthcare and their importance for understanding their problems, the reforms implemented in these systems have tackled three main issues: the health insurance financial deficits, the cost containment of healthcare expenditure and the governance of the system by the state. Hassenteufel and Palier (2007:586–7) recognise that the reforms adopted to deal with these issues in the cases of Germany, France and Netherlands have produced 'hybridisation' of their systems:

> It is possible to characterize as path-breaking some of the changes that occurred from the 1990s, since they introduced new principles and new instruments to the health insurance systems, some of them being close to the national health service systems (especially to the British one . . .), namely more universal coverage, more taxes to finance health expenditure, the development of New Public Management devices and more control over the patients' circulation within the system.

However, Hassenteufel and Palier (2007:590–3) conclude, 'Even so, despite the similarities in the instruments utilized, these evolutions have not ended the gap between health insurance and national health service systems' since

> until now and despite the institutional reforms, continental health insurance systems have remained Bismarckian (they are still mainly financed by social contributions, managed by health insurance funds, delivering public and private health care, and freedom is still higher than in national health services).

These 'structural changes without revolution' based on incremental strategies changing the logic of the institutions and not the institutions themselves have therefore produced hybrid 'neo-Bismarckian' healthcare systems combining universalisation through more state control and marketisation with regulated competition.

The ensuing debate on hybridisation

In the following years in the new millennium, the idea of 'hybridisation' raised a debate among scholars about the 'convergence hypothesis', namely

> a certain macro process in which a narrowing of system options takes place, compared with those theoretically possible, due to forces that generally lie beyond the control of particular national actors or institutions and to which more and more societies are being exposed.
> (Mechanic and Rochefort, 1996:242–3)

These new forces could be traced to the process of globalisation, which 'produced a wave of new convergence research that emphasized international policy diffusion, the old convergence forces of aging populations, economic decline (or at least slower growth in the rich democracies), and maturing welfare states' as 'the "common pressures" argument for convergence'. This led Beckfield, Olafsdottir and Sosnaud (2013:132) to conclude that 'because the rich democracies face similar challenges, they will tend to adopt similar responses'. Policy borrowing from other healthcare systems was considered a driving force leading to hybrid systems: consequently, even a system representing an ideal-typical category of NHS such as the UK was considered as transformed into a national hybrid by a policy of redesign, different from earlier phases of establishment and retrenchment (Tuohy, 2012).

On the other hand, although Western healthcare systems faced 'common pressures' and in reaction to them policymakers looked abroad for promising solutions to domestic problems, other scholars suggested that healthcare systems remain tightly embedded within their national social, economic and cultural systems, thus introducing the problem of path dependence into efforts to enhance cross-national policy learning (Marmor, Freeman and Okma,

2005; Saks, 2015b). This raised the interesting issue of the historical interplay of structure and conjuncture, social system and agency to explain both 'path dependence' and 'path deviance' (Wilsford, 1994). In the first case, we can hypothesise that structural forces dominate, therefore making social change most likely to only be incremental. In the second case, more radical reforms are feasible due to policy choices, making structural change of institutions a concrete option. An interesting attempt to explain the emergence of hybrid healthcare systems in this way was proposed by Schmid and colleagues (2010). They argued:

> [H]ealth care systems tend to feature specific, type-related deficiencies, which cannot be solved by routine mechanisms. As a consequence, non-system-specific elements and innovative policies are implemented, which leads to the emergence of 'hybrid' systems and indicates a trend toward convergence, or increasing similarities.
>
> (Schmid et al., 2010:455).

According to their analysis, hybridisation is thus a soft form of convergence resulting from the interplay of the structural forces in each system (path dependence) with the political actors' interpretation of problems pressure leading to the implementation of new policies (path deviance) towards service financing, provision and regulation.

This mix of structural and sociocultural factors (Béland, 2005) to explain mechanisms of change is applied by researchers to the state-led NHSs, corporatist social health insurances and market-driven private health insurances as the three system types of OECD countries. The system-specific problems of NHS systems based on state hierarchy (the UK, Ireland, Nordic and Mediterranean countries, Australia and New Zealand) were identified by Schmid and colleagues (2010:466) as having 'long waiting lists for certain treatments, insufficient investment in healthcare facilities, poor responsiveness, and low productivity or low motivation of providers'. The framing of these 'problem pressures' as 'inefficiencies' due to 'state failure' by relevant policy actors (governments) triggered market reforms based on non-system-specific elements in financing, service provision and regulation such as private financing, internal market, managed competition and privatisation of services. However, as Schmid and colleagues (2010:466–8) note, the increasing salience of marketisation and privatisation did not imply a structural change in the state-led systems; funding has remained mostly public; and since markets need to be regulated, 'market-oriented reforms tend to go hand in hand with intensified state hierarchy (the seesaw effect)'. Therefore, 'since the late 1980s, NHS systems have supplemented state hierarchy with market-style modes of regulation', so that 'the implementation of market-oriented reforms has entailed further state interventions to guarantee the functioning of markets, while intervening variables such as political conflicts help to explain the extent to which NHS-type systems have implemented competition as a coordination mechanism'.

Schmid and his collaborators (2010) go on to claim that social health insurance systems based on the collective bargaining of corporate actors (Austria, Belgium, France, Germany, Luxembourg, The Netherlands, Switzerland and, after 1996, Japan) have faced an eroding financial basis of their schemes due to decreasing wages and world competition because of economic globalisation, involving increasing difficulties in raising social health insurance contributions from both workers and entrepreneurs. Governments reacted to this major system-specific deficiency by attempting to broaden the financial basis of their insurance systems with the introduction of general taxes, flat-rate contributions and patient co-payments as non-system specific elements typical of a state hierarchy. At the same time, the common trend in service provision was towards privatisation, especially of hospitals, mainly driven by public opinion, shared fiscal austerity and perceived inefficiencies in the inpatient sector. As regards the regulation of the systems, Schmid and colleagues (2010:470–1) observed that there was 'a decreasing role of corporatist self-government in favor of state hierarchy and market competition'. On the one hand, there were 'state-driven cost containment policies in all social health insurance system countries since the late 1970s' involving 'hierarchical control manifested in hospital planning, sectoral budgets, and tariffs authorization'. On the other hand, since 'coverage based on employment status caused increasing imbalances within and between the schemes for different social groups', despite strong institutional constraints against structural reforms, 'a commonly perceived lack of cost-effectiveness and responsiveness facilitated the introduction of market mechanism in the early 1990s', with the implementation by governments of legal frameworks for competition among sickness funds.

Competition-driven healthcare systems dominated by private actors where healthcare is an industry (the US before the Obama reforms and Switzerland before the mid-1990s) are said by Schmid and colleagues (2010:472–3) to 'suffer from market failure rooted in information asymmetries, which causes adverse selection and leads to overutilization of services'. To tackle these system-specific deficiencies, they hold that increased cost-sharing was introduced on the demand side, but 'overutilization is a problem requiring supply-side management. In private, fee-for-service based health care systems, however, typically no such instruments for managing provider behavior exist'. Therefore, the lack of instruments for hierarchical control was compensated in service financing by increasing public funding supporting public insurances for the uninsured and underinsured (Medicare and Medicaid in the US) which also meant a significant rise in hierarchical state regulation, at least in relation to public programmes. Yet, since in the area of private insurance, government regulation was weak, especially in relation to providers, as a functional equivalent to government regulation vertically integrated Health Maintenance Organisations (HMOs) gained popularity from the late 1980s. Due to their hierarchical structure, HMOs were able to impose instruments for steering the behaviour of both providers and patients. While HMOs have recently declined due to bankruptcy and other factors (Saks, 2015b), the situation has changed again, and 'virtually' integrated networks now dominate, where provider management is based on long-term contracts. Although private providers dominate in the outpatient sector, in the inpatient sector, this is more differentiated, with a decreasing share of public hospitals and a growing share of both for-profit and non-profit (receiving tax subsidies) facilities. Schmid and colleagues (2010:473) therefore conclude that 'in coping with system deficiencies, hierarchical elements have increased considerably in private healthcare systems, from both public and private actors', even though profitability remains as a strong driver.

New classifications of healthcare systems

If the integration of non-system specific policy elements has led to the hybridisation of healthcare systems, this has implications for their comparative classification. The growing complexity of hybridised healthcare systems has challenged the canonised tripartite classification increasingly considered insufficient to account for real-world systems. This did not make comparison meaningless, but fostered, during the second decade of 2000s, the emergence of new models and classifications of the different systems. Among these, one of the most original is that elaborated by Reibling, Ariaans and Wendt (2019), who provide an extended typology of 29 OECD healthcare systems on the basis of a comparative-institutional perspective conceptualising them as an integral part of welfare states and their different institutional logics, integrated with an international health policy perspective. The synthesised framework combines conventional indicators on supply, public–private mix and institutional access regulations with measures on primary care orientation and performance management in prevention and quality of care.

A nine-cluster analysis by Reibling, Ariaans and Wendt (2019) identified five new types of healthcare systems:

- The *supply- and choice-oriented public systems* (Austria, Germany, France, Ireland, Iceland, Belgium, Slovenia, Czech Republic and Australia), mostly based on social health insurance, characterised by a medium to high level of financial resources, high level of human resources, free choice of providers, fee-for-service for specialists, the highest share of general practitioners, and low performance in terms of both prevention and quality of care.
- The *performance- and primary-care-oriented public systems* (Finland, Norway, Sweden, Portugal, New Zealand, Japan and South Korea), mostly based on NHSs, characterised by medium-level financing (mostly public), access to specialists limited by gatekeepers, regulated choice among providers, salaried specialists, strong primary care orientation, and high performance in prevention and quality of care.
- The *regulation-oriented public systems* (Denmark, The Netherlands, UK, Spain, Italy and Canada), mostly based on NHSs and medium levels of

financing (largely public), but with the highest levels of access regulations, limited choice of providers, absence of formalised cost-sharing, the lowest level of out-of-pocket expenditures, a low level of primary care orientation, and low performance in both prevention and quality of care.

- The *low-supply and low-performance mixed systems* (Estonia, Hungary, Poland and Slovakia), mostly based on social health insurance, characterised by low levels of financial (largely public) and human resources, high out-of-pocket payments, strong access regulations, no institutionalised cost-sharing, the lowest primary care orientation, and low performance in both prevention and quality of care.
- The *supply- and performance-oriented private systems* (Switzerland and the US), mainly based on private health insurance, characterised by high levels of financing (mostly private), high out-of-pocket expenditures, no access regulations, cost-sharing regulations, high primary care orientation, and medium to high levels of performance in prevention and quality of care.

As can be seen, this new typology does not fit with the standard tripartite typology and is strongly empirically based on cluster analyses of OECD indicators. Moreover, Reibling, Ariaans and Wendt (2019:618) argue that the five types should not be considered as stable since 'instead of assuming the existence of "frozen" regimes that are built on long path-dependent historical trajectories, system types are in fact the result of institutional stabilities and ongoing policy change'. It is thus concluded that 'any typology of welfare regimes therefore remains valid only as long as history stands still' (Esping-Andersen, 1999:73).

In the above classification, the NHS ideal-type no longer exists, being disaggregated between types 2 and 3. As Reibling, Ariaans and Wendt (2019:618) claim:

> [T]he dividing line between Social Insurance and National Health Service systems is also of little relevance for other dimensions, such as primary care orientation or performance . . . which suggests that the hybridization of healthcare systems through the health policy reforms of the past three decades has in many ways fractured old institutional systems.

However, the deductive classification of 30 OECD healthcare systems proposed by Böhm and colleagues (2013) appears to be more conventionally based on the canonic tripartite typology enriched by two new types. By further developing and testing the empirical applicability of the taxonomy originally proposed by Rothgang and colleagues (2005) – based on the participation levels of three types of actors (state, societal and private) and a hierarchical relationship between the three core dimensions of regulation, financing and service provision, led by regulation, followed by financing and finally service provision – they found that most of them were not identifiable in practice, resulting in five system types beyond the classic three types, with the two additional types defined as *etatist social health insurance* and *national health insurance*.

The first of these is the only completely mixed healthcare type that exists and is characterised by a clear hierarchy of the three dimensions, with the state responsible for regulating the system, financing organised by societal actors and provision delegated to private actors. This hybrid type is present in 11 OECD countries: Central and Eastern European countries (Czech Republic, Estonia, Hungary, Poland and Slovakia), Asian countries (Japan and South Korea), and a group of Western countries (Belgium, France, Israel and The Netherlands) that in canonic tripartite typologies were categorised under social health insurance systems, and not considered as Bismarckian because of the minor role of societal actors in regulation, dominated by the state. The second type, national health insurance (NHI), combines NHS regulatory structures and tax financing with dominantly private service provision, including Australia, Canada, Ireland, Italy and New Zealand. Some of these countries were referred to as NHS or social health insurance systems, but since service provision remains for the most part in private hands, they are placed in the latter category. However, this may be questioned because other Mediterranean countries, such as Portugal and Spain, where private insurance and out-of-pocket spending as well as private provision are also significantly pronounced, may be best considered as NHSs.

Moreover, the same utilisation of the category of 'national health insurance' appears questionable, since, contrary to Lee and colleagues (2008), it is not applied to the cases like South Korea (considered instead as *etatist social health insurance*) on the basis that their typology distinguishes not between multi-payer and single-payer systems, but between contribution and tax financing. As Cuadrado and colleagues (2019:624) point out, this shows that, even though in the last decade the 'national health insurance' type has emerged and become consolidated as an independent health financing arrangement, 'substantial differences concerning the definitions and boundaries that diverse authors proposed for a National Health Insurance remains'. The most recent definition of this proposed ideal-type sounds more convincing, because it adequately differentiates between NHI and NHS systems on the basis of the purchasing function:

> Whereas the NHI celebrates contractual agreements with both public and private (non-for-profit and for-profit) providers as a single payer, there is no vertical integration between the NHI and these providers. This is a clear distinction with the NHS-type model, where there is common ownership between the payer and the providers, particularly at a hospital level.
>
> (Cuadrado et al., 2019:625–6)

In this way, they include, in the NHI-type model, not only South Korea but also Canada and Australia up to 1984 and Estonia and Uruguay as the most recent single-payer systems.

The discrepancies, inconsistencies and controversies among the most recent attempts of classification of healthcare systems highlight the complexity of developing this because the hybridisation process has blurred historical boundaries of the national political, economic, cultural and epidemiological contexts that originally gave rise to different healthcare system trajectories. With specific reference to the NHS-type model, we can wonder whether it is still helpful or it is best to differentiate new types, as Reibling, Ariaans and Wendt (2019) suggest. And if the answer is positive, how many of the original principles of the NHSs are actually still valid for these systems after four decades of neo-liberal health reform in Western countries? To what extent have these policies seriously affected and significantly changed the nature of these systems? In particular, has the role of the state significantly changed? Finally, ahead of the common challenges to contemporary healthcare systems after the Covid-19 pandemic, how different or convergent is the shape of NHSs compared with other healthcare systems in the West and beyond (including in social health insurance, national health insurance and private insurance systems)? In summary, can we perhaps redefine the NHS systems as 'neo-Beveridgian', in the sense that the role of the state in the healthcare arena remains central but with a changed logic, similar to what Hassenteufel and Palier (2007) proposed for 'neo-Bismarckian' health insurance systems?

Conclusion: the scope of the book

These are the main issues this book will try to answer by adopting primarily neo-Weberian and neo-institutionalist perspectives based on competing interest groups under capitalism – state policymakers and managers, medical and health professions, the medical–industrial complex, citizens and civil society associations – in the context of late Western European democracies. As Saks (2021) relates, the neo-Weberian approach is centrally based on doctors and other professions establishing exclusionary social closure against outsiders, legally underwritten by the state. This brings market advantages in terms of income, status and power and a concomitant conceptualisation of professions as interest groups in a competitive marketplace. The neo-Weberian framework is broadened further in the book with reference to the complementary neo-institutionalist approach which synergistically sees professions and other institutional forms, from transnational corporations to managers, competing for jurisdiction and social position. As such, it is distinguished from mainstream macro-theoretical approaches like the rather more class-conflict-based Marxist and consensual structural functional perspectives (Saks, 2016). Already successfully applied in the field of professions in organisational contexts in Europe (Saks and Brock, 2018), this blended perspective has not yet been adequately employed in the study of comparative healthcare systems by analysing how institutional structures, rules, norms and cultures influence the policy choices and actions of competing interest groups – as well as the extent to which the ideas and the actions of such groups can significantly shape and change such systems according to self-interests and other factors.

While there are some relatively recent books following these neo-Weberian and neo-institutionalist models in specific NHSs – such as the overview by Klein (2013) on the British NHS – there is no recent comprehensive comparative book about NHSs in Western Europe, their history, current challenges and reform policies. Instead, readers must normally make do with single chapters or short paragraphs in comparative social and health policy handbooks like that of Johnson, Stoskopf and Shi (2017) which generally place healthcare systems within a broader typology, comparing them with other kinds of healthcare systems without much comparative analysis of their strengths, weaknesses in different historical contexts and analysis of their prospective futures. Books which take a wider and more incisive berth like that of Chamberlain, Dent and Saks (2018) on international professional health regulation are certainly the exceptions that prove the rule. In the context of the research agenda of this volume, therefore, we hope to be able to better understand the degree to which hybridisation (Powell and DiMaggio, 1991) has been the outcome of the neo-liberal approach pursued in Western NHSs, particularly since the 1980s.

The reason for focusing on the development of NHSs in Western Europe to answer this question lies in a limitation grounded in middle-range-controlled comparison based on similar system design; given the importance of the societal and welfare contexts in which the NHSs are embedded, the more similar they are, the less the influence may be of intervening variables. For this purpose, the other key concept we have adopted in the organisation of this book is that of a 'health macro-region' as a family of similar healthcare systems considered in the context of the complex of multidimensional factors – political, economic, social, cultural and epidemiological – that influence the health and disease of a population (Giarelli, 2022). In these terms, we have identified three different Western European health macro-regions in this book: the *British health macro-region*, including England, Scotland and Wales in the UK; the *Scandinavian health macro-region*, encompassing the illustrative cases of Norway, Denmark and Sweden; and the *Mediterranean health macro-region*, including the societies of Italy, Spain, Portugal and Greece.

For each macro-region, the nine chapters of Part I cover the main national case studies with similar structures, both historically and contemporaneously. Here a range of expert contributors have been asked to address the following questions within the parameters of the book:

- a short historical reconstruction of the origins of the NHS;
- the main health reform policies of the last 40 years according to their objectives, content and implementation, including in public health which is so central in combatting Covid-19;

- their impact on the architecture of the system and on the population's health according to statistical indicators, official documents and published field research;
- an evaluation of the future sustainability of the NHS on the basis of demographic and epidemiological trends, policy evolution and the cultural and socio-political context;
- an assessment of how far the neo-liberal health reforms of the last four decades have significantly changed the NHS and whether it remains as such.

The four chapters of Part II concentrate on deepening the comparative analyses of the above case studies according to the neo-Weberian and neo-institutionalist perspective by focusing on the changing role of the four main actors involved in the healthcare arena with regard to the evolution and future sustainability of the NHSs: the state, the medical and health profession, patients and the public and the medical–industrial complex. Here the brief included:

- a specific analysis of the role historically played by the actors concerned in the NHSs in comparison with the other different healthcare systems;
- a comparative analysis of the way this role, has or has not, changed during the last four decades as a consequence of neo-liberal reform policies;
- some insights about the possible direction of evolution of this role in future years.

The Conclusion meanwhile attempts to synthesise the outcomes in comparative terms by proposing insights on the possible future direction of the development of the Western European NHSs and their sustainability in comparison with other healthcare systems based on social insurance and private insurance, and selected comparators beyond the neo-liberal area considered here. As one of the first books of its kind to take this approach at the time of the devastating Covid-19 outbreak, when the NHSs of Western Europe are a critical aspect of our defence against the virus, we trust that it will offer readers – from higher-level undergraduate students and postgraduates through lecturers and researchers to policymakers and professionals themselves – a relevant and meaningful contribution to understanding the past, present and future development of the healthcare systems considered.

Notes

1 According to Marradi (1990), they are two different types of classification: typologies are typically produced when more than one *fundamentum divisionis* is simultaneously taken into account, whereas a taxonomy is produced when *fundamenta* are considered in succession, establishing a hierarchical order, a rank-based scientific classification (for instance, the Linnean taxonomy).

2 Decommodification refers to the degree to which individual, or families, can uphold a socially acceptable standard of living independent of market participation;

destratification is related to the reduction of inequality of the class relationships in the social stratification system (Esping-Andersen, 1990).

References

Abel-Smith, B. (1992) 'The Beveridge report: Its origins and outcomes', *International Social Security Review* 45(1–2): 5–16.

Allsop, J. (1995) *Health Policy and the NHS*, 2nd edition, London: Longman.

Anderson, O. W. (1963) 'Medical care: Its social and organizational aspects. Health services systems in the United States and other countries', *New England Journal of Medicine* 269: 839–43.

Bambra, C. (2005) 'Cash versus services: "Worlds of welfare" and the decommodification of cash benefits and health care services', *Journal of Social Policy* 34(2): 195–213.

Beckfield, J., Olafsdottir, S. and Sosnaud, B. (2013) 'Healthcare systems in comparative perspectives: Classification, convergence, institutions, inequalities, and five missed turns', *Annual Review of Sociology* 39: 127–46.

Béland, D. (2005) 'Ideas and social policy: An institutional perspective', *Social Policy and Administration* 39: 1–18.

Berridge, V., Webster, C. and Walt, G. (1993) 'Mobilisation for total welfare, 1948 to 1974', in Webster, C. (ed) *Caring for Health: History and Diversity*, Buckingham: Open University Press.

Blank, R. H. and Burau, V. (2007) *Comparative Health Policy*, 2nd edition, New York: Palgrave Macmillan.

Böhm, K., Schmid, A., Götze, R., Landwehr, C. and Rothgang, H. (2013) 'Five types of OECD healthcare systems: Empirical results of a deductive classification', *Health Policy* 113(3): 258–69.

Cant, S. and Sharma, U. (1999) *A New Medical Pluralism? Alternative Medicine, Doctors, Patients and the State*, London: Routledge.

Chamberlain, J. M., Dent, M. and Saks, M. (eds) (2018) *Professional Health Regulation in the Public Interest: International Perspectives*, Bristol: Policy Press.

Conrad, P. (2007) *The Medicalization of Society: On the Transformation of Human Condition Into Treatable Disorders*, Baltimore, MA: The Johns Hopkins University Press.

Cuadrado, C., Crispi, F., Libuy, M., Marchildon, G. and Cid, C. (2019) 'National health insurance: A conceptual framework from conflicting typologies', *Health Policy* 123: 621–9.

Ehrenreich, J. (ed) (1978) *The Cultural Crisis of Modern Medicine*, New York: Monthly Review Press.

Elston, M. A. (1991) 'The politics of professional power: Medicine in a changing health service', in Gabe, J., Calnan, M. and Bury, M. (eds) *The Sociology of the Health Service*, London: Routledge.

Enthoven, A. (1993) 'The history and principle of managed competition', *Health Affairs* 12: 24–48.

Esping-Andersen, G. (1990) *The Three Worlds of Welfare Capitalism*, Cambridge: Polity Press.

Esping-Andersen, G. (1999) *Social Foundations of Postindustrial Economies*, Oxford: Oxford University Press.

Field, M. G. (1973) 'The concept of the "health system" at the macrosociological level', *Social Science and Medicine* 7(19): 763–86.

Field, M. G. (1980) 'The health system and the polity: A contemporary American dialectic', *Social Science and Medicine* 14A: 397–413.

Freeman, R. and Frisina, L. (2010) 'Health care systems and the problem of classification', *Journal of Comparative Policy Analysis: Research and Practice* 12(1): 101–15.

Gabe, J. (1997) 'The Americanization of British health care?', *Discussion Paper DP97/1*, Department of Social Policy and Social Science, Royal Holloway University of London.

Gabe, J. (2016) 'Pharmaceuticalisation as an evolving concept', in Giarelli, G., Jacobsen, B., Nielsen, M. and Reinbacher, G. S. (eds) *Future Challenges for Health and Healthcare in Europe*, Aalborg: Aalborg University Press.

Giaimo, S. and Manow, P. (1999) 'Adapting the welfare state. The case of health care reform in Britain, Germany and the United States', *Comparative Political Studies* 32(8): 967–1000.

Giarelli, G. (2022) 'The European health systems facing the Covid-19 outbreak: A macro-regional approach', *Forum for Social Economics* 51(2): 161–74.

Goodyear-Smith, F. and Ashton, T. (2019) 'New Zealand health system: Universalism struggles with persisting inequities', *Lancet* 394: 432–42.

Hassenteufel, P. and Palier, B. (2007) 'Towards neo-Bismarckian health care states? Comparing health insurance reforms in Bismarckian welfare systems', *Social Policy and Administration* 41(6): 574–96.

Hughes, D. (1991) 'The reorganization of the national health service: The rhetoric and the reality of the internal market', *The Modern Law Review* 54: 88–103.

Illich, I. (1976) *Medical Nemesis. The Expropriation of Health*, New York: Pantheon Books.

Johnson, J. A., Stoskopf, C. and Shi, L. (2017) *Comparative Health Systems: A Global Perspective*, 2nd edition, Burlington, MA: Jones & Bartlett Learning.

Kennet, P. (2004) 'Introduction: The changing context of comparative social policy', in Kennet, P. (ed) *A Handbook of Comparative Social Policy*, Cheltenham: Edward Elgar.

Klein, R. (2013) *The NHS: From Creation to Invention*, 7th edition, London: CRC Press.

Lee, S.-Y., Chun, C.-B., Lee, Y.-G. and Seo, N. K. (2008) 'The national health insurance system as one type of new typology: The case of South Korea and Taiwan', *Health Policy* 85: 105–13.

Le Grand, J. and Bartlett, W. (1993) *Quasi-markets and Social Policy*, London: Palgrave Macmillan.

Marmor, T., Freeman, R. and Okma, K. (2005) 'Comparative perspectives and policy learning in the world of health care', *Journal of Comparative Policy and Analysis: Research and Practice* 7: 331–48.

Marradi, A. (1990) 'Classification, typology, taxonomy', *Quality and Quantity* XXIV(2): 129–57.

Marshall, T. H. (1950) *Citizenship and Social Class and Other Essays*, Cambridge: Cambridge University Press.

Maynard, A. (2005) 'European health policy challenges', *Health Economics* 14: S255–S263.

Mechanic, D. and Rochefort, D. (1996) 'Comparative medical systems', *Annual Review of Sociology* 22: 239–70.

Moran, M. (1988) 'Crises of the welfare state', *British Journal of Political Science* 18(3): 397–414.

Moran, M. (1999) *Governing the Health Care State: A Comparative Study of the United Kingdom, The United States and Germany*, Manchester: Manchester University Press.

Moran, M. (2000) 'Understanding the welfare state: The case of health care', *British Journal of Politics and International Relations* 2(2): 135–60.

Omran, A. R. (1971) 'The epidemiological transition: A theory of the epidemiology of population change', *The Milbank Quarterly* 49: 509–38.

Organization for Economic Cooperation and Development (1987) *Financing and Delivery of Health Care: A Comparative Analysis of OECD Countries*, Paris: OECD.

Pescosolido, B. A. and Kronenfeld, J. J. (1995) 'Health, illness and healing in an uncertain era: Challenges from and for medical sociology', *Journal of Health and Social Behavior* (Special Issue): 5–33.

Pettigrew, A., Ferlie, E. and McKee, L. (2009) 'Shaping strategic change. The case of the NHS in the 1980s', *Public Money and Management* 12(3): 27–31.

Powell, W. W. and DiMaggio, P. J. (eds) (1991) *The New Institutionalism in Organizational Analysis*, Chicago, IL: University of Chicago Press.

Reibling, N., Ariaans, M. and Wendt, C. (2019) 'Worlds of healthcare: A healthcare system typology of OECD', *Health Policy* 123: 611–20.

Rico, A., Saltman, R. B. and Boerma, W. G. W. (2003) 'Organizational restructuring in European health systems: The role of primary care', *Social Policy and Administration* 37(6): 592–608.

Roemer, M. I. (1991) *National Health Systems of the World. Volume One: The Countries*, Oxford: Oxford University Press.

Rothgang, H., Cacace, M., Grimmeisen, S. and Wendt, C. (2005) 'The changing role of the state in health care systems', *Transform State* 13(1): 187–212.

Saks, M. (2003) *Orthodox and Alternative Medicine. Politics, Professionalization and Health Care*, London: Sage.

Saks, M. (2015a) 'Health policy and complementary and alternative medicine', in Kuhlmann, E., Blank, R., Bourgeault, I. and Wendt, C. (eds) *The Palgrave International Handbook of Healthcare Policy and Governance*, Basingstoke: Palgrave Macmillan.

Saks, M. (2015b) *The Professions, State and the Market: Medicine in Britain, the United States and Russia*, Abingdon: Routledge.

Saks, M. (2016) 'Review of theories of professions, organizations and society: Neo-Weberianism, neo-institutionalism and eclecticism', *Journal of Professions and Organization* 3(2): 170–87.

Saks, M. (2018) 'Regulation and Russian medicine: Whither medical professionalisation?', in Chamberlain, J. M., Dent, M. and Saks, M. (eds) *Professional Health Regulation in the Public Interest: International Perspectives*, Bristol: Policy Press.

Saks, M. (2021) *Professions: A Key Idea for Business and Society*, Abingdon: Routledge.

Saks, M. and Brock, D. (2018) 'Professions and organizations in Europe', in Siebert, S. (ed) *Management Research: European Perspectives*, Abingdon: Routledge.

Schmid, A., Cacace, M., Götze, R. and Rothgang, H. (2010) 'Explaining health care system change: Problem pressure and the emergence of "hybrid" health care systems', *Journal of Health Politics, Policy and Law* 35(4): 455–86.

Terris, M. (1978) 'The three world systems of medical care: Trends and prospects', *American Journal of Public Health* 68(11): 1125–31.

Titmuss, R. (1958) *Essays on the Welfare State*, London: Allen & Unwin.

Tuohy, C. H. (1999) *Accidental Logics: The Dynamics of Change in the Health Care Arena in the United States, Britain and Canada*, New York: Oxford University Press.

Tuohy, C. H. (2012) 'Reforms and the politics of hybridization in mature health care states', *Journal of Health Politics, Policy and Law* 37(4): 611–32.

Wendt, C., Frisina, L. and Rothgang, H. (2009) 'Healthcare systems types: A conceptual framework for comparison', *Social Policy and Administration* 43(1): 70–90.

Wilensky, H. (1975) *The Welfare State and Equality: Structural and Ideological Roots of Public Expenditures*, Berkeley, CA: University of California Press.

Wilkinson, R. G. (1994) 'The epidemiological transition: From material scarcity to social disadvantage?', *Daedalus* 123(4): 61–77.

Wilsford, D. (1994) 'Path dependency, or why history makes it difficult but not impossible to reform health care systems in a big way', *Journal of Public Policy* 14: 251–83.

Part I

Case studies

The British macro-region

1 England

Rob Baggott

Introduction

As the pioneer of the comprehensive National Health Service (NHS) model, the British case is likely to provide valuable insights into how such systems have responded to economic, political and social pressures, and policy changes. The central aim of this chapter is to assess how far the neo-liberal/new public management reforms of the last four decades have significantly changed the NHS and whether it remains as such. In line with the neo-Weberian/neo-institutionalist frame of this book, it considers whether there has been a shift towards a more responsible state that seeks to meet citizens' needs without recourse to a commercial ethos (Mazur and Kopycinski, 2020; Pollitt and Bouckaert, 2011). Furthermore, it sheds light on two major issues of relevance to the neo-Weberian perspective: state capacity to deliver key services, in this case health services, to its population; and state legitimacy, related to its effectiveness and fairness in meeting needs.

This chapter begins by briefly outlining the creation of the NHS and its early years. The remaining sections focus on subsequent reforms in three periods: the Conservative governments of Margaret Thatcher and John Major (1979–97); the New Labour governments of Tony Blair and Gordon Brown (1997–2010); and finally, the governments of the 2010s – the Conservative-Liberal Democrat Coalition led by David Cameron (2010–15) and the Conservative administrations of Cameron, Theresa May and Boris Johnson (2015–22). The chapter focuses wholly on England (Scotland and Wales are covered in the following chapter) and concentrates on health policy, including public health and prevention policies. It does not explore social care in any depth but acknowledges the importance of this sector for healthcare and wider public health.

The creation of the NHS and its early years

Although the idea of a comprehensive NHS was around for many years prior to its creation, political opposition (including from the medical profession as well as vested interests in insurance-based financing and voluntary hospitals) blocked progress (see Webster, 1988). Some health reforms were possible,

DOI: 10.4324/9781003139799-4

including the public health measures of the Victorian and Edwardian periods, the development of local authority health and welfare services, and the system of National Health Insurance for workers introduced in 1912. However, the health system was highly fragmented and poorly coordinated. Access was inequitable and, for many, dependent on ability to pay. These problems were well known by the outbreak of war in 1939. Indeed, the Ministry of Health was already exploring the feasibility of a more comprehensive system. The experience of state intervention in healthcare during wartime, coupled with the endorsement of a NHS by the 1942 Beveridge report, was a catalyst in mobilising public support and political commitments for a comprehensive NHS.

The form of the NHS was finally determined following the 1945 General Election, which the Labour Party won with a large majority. Aneurin Bevan, the minister of health, nationalised both the voluntary and local authority hospitals. Local authorities retained responsibility for community health and welfare services, as well as public health. General practitioners (GPs) and other independent contractors were corralled into a separate administrative division under local Executive Councils. The existing national health insurance system was abolished, though a proportion of the new health service budget was (and still is) funded by national insurance contributions.

Although the NHS was popular, several problems emerged (see Webster, 1988; Klein, 1983). These included rising costs, exceeding initial estimates. Both Conservative and Labour governments responded by imposing charges for prescriptions and other services, such as spectacles and dentures (Labour briefly abolished prescription charges in the 1960s only to reimpose them later due to economic constraints). They also explored the potential for other ways of raising revenue, such as charges for hospital boarding costs. In the 1950s, the Conservative government considered, but did not take forward, a contribution-based health service funding scheme. The Conservatives also established an inquiry into the cost of the NHS which found that spending was not actually excessive but had actually fallen as a percentage of General Domestic Product. After this, the trajectory of health spending began to rise.

Despite the extra resources allocated to the NHS, capacity problems were indicated by longer waiting lists and waiting times, which became a key political issue. Furthermore, NHS resources depended on historical allocations rather than being based on population need. In the 1970s, indicators of health need (such as mortality rates) were used to inform allocations, but inequities persisted. Added to this were concerns about inadequate (and in some cases, inhumane) care for disadvantaged groups, notably people with mental illness, with physical or mental disabilities and older people. A series of scandals came to light, leading to more scrutiny of these services and new priorities for these groups. This also led to other, wider changes such as the reform of complaint systems, the introduction of a health ombudsman and the establishment of Community Health Councils to monitor health services. Furthermore, concern about wider inequalities in health began to grow. An official inquiry by Sir Douglas Black (Department of Health and Social

Security, 1980) found significant inequalities in mortality rates between the professional and unskilled social classes as well as inequalities between Northern and Southern regions. The Black report called for a sustained programme of expenditure and reform to address this issue, but this was rejected by the incoming Conservative government.

Another problem was that health services lacked strategic planning which, combined with weak upward accountability, inhibited the implementation of national priorities. National plans were formulated but it was increasingly acknowledged that structures and planning processes must be strengthened in order to implement them. Related to this were questions about the appropriate balance of central and local priorities, as well as accountability between the Ministry of Health and the various tiers of the NHS (initially the Regional Hospital Boards, the local Hospital Management Committees and the Executive Councils). Several attempts to restructure the NHS culminated in a reorganisation in 1974 which created new health authorities at regional and area level and local district management teams. Family Practitioner Committees replaced Executive Councils (though they had much the same function). This structure was accompanied by a new planning system which operated within clearer central priorities and involved regional, area and local plans. However, this was criticised for being overly bureaucratic (Klein, 1983).

The 1974 reorganisation also sought to address the 'tripartite' division of hospital, primary care and local authority services in the original structure, which had been problematic especially for those patients needing services across organisational boundaries. The reorganisation led to most local authority health functions being transferred to the new health authorities. However, these changes created further problems, as services that were retained – environmental health and social care services – became isolated from NHS public health- and community-based services. The reorganisation was also seen as an opportunity to redress the imbalance between public health and healthcare services, emphasising the importance of disease prevention (Baggott, 2010). But although the 1974 reorganisation brought public health practitioners under the new NHS health authorities, it did not improve their status or influence over resources.

The Thatcher and Major governments 1979–97

Strongly influenced by neo-liberal ideology, the Conservative governments of Thatcher and Major sought to transform the post-war welfare state by reducing the public sector and encouraging private sector provision, the use of market forces and greater individual responsibility. They favoured policies such as privatisation, public spending retrenchment and greater efficiency, competitive tendering for public service provision and business-style approaches to management.

The Thatcher governments initially explored radical options for the NHS, including the extension of user charges and private insurance. However, these ideas were unpopular, even among Conservatives and even Thatcher herself was forced to retreat, reassuring the public that the NHS was safe under her government. Nonetheless, non-clinical services such as laundry, catering and cleaning services were exposed to competitive tendering, and the private healthcare sector was increasingly used to reduce NHS waiting lists, paid for out of public funds. The 1980s also saw the NHS receive its lowest average annual real-term increase of 2% (Health Foundation, 2015). Prescription and other charges were raised well above the rate of inflation, and new charges for dental and sight tests were introduced. Revenue from charges rose to 4% of the NHS budget in 1990. Private health insurance was encouraged through tax relief. The percentage of people with private insurance rose from 4% on 1979 to 13% in 1989, and the share of private and voluntary spending in total health expenditure also increased in the 1980s, by 6% (Organisation for Economic Cooperation and Development, 2021).

The Thatcher governments established a more streamlined system of administration and planning, replacing existing area health authorities with district authorities. The planning system was initially decentralised, though central government later reasserted its grip. Following the Griffiths Report (Department of Health and Social Security, 1983), the government introduced a new planning and review process and a system of general management, designed to make regional and local health bodies more responsive to central priorities. This step towards a more corporate-style NHS was followed, in 1990, by the replacement of traditional health authority bodies by boards comprising both executive and non-executive directors. This managerial style focused heavily on reducing costs. During the 1980s, cost improvement programmes were introduced, followed by efficiency targets for NHS bodies.

In the late 1980s, following a financial crisis in the NHS, the Thatcher government launched a review. This culminated in a White Paper *Working for Patients* (Department of Health, 1989), which proposed an internal market in healthcare. NHS organisations were divided into purchasers (or as now more commonly known, commissioners) and providers of services. It was envisaged that providers (hospitals and community health services, which were reconstituted as NHS trusts) would generate income through contracts, while commissioners (health authorities and GP fundholders – GP practices permitted to hold their own budgets) would set strategic priorities and secure better value for money. However, this never worked as intended. John Major, Thatcher's successor, sought to distance himself from the market-style reforms. The internal market was introduced but gradually and with caution. Competition was managed and the worst effects of the market curbed through planning, regulation and the reorganisation of services.

Major presented himself more convincingly as a supporter of the NHS, ruling out charges for hospital treatment and GP visits. He championed a consumer-responsive public service approach within the NHS, introducing a *Patient's Charter* (Department of Health, 1991) which strengthened performance management, setting standards and targets (for example, on waiting times). His record on funding the NHS was more generous than Thatcher's, and taking the Thatcher–Major period together, the real-term average annual increase in the budget at 3.3% was only marginally lower than the average for previous post-war governments (3.5%) (Stoye and Zaranko, 2019). The share of NHS funding raised by charges fell under Major, to 2% (King's Fund, 2021). The percentage of people with private insurance also slightly declined, to around 11%. Nonetheless, the Major governments continued to utilise the private health sector as a means of reducing NHS waiting lists and in the supply of non-clinical services, and extended the Private Finance Initiative (PFI) to hospital capital programmes, discussed further later.

It is also important to examine Thatcher's and Major's records on public health and prevention. Although instinctively against state intervention, Thatcher's governments were forced to respond to a range of high-profile public health issues such as food safety, public drunkenness and the HIV/AIDS pandemic. In addition, inquiries into systemic failures in the English public health system led to efforts to strengthen leadership and coordination (Baggott, 2010).

Nonetheless, Thatcher's policies exacerbated public health problems by widening inequalities in income and wealth and by increasing the proportion of people in poverty (Baggott, 2010). Mass unemployment, cuts to social security entitlements and the privatisation of essential public services damaged the infrastructure of social protection. Thatcher's policies had a disproportionate effect on different regions, as the declining industrialised areas of the north suffered greatly while many areas in the south prospered. The Thatcher government also rejected the recommendations of aforementioned Black inquiry (Department of Health and Social Security, 1980).

In contrast, the Major government introduced a national public health strategy titled *The Health of the Nation* (Department of Health, 1992), with targets to address the key causes of death and illness such as cancer and heart disease. However, the strategy failed to provide sufficient resources and a coherent framework to coordinate efforts to improve health. It did not tackle the socio-economic determinants of ill health and failed to address powerful vested interests in alcohol, tobacco and food policy (Baggott, 2010).

What was the impact of Thatcher and Major governments' policies? Cost-efficiency in the NHS improved by 1.54% between 1980–81 and 1991–92 (when the internal market was introduced) and by 1.95% from then until 1995–96 (Le Grand, Mays and Mulligan, 1998). However, studies of efficiency were criticised for inaccurate measures, poor quality data and for failing to acknowledge the full cost of reforms. The effect of the Conservatives' reforms on service quality was mixed. A study of GP fundholders found that, for most conditions, quality was maintained (Howie, Heaney and Maxwell, 1995). But competition between hospitals appeared to have an adverse effect on quality (Propper, Burgess and Abraham, 2002). Regarding patient choice, some studies found that GP fundholders seemed more willing to take patients' preferences into account compared with non-fundholders (see Howie, Heaney and Maxwell, 1995; Glennerster, Matsaganis and Owens, 1994), while others found a reduction in choice of provider (Fotaki, 1998).

One of the major concerns about the fundholding scheme was that their patients could get quicker access to treatment than non-fundholders' patients (Kammerling and Kinnear, 1996). Others, however, suggested that was not a significant issue, at worst a temporary effect (Glennerster, Matsaganis and Owens, 1994). There was also evidence that 'high-cost' patients, such as those with chronic illnesses, fared worse under fundholding (Howie, Heaney and Maxwell, 1995). However, this effect was thought to be small largely, as the scheme excluded high-cost treatments.

What effect did the Conservative's policies have on health outcomes? Overall life expectancy at birth in the UK rose between 1979 and 1997, by an average annual increment of 0.24 years for men and 0.19 years for women (World Bank, 2021). As a comparison, under the previous Labour government (1974–79), these figures were 0.16 and 0.14 years, respectively. Infant mortality (per 1,000 live births) fell by 0.38 per annum on average between 1979 and 1997. This is compared with a 0.66 annual reduction under the previous Labour government. Although, in terms of these headline indicators, health continued to improve, health inequalities widened substantially in this period. In men, the gap in life expectancy between professional and unskilled social classes grew from 5.5 years (in 1972–76) to 9.5 (in the period 1992–96). In women, the gap grew from 5.3 to 6.4 years (Hattersley, 1999).

New Labour: Blair and Brown

Following the Conservatives defeat at the 1997 General Election, the NHS was under the stewardship of Labour governments, led by Blair (1997–2007) and Brown (2007–10). The Labour Party rebranded itself as New Labour, reflecting a 'third way' in public policy between state ownership and the free market. Governments in this period were more receptive to neo-liberal ideas than their Labour predecessors but retained some traditional principles such as concern for social injustice and inequality.

After initially imposing spending constraints, the first Blair government committed to higher funding levels. This was linked to its NHS Plan (Department of Health, 2000), which promised increased staffing, service improvement and modernisation, reduced waiting times, a reduction in health inequalities, extended choice and improved collaboration between the health and social care sectors. Between 1997 and 2010, the Blair and Brown governments increased the NHS budget by an annual average of 6% in real terms (1997–2010) (Stoye and Zaranko, 2019) – well above the historical average. Charges declined as a percentage of health spending and tax reliefs on private health insurance were abolished. Notably, the percentage of healthcare in the UK funded through private or voluntary sources fell by 6.5% between 1997 and 2010 (Organisation for Economic Cooperation and Development, 2021).

Even so, New Labour was prepared to involve the private sector in its plans. The Conservative's PFI scheme was used to modernise the NHS estate. Under this scheme, consortia of commercial organisations supplied finance for capital developments, as well as maintenance and other support services. PFIs made large profits for companies and investors but saddled NHS trusts with enormous debts, in some cases rendering their finances unsustainable (Centre for Health in the Public Interest, 2017).

The Blair governments also encouraged the 'independent health sector', a term that included third sector organisations such as voluntary organisations and social enterprises as well as the 'for-profit' private sector. Independent-sector treatment centres were established to increase capacity for elective procedures for NHS patients. There was a broader policy of outsourcing care and support services, and many of the beneficiaries were overseas corporations (Davis, Lister and Wrigley, 2015). The policy of using independent providers led to an increase in their share of the NHS budget, from 2.8% in 2006–07 to 4.4% in 2009–10 (Full Fact, 2017). However, if one includes other non-NHS providers, including independent contractors such as GPs, just over 20% of NHS spending was on independent provision in 2009–10 (Buckingham and Dayan, 2019).

Although GP fundholding was abolished by New Labour, the division between commissioners and providers was retained. Initially, GPs were corralled into local Primary Care Groups (PCGs) as a means of influencing health authority commissioning. PCGs were later replaced by Primary Care Trusts (PCTs) with health authorities consequently abolished. On the supply side, the Blair government enabled NHS providers to become Foundation Trusts with greater freedoms to manage their own activities and generate income (including from private sources). They even had their own regulatory body (Monitor), though remained part of the NHS and subject to national standards.

In 2003, a system of 'payment by results' was introduced to encourage competition between providers. Related to this, 'Choose and Book' was introduced in 2005, allowing GPs to offer patients appointments from a range of available hospitals or clinics, including independent providers. In addition, practice-based commissioning was piloted, with the aim of giving GPs and other primary care professionals more influence over commissioning budgets.

The Blair government initially pledged to reduce hospital waiting lists by 100,000. This focus later shifted to waiting-time targets for specific services, such as elective treatment for inpatients and outpatients, primary care appointments, accident and emergency (A&E) visits, diagnostic tests and cancer treatment. Performance management was reinforced by a robust process of monitoring and review, which became known as 'targets and terror' (Bevan and Hood, 2006). Performance management processes were extended into primary care and community health services. Star ratings were also introduced for NHS organisations, with those rated highly promised greater autonomy with lower rated organisations subjected to detailed scrutiny and intervention.

The use of efficiency targets continued under New Labour, though with greater acknowledgement that cost reduction must not compromise quality. Increasingly, quality of service and patient safety criteria (notably concerning hospital-acquired infections) were included in performance reviews, though waiting times and financial targets remained the highest priorities. A new approach to assessing costs and benefits of healthcare interventions was adopted with the creation of the National Institute for Clinical Excellence (NICE) in 1999, which produced guidance on the cost-effectiveness of healthcare technologies. Its role has since expanded to include guidance on public health interventions, health service quality standards and social care (and is now known as the National Institute for Health and Care Excellence).

NHS quality and safety issues became prominent following well-publicised cases of medical negligence, such as the Bristol Royal Infirmary scandal (Bristol Royal Infirmary Inquiry, 2001). Other measures included strengthening professional regulation, the formulation of national service frameworks for specific areas of care and treatment, a modernisation programme to improve the quality and safety of care and a new system of clinical governance and audit in the NHS. New regulatory bodies were introduced with ever-expanding remits, beginning with the Commission for Health Improvement in 1999, replaced by the Healthcare Commission in 2004 and subsequently by the Care Quality Commission (CQC) in 2009. Meanwhile in primary care, new services such as Walk in Centres and NHS Direct (a remote triage service) aimed to improve access, and a new incentive scheme to improve GP services, the Quality and Outcomes Framework (QOF), was introduced.

To address the long-standing problem of poor collaboration between services, new statutory duties were placed on health authorities (and later, PCTs), NHS Trusts and local authorities. In addition, joint plans were formulated for groups that needed both health and social care, such as older people. Financial rules were also changed to allow NHS bodies and local authorities to pool and delegate budgets for these groups. Local authorities and PCTs were required to undertake joint-needs assessments of their populations. In addition, local authorities were given additional scrutiny powers over health services.

National targets were set to reduce mortality from specific diseases (such as cancer and cardiovascular disease) and their risks (such as smoking). Changes were made to incorporate public health within NHS planning processes, though it remained marginalised. The Blair governments strengthened policy in some areas: notably smoking where it introduced higher taxes, marketing and sponsorship bans, a ban on smoking in public places and a national smoking cessation programme. It also introduced important food policies such as the establishment of the Food Standards Agency, restrictions on the marketing of product high in fat salt and sugar, a reformulation programme to reduce salt levels and improvements in school meals (Baggott, 2010).

The Blair governments adopted national inequality targets to bring life expectancy and infant mortality rates for the most deprived areas and people closer to the national average. Attempts to narrow inequalities were also reflected in programmes to reduce poverty and social exclusion, to regenerate disadvantaged areas and to improve housing, education and child welfare services (including Sure Start, a flagship scheme for families with young children). Health inequality was identified as a key priority for the NHS with changes to address the historical underfunding of poorer areas. These areas were also chosen to pilot new public health initiatives.

Under Gordon Brown, government placed less emphasis on open external competition for NHS services. Brown appointed Lord Darzi (an eminent surgeon) as a health minister. Darzi's review of the NHS recommended a range of improvements including better information on quality, the inclusion of patients' views, personal care plans for people with chronic illness, personal health budgets, more autonomy for local health services, integration of health and social care, a greater emphasis on preventing illness and consistent quality standards. Darzi wanted to strengthen primary care, increasing the choice of GP, extending practice-based commissioning and creating new primary care centres. He also recommended an NHS Constitution, setting out the rights and responsibilities of citizens, which was introduced in 2009.

The New Labour governments had some major successes in health policy (see Thorlby and Maybin, 2010; Mays, Dixon and Jones, 2011). The median waiting time for elective treatment fell from around 13 weeks in March 1997 to four weeks in 2009. The 18-week 'referral to treatment' (RTT) targets (that 90% of inpatients and 95% of outpatients be treated within this time) were achieved, and the A&E 4-hour waiting-time target (to be met by 98% of patients) was also attained. Most people were seen within the primary-care waiting-time targets, though access was reduced by contractual changes which enabled GPs to end their responsibility for out-of-hour care.

There was evidence of improvements in the quality and safety of care, such as the reduction in major hospital-acquired infections and improvements in cardiac surgery, stroke care and cancer treatment. Improvements also occurred in primary care, though these may have occurred in the absence of the QOF incentive scheme mentioned earlier (Doran et al., 2008). Moreover, areas of care not subject to additional incentive payments tended to get neglected. NHS productivity grew by 0.5% per annum under New Labour (Vizard et al., 2021), though this did not fully account for improvements in the quality of services. Moreover, there are other additional costs which are not fully incorporated in calculations, such as NHS reorganisation, the creation of regulatory bureaucracies, the transaction costs of the internal market system and the high costs of PFIs.

Changes to commissioning under New Labour were regarded as insufficient to alter providers' behaviour significantly (Mays, Dixon and Jones, 2011). Practice-based commissioning pilots showed some promise but were not rolled out. Patient choice initiatives did not improve efficiency and had no apparent effect on quality. However, payment by results was believed to have helped reduce unit costs while not harming service quality. Competition is believed to have increased in the second half of the 2000s, and this was linked to quality improvement by some studies (Mays, Dixon and Jones, 2011; Cooper et al., 2011) though this was challenged by others (Pollock, 2011).

Foundation Trusts were associated with better quality services, though there was an element of self-selection as poorer quality and financially stretched providers were unable to join the scheme (Mays, Dixon and Jones, 2011). However, Foundation Trusts were blamed for blocking systemwide improvements which they perceived to be against their interests – such as a shift in services from hospital to the community. Meanwhile, star ratings appeared to be a powerful motivator for improved performance, but encouraged a crude 'league table' mentality and had a demoralising effect on those providers facing problems outside their control. Performance indicators and targets did not necessarily improve care and could produce unintended consequences, distorting clinical priorities to the disadvantage of patients.

Turning to health outcomes, overall life expectancy for men and women continued to improve under New Labour. The average rise in male life expectancy (0.29 years per annum) was slightly higher in the period 1997–2010 than in the Thatcher–Major era, while for women, the improvement was the same (0.19 years per annum). Infant mortality rate fell by an average of 0.12 per 1,000 live births per year in the Blair–Brown era, smaller than the decline during the Thatcher–Major period (World Bank, 2021). Labour achieved its infant mortality inequality target (Vizard and Obolenskaya, 2013) and the targets for reducing inequalities in male and female life expectancy (Barr, Higgerson and Whitehead, 2017). Nonetheless, an inquiry into New Labour's policies on health inequalities (Marmot, 2010) argued that more could have been done to address the problem.

Regarding specific risk factors, there was a mixed picture (Vizard and Obolenskaya, 2013). There was a major decline in heart and circulatory disease mortality rates and a substantial fall in cancer death rates, enabling the governments to meet its targets. The suicide death rate and the accidental death rates also declined, but not sufficiently to meet their targets. There was some progress in tackling the key risk factors for disease (Vizard and Obolenskaya, 2013). Labour met its target of reducing smoking prevalence to 21% or less by 2010, and child obesity rates fell by three percentage points between 2004 and 2009. Adult obesity, however, continued to rise. There was a mixed picture in alcohol consumption where drinking over recommended limits remained stable for men but decreased for women after 2006 while children's alcohol consumption also decreased in the 2000s.

Coalition and Conservatives 2010 onwards

In 2010, Labour was replaced by a Conservative-Liberal Democrat Coalition government led by David Cameron. The new secretary of state for health, Andrew Lansley, initiated a comprehensive reorganisation of the NHS. PCTs were abolished and replaced by local clinical commissioning groups (CCGs) led by GPs and other clinicians. The Health Secretary's responsibilities and powers were limited to setting health strategy and the overall NHS budget. NHS England (NHSE), a new national commissioning body separate from the Department of Health, would issue implementation plans and guidelines, allocate budgets and commission some services. Foundation Trusts were given more leeway to generate private income. Competition and choice were enshrined in law, and Monitor (the Foundation Trust regulator) became the joint regulator of competition, alongside the Competition and Markets Authority.

Lansley assumed that greater competition and an increased role for the independent sector would improve health services, but compromised in the face of strong opposition, including from within his own party (Timmins, 2012). Price competition was ruled out and only 'qualified providers' were allowed to compete for contracts. Other concessions included allowing service integration even if this limited competition. In addition, there was a strengthening of duties and responsibilities in the legislation to ensure greater accountability, improvements in the quality and safety of services and equitable access to services. Lansley also changed his position on abolishing New Labour's targets: many were retained or modified, including the RTT targets for elective treatment, cancer referral and treatment, and A&E waiting times.

Despite these concessions, the reforms continued to attract criticism, especially for encouraging privatisation. Using a narrow measure (as stated earlier), independent provision of NHS services rose from 4.4% in 2009–10 to 7.6% in 2015–16 (Full Fact, 2017). From this point, this percentage remained around the same level. Using a wider measure, the proportion of healthcare spending on independent providers and non-NHS providers remained fairly stable up to 2019, fluctuating around the 22% mark (Buckingham and Dayan, 2019).

Private spending as a proportion of total health expenditure rose by 2.3% between 2010 and 2015 (OECD, 2021). It increased by a further 1.7% between 2015 and 2018, making an aggregate increase of 4% for the period 2010–18. NHS expenditure in real terms rose only 1.1% per annum during the Coalition years, far lower than the 4.4% annual average between 1955–56 and 2009–10 (Vizard et al., 2021). Subsequently, the Conservative governments of Cameron (2014–15 to 2016–17) and May (2016–17 to 2018–19) provided below-average annual increases of 2.5% and 1.3%, respectively. However, under Johnson (2018–19 to 2019–20), spending rose by 5.2% per annum. In 2020 and 2021, the Covid-19 pandemic led to a huge increase in spending, though, given the unprecedented circumstances, this was not comparable with previous settlements.

The 2010s also saw a renewed effort to increase efficiency. Prior to the Coalition taking office, NHS leaders had set a target of £20 billion of efficiency savings to be achieved by 2014–15. This was adopted by the Coalition, which sought to drastically reduce management costs and implemented an NHS pay freeze. From 2015, the Conservative government set a new target for efficiency, pursuing a goal of £22 billion savings by 2020.

Lansley was succeeded as Health Secretary by Jeremy Hunt in 2013. Hunt was less focused on competition and choice, focusing more on improving access to and quality of services. He presided over regulatory changes, inspired by service failures revealed by the Mid-Staffordshire NHS Foundation Trust Inquiry (2013) and other scandals during this period. A special measures regime was introduced in 2013 for trusts with serious shortcomings in care quality, later extended to those with major financial problems, under which they received support and closer oversight. Additional regulations were introduced, including a new statutory duty of candour for NHS providers, penalties for misleading regulators and a 'fit and proper persons' test for NHS Trust board members. New fundamental standards were established along with greater independence and powers for the CQC. A revised quality-assessment framework was also introduced (with graded performance ratings as used in the education sector: Outstanding; Good; Requires Improvement and Inadequate). Hunt also established the Healthcare Safety Investigation Branch, to conduct independent investigations into patient safety in NHS-funded care.

NHS England (2014) and other national bodies set out a Five Year Forward View, which aimed to improve care quality and safety while making further efficiency gains. This emphasised disease prevention and public health. It also proposed new models of care with greater integration of health services between mental and physical health, community-based and hospital care and health and social care. Meanwhile, a greater degree of control was imposed on the NHS market, leading to constraints on Foundation Trusts. New Sustainability and Transformation Plans were developed in 44 areas across England bringing together CCGs, Trusts and Foundation Trusts and local authorities. These were expected to address the needs of the local area within financial constraints, to improve quality and efficiency and to develop integrated models of care, health and well-being. Although greater integration was the buzzword, movement towards this was slow (Vizard et al., 2021; National Audit Office, 2020c).

In 2019, a long-term plan for the NHS was produced (NHS England, 2019), which again endorsed prevention and signalled the rollout of integrated care systems across England. It also acknowledged the constraints of the existing statutory framework and that more could be done to improve integration, efficiency and accountability. The Covid-19 pandemic hastened this process, prompting a more centrally planned and collaborative system. In the light of this experience, a White Paper (Department of Health and Social Care, 2021) proposed to reorganise the NHS with an explicit focus on service integration and greater central control.

Throughout the 2010s, collaboration between health and social care remained a problem. One of the key problems was funding. The Coalition's austerity policies limited the capacity needed to transform services. This funding gap was not addressed sufficiently in the second part of the decade. Some piecemeal changes were made – for example, the Better Care Fund provided a funding stream for integrated services (Harlock et al., 2019), and local authorities were permitted to raise additional council tax funds for social care. Extra funding was also provided by central government between 2016 and 2019, but did not bridge the shortfall, estimated at least £8 billion. The Johnson government has since adopted changes to social care funding that seeks to cap costs for individuals, alongside a new national insurance levy to raise additional resources for health and social care.

The 2010s saw wide-ranging reform of public health. The Coalition created a new national body, Public Health England, and local public health teams were transferred from the NHS to upper-tier local authorities, to commission public health services. These local authorities also hosted statutory health and well-being boards, whose membership was drawn from the NHS, local authorities and the voluntary sector, to produce strategic plans for their area. These bodies were also given key roles in coordinating health and care services (and other relevant services), promoting health and well-being and reducing inequalities. They were also expected to coordinate local efforts to improve health and well-being. Although these bodies emphasised the importance of public health and prevention and provided a useful forum for discussing collaboration, they were marginalised and lacked clout (Buck, 2020).

A central, ring-fenced public health grant was allocated to each public health authority. However, from 2015–16 up to 2019–20, this declined by 8% in real terms. It increased by 1% in 2020–21, much less than the NHS budget increase. Despite emphasising the importance of public health and prevention, the Coalition and Conservative governments neglected key public health priorities and opted for a narrow focus on individual responsibility rather than addressing environmental or structural factors (see National Audit Office, 2020b).

The health implications of austerity were ignored (Marmot et al., 2020). Council budget cuts disproportionately affected those living in poorer areas (Hastings et al., 2015). Social security reforms – notably universal credit and changes to disability benefits – were damaging to claimants' health and well-being. Existing programmes that addressed social disadvantage were scaled down – such as Sure Start Children's Centres – despite evidence of effectiveness (Cattan et al., 2021). In addition, Labour's health inequality targets were abandoned.

However, the Coalition introduced free lunches for all infant schoolchildren, which continued under May and Johnson. May committed to reducing the gap in healthy life expectancy between richest and poorest, though little was done to achieve this. The *Long Term Plan for the NHS* acknowledged the need for local health systems to set action plans for health inequalities (NHS England, 2019). It also stated that funding allocations to local areas would be based on a more accurate assessment of health inequalities. Even so, there was little detail on how socio-economic inequality and deprivation would be addressed and the so-called 'levelling up agenda' of Boris Johnson, supposedly to increase investment in less affluent areas, fell well short of a systematic assault on socio-economic and health inequalities.

The Coalition encouraged 'public health responsibility deals' with business, enabling alcohol and food companies to present themselves as responsible businesses, while at the same time lobbying against potentially effective policies. Food policy was significantly weakened – for example, the salt reduction scheme introduced by Labour was diluted. A new but weaker obesity policy was introduced in 2011. Five years later, the Conservative government introduced a revamped strategy to halve childhood obesity by 2030, while reducing inequalities between children in the most and least deprived areas. Although criticised for not sufficiently restricting marketing of unhealthy foods and relying too much on voluntary targets to reduce salt and sugar, it did commit to a soft drinks levy, implemented in 2018. The Coalition initially endorsed minimum alcohol pricing but backed down following industry pressure. Tough policies on tobacco continued, however, with the Coalition banning retail display of tobacco products and the Conservative governments backing measures to ensure that tobacco products can only be sold in plain packaging (introduced in 2017).

Subsequently, the Covid-19 pandemic exposed the greater vulnerability to infection and death among those with existing chronic illness, especially smoking and obesity, and also in deprived populations (Raleigh, 2021). It also led to structural changes in the governance of public health, criticism of Public Health England leading to its replacement by the UK Health Security Agency and the Office for Health Improvement and Disparities. In addition, new commitments on public health were also made in the light of concerns about chronic disease risks, including a ban on unhealthy food TV advertisements prior to 9 pm and a pledge to achieve a smoke-free society by 2030.

What was the impact of the Coalition's and Conservatives' health policies? The smaller increments in the NHS budget in the 2010s, coupled with real-term cuts in social care and public health, made it difficult to meet the rising demands of an ageing population. From 2010 onwards, waiting times for treatment increased. By May 2015, although some outpatient and inpatient waiting-time targets were met, others were missed, including the 62-day RTT for cancer, the A&E 4-hour target and one of the main elective RTT targets. After 2015, the situation deteriorated further with all the main targets missed (Thorlby, Gardner and Turton, 2019; Vizard et al., 2021). A few statistics illustrate this decline. The percentage of patients spending over four hours in A&E rose from 4% in December 2011 to 20% in December 2019. 4% of patients waited more than six weeks for a diagnostic test in 2019 compared with 1.5% in 2010. The 18-week RTT target for people on the waiting list was not met after March 2016, and by December 2019, 92% of people had been waiting for almost 25 weeks (House of Commons, 2020). There was also deterioration in primary care – surveys reported increasing difficulties in making a timely appointment (Thorlby, Gardner and Turton, 2019).

However, NHS productivity under the Coalition grew by an annual average of 1.8%, falling slightly to 1.3% under the Conservative governments during 2015–17 (Vizard et al., 2021). Productivity growth was 0.8% in

2017–18 but was negative (–0.5%) in 2018–19. But even the increase in productivity in the early 2010s was partly due to the pay restraint imposed on the NHS, increased job vacancies and 'one off' savings, rather than long-term improvements in efficiency (National Audit Office, 2020c).

Regarding the impact in health outcomes, infant mortality in the UK continued to fall but at a much lower rate, especially from 2015. It fell by 0.08 per 1,000 per annum between 2010 and 2019. The average annual increase in male life expectancy was reduced to a third of that in the New Labour era, while for women, the rate of growth more than halved. These trends are reflected in deaths from specific diseases. The reduction in heart disease deaths slowed down in the 2010s compared with the previous decade (Vizard et al., 2021) and the same was true of cancer death rates (Cancer Research Campaign, 2020).

Inequalities in health widened. Notably the life expectancy of women living in the most deprived areas actually fell between 2011–13 and 2016–18, while the gap between these women and those living in the least deprived areas increased from 6.88 to 7.69 years (Vizard et al., 2021). Inequalities in healthy life expectancy for both men and women have widened since 2011–13, while the gap between local government areas in the UK with the highest and lowest life expectancy widened for both men and women between 2013–15 and 2016–18.

The major risk factors for ill health persisted, though there were some improvements. The 2010s saw a substantial decline in cigarette smoking – from 20% to 14% of adults (NHS Digital, 2019) while the percentage of children smoking halved. Alcohol consumption per capita in the UK slightly declined in the early part of the decade but rose thereafter, returning to 2010s levels while the downward trend in alcohol consumption in children continued.

Adult obesity increased slightly over the period 2010–18, while child obesity was stable in 4–5 year olds but rose slightly in 10–11 year olds (NHS Digital, 2020). The sugar tax appears to have had some impact on reducing consumption in soft drinks (Pell et al., 2021), but overall sugar consumption fell only marginally (National Audit Office, 2020b).

Covid-19

Even before the Covid-19 pandemic, the NHS struggled to meet needs (Vizard et al., 2021). Despite warnings about challenges, such as health inequalities, an ageing population and the challenges of chronic illness, the 2010s saw historically low funding for the health and social care system. Nonetheless, prior to the Covid-19 pandemic, the UK health system was ranked high for its resilience to an epidemic (Global Health Security Index, 2019). In the initial outbreak, the UK had one of the highest levels of excess deaths compared with similar countries (Kontis et al., 2020). As the pandemic continued, the UK was ranked seventh in Europe for excess deaths (Raleigh, 2021).

The NHS was overwhelmed and its lack of capacity harshly exposed, though was not alone in facing overload.

In the early stage of the pandemic, many old and vulnerable people were discharged from hospital to care homes without being tested (National Audit Office, 2020a). People in medical need became more reluctant to access urgent and emergency care; attendance at A&E fell initially by almost half (NAO, 2020a). Access to GPs became more difficult, and there was a major shift towards remote forms of triage, especially for initial contact (Healthwatch, 2021). Elective treatments were postponed, waiting lists grew and waiting times increased (O'Dowd, 2021). Referrals fell, increasing the hidden backlog of illness. Furthermore, long-term chronic illness from Covid-19 (so-called 'Long Covid') affected many people (Whitaker et al., 2021), imposing additional future demands on the NHS. There was also a rise in mental health problems linked to the pandemic and its associated social restrictions.

One of the consequences of Covid-19 was a strengthening of central planning, as the NHS was put on a war footing. There was a weakening or suspension of some neo-liberal reforms, such as payment by results. There was also greater collaboration between different parts of the NHS and to some extent between health and social care. These changes were consolidated in the 2021 White Paper, which includes the abolition of CCGs and the establishment of integrated care systems in law, though some form of commissioning, contracting, payment by results and outsourcing will likely continue. Furthermore, as noted earlier, the era of Covid brought prevention and public health considerations to the fore and has already influenced policy in areas such as obesity as well as inducing structural changes to the public health system.

Conclusion

The NHS in England has been resilient institution. It has generally responded well to major challenges such as scarce resources, rising costs and the increasing demands as well as rising expectations. It has also been successful in moderating neo-liberal policies – its popularity has protected it more than most public services. But it has been unable to completely resist these forces. Although the NHS remains a public service, and the English healthcare system is still mostly free at point of use and funded out of public revenues, the private sector plays a much bigger role in healthcare than 40 years ago and will continue to do so. Furthermore, the NHS is managed more like a corporate business entity today and has provided a rich seam of profits for capitalist enterprises in a way that would have appalled its architects. Even so the NHS has not been privatised to the extent of other UK public services, and there has been a limit to the neo-liberal/New Public Management insurgency in health.

But the threat remains. Although the original principles of the NHS are still valued, the Covid-19 pandemic has exposed the weaknesses of the health system. The public literally applauded the NHS during the early stages of the pandemic. But there is currently much criticism of the service due to its lack of capacity and continuing difficulties in accessing services, exacerbated by recent strikes by health workers. More than six million people are currently waiting for treatment, with over 300,000 waiting for over 52 weeks. Not surprisingly, this has raised questions about the sustainability of the NHS. Even before now, pandemic concerns were being raised about the pressures on health services from demographic issues, such as the ageing population, and from population health factors, such as obesity and health inequalities.

Additional funding has been promised for the NHS, and (yet another) restructuring is underway, but it remains to be seen whether public concern will be alleviated. Added to this mix, we also now have a global economic crisis, an energy crisis, war in Ukraine and the threat of severe food shortages, all of which carry adverse implications for health in Europe and the wider world. The danger for the NHS is that additional demands upon it and continued public dissatisfaction with it will undermine its legitimacy. This could create an environment for further reform of the health system, reinvigorating a shift towards a more radical neo-liberal health agenda.

References

Baggott, R. (2010) *Public Health: Policy and Politics*, Basingstoke: Palgrave.

Barr, B., Higgerson, J. and Whitehead, M. (2017) 'Investigating the impact of the English health inequalities strategy: Time trend analysis', *British Medical Journal* 358: j3310.

Bevan, G. and Hood, C. (2006) 'Have targets improved performance in the English NHS?', *British Medical Journal* 332: 419–22.

Beveridge, W. (1942) *Social Insurance and Allied Services*, London: HMSO.

Bristol Royal Infirmary Inquiry (2001) *The Inquiry Into the Management of Care of Children Receiving Complex Heart Surgery at the Bristol Royal Infirmary – Final Report*, London: HMSO.

Buck, D. (2020) *The English Local Government Public Health Reforms: An Independent Assessment*, London: King's Fund.

Buckingham, H. and Dayan, M. (2019) 'Privatisation in the English NHS: Fact or fiction?', *Blog*, 15 November. Available at: www.nuffieldtrust.org.uk

Cancer Research Campaign (2020) *Cancer Mortality Statistics*. Available at: www.cancerresearchuk.org

Cattan, S., Conti, G., Farquharson, C., Ginja, R. and Pecher, M. (2021) *The Health Impacts of Universal Early Childhood Interventions: Evidence From Sure Start*, London: Institute for Fiscal Studies.

Centre for Health in the Public Interest (2017) *Profiting From Infirmaries*. Available at: www.chpi.org.uk

Cooper, Z., Gibbons, S., Jones, S. and McGuire, A. (2011) 'Does hospital competition save lives?', *Economic Journal* 121: 228–60.

Davis, J., Lister, J. and Wrigley, D. (2015) *NHS for Sale*, London: Merlin Press.

Department of Health (1989) *Working for Patients*, London: HMSO.

Department of Health (1991) *The Patient's Charter*, London: HMSO.

Department of Health (1992) *The Health of the Nation*, London: HMSO.

Department of Health (2000) *The NHS Plan: A Plan for Investment. A Plan for Reform*, London: HMSO.

Department of Health and Social Care (2021) *Integration and Innovation: Working Together to Improve Health and Social Care for All*, London: DHSC.

Department of Health and Social Security (1980) *Report of the Working Group on Inequalities in Health*, London: DHSS.

Department of Health and Social Security (1983) *NHS Management Inquiry*, London: HMSO.

Doran, T., Fullwood, C., Kontopantelis, E. and Reeves, D. (2008) 'Effect of financial incentives on inequalities in the delivery of primary care in England', *Lancet* 372: 728–36.

Fotaki, M. (1998) 'The impact of market-oriented reforms on patients choice and information: A case study of outer London and Stockholm', *Social Science and Medicine* 48: 1415–32.

Full Fact (2017) *How Much More Is the NHS Spending on the Private Sector?* Available at: www.fullfact.org

Glennerster, H., Matsaganis, M. and Owens, P. (1994) *Implementing GP Fundholding: Wild Card or Winning Hand?*, Buckingham: Open University Press.

Global Health Security Index (2019) Available at: www.ghsindex.org

Harlock, J., Caiels, J., Marczak, J., et al. (2019) 'Challenges in integrating health and social care: The Better Care Fund in England', *Journal of Health Services Research and Policy* 25(2): 86–93.

Hastings, A., Bailey, N., Bramley, G., Gannon, M., Watkins, D., et al. (2015) *The Cost of the Cuts; The Impact on Local Government and Poorer Communities*. York: Joseph Rowntree Foundation, Available at: www. jrf.org

Hattersley, L. (1999) 'Trends in life expectancy by social class – an update', *Health Statistics Quarterly* 2: 16–24.

Health Foundation (2015) *How Funding for the NHS Has Changed Over a Rolling Ten Year Period*. Available at: www.health.org

Healthwatch England (2021) *GP Access During COVID*. Available at: www.healthwatch.co.uk

House of Commons (2020) *NHS Key Statistics*, London: House of Commons Library.

Howie, J., Heaney, D. and Maxwell, M. (1995) *General Practice Fundholding Shadow Project and Evaluation*, Edinburgh: University of Edinburgh.

Kammerling, R. and Kinnear, A. (1996) 'The extent of the two-tier service for fundholders', *British Medical Journal* 3212: 1399–401.

King's Fund (2021) *How the NHS Is Funded*. Available at: www.kingsfund.org.uk

Klein, R. (1983) *The Politics of the National Health Service*, London: Longman.

Kontis, V., Bennet, J. E., Rashid, T., et al. (2020) 'Magnitude, demographics, and dynamics of the effect of the first wave of COVID-19 pandemic on all-cause mortality in 21 industrialised countries', *Nature Medicine* 26: 1919–28.

Le Grand, J., Mays, N. and Mulligan, P. (eds) (1998) *Learning From the NHS Internal Market: A Review of the Evidence*, London: King's Fund.

Marmot, M. (2010) *Fair Society Healthy Lives*, London: Institute for Health Equity.

Marmot, M., Allan, J., Boyce, T., et al. (2020) *Health Equity in England: The Marmot Review Ten Years On*, London: Institute for Health Equity.

Mays, N., Dixon, A. and Jones, L. (2011) *Understanding New Labour's Market Reforms of the English NHS*, London: King's Fund.

Mazur, S. and Kopycinski, P. (2020) *Public Policy and the Neo-Weberian State*, London: Routledge.

Mid-Staffordshire NHS Foundation Trust Public Inquiry (2013) *Report*. Available at: www.gov.uk

National Audit Office (2020a) *Readying the NHS and Adult Social Care in England for COVID-19*, London: NAO.

National Audit Office (2020b) *Childhood Obesity*, London: NAO.

National Audit Office (2020c) *NHS Financial Management and Sustainability*, London: NAO.

NHS Digital (2019) *Health Survey for England 2019*, London: NHS England.

NHS Digital (2020) *Statistics on Obesity, Physical Activity and Diet, England 2020*, London: NHS England.

NHS England (2014) *The NHS Five Year Forward View*, London: NHSE.

NHS England (2019) *The NHS Long Term Plan*, London: NHSE.

O'Dowd, A. (2021) 'NHS waiting list hits 14 year record high of 4.7 million', *British Medical Journal* 373: n995.

Organisation for Economic Cooperation and Development (2021) *Health Statistics: Health Expenditure and Financing*. Available at: www.stats.oecd.org

Pell, D., Mytton, O., Penney, T. L., et al. (2021) 'Changes in soft drinks purchased by British household associated with UK soft drinks industry levy', *British Medical Journal* 372: n254.

Pollitt, C. and Bouckaert, G. (2011) *Public Management Reform: A Comparative Analysis – New Public Management, Governance and the Neo-Weberian State*, Oxford: Oxford University Press.

Pollock, A., Macfarlane, A., Kirkwood, G., et al. (2011) 'No evidence that patient choice saves lives', *Lancet* 378: 2057–60.

Propper, C., Burgess, S. and Abraham, D. (2002) 'Competition and quality: Evidence from the internal market 1991–99', Paper presented at Conference of the National Institute of Economic and Social Research, London, November.

Raleigh, V. (2021) *Deaths From Coronavirus: How Are They Counted and What Do They Show?* Available at: www.kingsfund.org.uk

Stoye, G. and Zaranko, B. (2019) *UK Health Spending*, London: IFS.

Thorlby, R., Gardner, T. and Turton, C. (2019) *NHS Performance and Waiting Times: Priorities for the New Government Health Foundation*. Available at: www.health.org.uk

Thorlby, R. and Maybin, J. (eds) (2010) *A High Performing NHS: A Review of Progress 1997–2010*, London: King's Fund.

Timmins, N. (2012) *Never Again? The Story of the Health and Social Care Act 2012*, London: King's Fund.

Vizard, P. and Obolenskaya, P. (2013) *Labour's Record on Health*. Available at: www.sticerd.lse.ac.uk

Vizard, P. and Obolenskaya, P. with Hughes, J., Treebhoohun, K. and Wainwright, I. (2021) 'Health from May 2015 to pre-Covid 2020: Policies spending and outcomes', in Vizard, P. and Hills, J. (eds) *Social Policies and Distributional Outcomes in a Changing Britain: The Conservative Governments Record on Social Policy from May 2015 to pre-COVID 2020*. Available at: www.sticerd.lse.ac.uk

Webster, C. (1988) *The Health Services Since the War Volume I: Problems of Healthcare the NHS Before 1957*, London: HMSO.

Whitaker, M., Elliott, J., Chadeau-Hyama, M., Riley, S., Darzi, A., Cooke, G., Wards, H. and Elliott, P. (2021) *Persistent Symptoms Following SARS-CoV-2 Infection in a Random Community Sample of 508,707 People*, London: Imperial College.

World Bank (2021) *DataBank*. Available at: www.data.worldbank.org

2 Scotland and Wales

David Hughes

Introduction: devolved governments and divergent health policies

As with other country's case studies in this volume, change in the healthcare systems of England and Wales has been shaped by professionally dominated divisions of labour of the kind described by neo-Weberian theory (Saks, 2010) and affected by pre-existing institutional structures, norms and cultures (see Hughes and Vincent-Jones, 2008). This is a story about how devolved governments that opposed market reforms introduced in England created integrated systems closer to the 1948 National Health Service (NHS) vision and developed distinctive health policies that meshed with the views of their professional elites, their service histories and political cultures, even while maintaining many common features shared with their larger English NHS neighbour.

Scotland and Wales are two of the four home countries making up the United Kingdom (UK), the nation state that also contains England and Northern Ireland. The UK's Westminster Parliament determines policy on matters such as the constitution, the civil service, defence and international relations. Under the provisions of the Scotland Act 1998 (amended by the Scotland Acts of 2012 and 2016) and the Government of Wales Act 1998 (amended by the Government of Wales Act 2006 and the Wales Acts of 2014 and 2017), assemblies were created and granted certain legislative powers. Thus the Scottish Parliament and the Welsh Senedd are able to use devolved powers to legislate in areas such as local government, agriculture and fisheries, education and health. This differs from a federal system in that the grant of powers is made, and could be rescinded, by the Westminster Parliament, thus preserving the UK's *de jure* status as a unitary state. Health became a devolved matter on 1 July 1999. Since then, each country has developed its NHS system in a distinctive way (Greer, 2004; Hughes and Vincent-Jones, 2008).

In retrospect, the Labour government devolution reforms, which at the time attracted only limited attention in health policy circles, were to have a more profound and lasting effect on the UK's healthcare system than other health reforms of that period. Following Labour's victory in the 1997 UK general election, the Blair Government initially appeared set to end the split between NHS purchasers and providers and to replace the NHS internal market with

DOI: 10.4324/9781003139799-5

an integrated system, but it quickly returned to policies favouring markets and competition. From 2003, it introduced a package of reforms that created a 'provider market' based on autonomous Foundation Trust hospitals, a role for independent-sector treatment centres, increased patient choice of provider, standard national tariffs for NHS treatments and system regulation via arm-length agencies in the form of the Care Quality Commission and Monitor. Under the internal market system, Scotland and Wales were already leaning towards greater system integration and cooperation rather than competition, and had moved to 'soften' the market by encouraging 'partnership' working between NHS purchasers and providers. Now dissident Labour-led administrations in the Scottish and Welsh assemblies decided to break from these Westminster New Labour policies. In 2004, Scotland created unified regional health boards, thus ending its purchaser/provider split. Wales continued for a few years with a soft version of the internal market in which Local Health Boards purchased services from NHS trusts, before abolishing its internal market in 2009 in favour of unified health boards. Thus the early post-devolution period heralded a striking divergence in policy, as Scotland and Wales explored alternatives to the English market approach.

A shared history?

The NHS began operation across the whole of the UK on 5 July 1948, based on common principles and entitlements. The aim was to provide universal and comprehensive health services, according to need rather than ability to pay to all residents. Although the title 'National Health Service' implies a single UK-wide health service, separate legislation was used to create one NHS for England and Wales, accountable to the secretary of state for health, and a separate NHS for Scotland, accountable to the secretary of state for Scotland. Similar health services in Northern Ireland were created through the Health Services Act (Northern Ireland) 1948.

During the early history of the NHS, the health systems of England and Wales were managed by the central government's main health department (initially the Ministry of Health and later the Department of Health and Social Security, the Department of Health and currently the Department of Health and Social Care [DHSC]), while Scotland and Northern Ireland were managed by the Scottish Office and Northern Ireland Office, respectively. In 1969, new legislation separated the Welsh NHS from the English NHS and put it under the control of a separate UK government department, the Welsh Office, rather than the Department of Health.

Scotland

Shortly after devolution in 1999, the Scottish Government, then a Labour-led coalition, began discussions on dismantling the internal market, dissolving trusts, promoting integration of care, strengthening primary care and improving public health. The NHS Reform (Scotland) Act 2004 abolished trusts and transferred their functions to 15 integrated regional Health Boards (later reduced to 14) (Robson, 2011). The Health Boards have been described as 'all-purpose organisations' that plan, commission and deliver a wide range of hospital and community health services, including managing contracts with general practitioners (GPs) and dentists who operate as independent contractors. A unique feature of the reform was that the Health Boards were given powers to create Community Health Partnerships (CHPs), networks in which frontline NHS staff worked closely with local authority and voluntary agency staff to improve health services in a geographical area (Forbes and Evans, 2008).

A further significant change occurred in 2007 when a minority Scottish National Party (SNP) government came to power. Its big idea was a 'mutual NHS' as outlined in the policy document *Better Health, Better Care*. The new policy emphasised cooperation and collaboration rather than market competition and outlined a vision of greater public involvement, improved quality driven by performance targets and strengthened partnership working. With the election of a majority SNP government in 2011, policies based on mutuality developed further. The report of the Christie Commission on the Future Delivery of Public Services published shortly after the election suggested a framework for further reform. The perceived need for improved integration of NHS and local authority services put a question mark against the CHPs, whose track record in achieving health improvement had been questioned in a 2011 Audit Scotland Report. The 2014 Public Bodies (Joint Working) (Scotland) Act replaced CHPs with Health and Social Care Partnerships, spanning the two sectors, which became operational from 2016 (Pearson and Watkins, 2018; Taylor, 2015).

In an analysis of the language of policy documents from the four countries, Prior, Hughes and Peckham (2012) point to a rhetorical emphasis in the Scottish documents on the nation and the 'people of Scotland' that gives them a more overtly nationalistic tone than the documents of the other countries. A narrative is constructed in which the Scottish population is ageing faster and dying quicker than 'any other industrial nation', that the 'Scottish people' must improve their healthcare system so that it compares with 'other European countries', that a change of the culture of both professionals and the public is needed, and that this should take a distinctively Scottish form, involving values of mutuality, co-ownership, partnership, and involvement, as well as a collective approach. In this narrative, the Scottish people and the staff of the NHS are seen as partners or co-owners of an NHS that relies on cooperation and collaboration rather than internal competition (Prior, Hughes and Peckham, 2012).

At the time of writing, the Scottish Government Directorate for Health and Social Care oversees 14 territorial Health Boards, connected to 31 integration partnerships that span the Health Boards and Councils. The Directorate also manages a number of special health authorities with discrete roles, such as Public Health Scotland, and central support departments within NHS National Services Scotland.

Wales

After devolution, the direction of Welsh policy initially involved a softening, rather than rejection of the NHS internal market, but in 2007, a Labour/Plaid Cymru coalition government published a *One Wales Delivery Plan* signalling the intention to end the purchaser/provider split and phase out use of the private sector for NHS work in Wales. Subsequently, seven unified health authorities were created to replace the then existing 22 Local Health Boards and seven NHS Trusts (Local Health Boards [Directed Functions] [Wales] Regulations 2009, SI 2009/1511). The Health Boards are responsible for a wide range of health services, including primary and specialised care for their populations, and they share responsibility for public health services with the national Public Health Wales and the local authorities. Currently the National Delivery Group within the Department of Health and Social Services oversees the seven Health Boards and three NHS Trusts, Public Health Wales, the Welsh Ambulance Service, and a specialist cancer and blood services trust.

Since the 2009 reorganisation, Welsh health policy has focused on such matters as improving population health, increased emphasis on prevention as opposed to curative services, improving joint working between health and social care, removing charges that might affect access (drug prescription charges and hospital parking charges) and reorganising structures to reduce waste. Riley (2016) identifies reduction of health inequalities as a key policy aim at this time. There was an attempt to coordinate policies targeting poverty reduction, community regeneration, early childhood support and integrated health services. The *1000 Lives* and *1000 Lives Plus* were two high-profile programmes that sought to save lives and reduce preventable morbidity.

The Welsh Government's big idea for improving services in a period of constrained budgets is 'prudent healthcare'. This concept was developed by the Bevan Commission (2013:3), an expert group convened to advise the health minister, and was defined as: 'healthcare which is conceived, managed and delivered in a cautious and wise way characterised by forethought, vigilance and careful budgeting which achieves tangible benefits and quality outcomes for patients'. Prudent healthcare is healthcare that is parsimonious but efficient; it seeks to get more for less by minimising waste and maximising clinical effectiveness. The initiative re-assembles familiar building blocks – co-production by professionals and patients, involving people in treatment and policy decisions, treating according to clinical need rather than targets, not over-treating, accelerating innovation, increased focus on patient safety and evidence-based treatments. A recent study identifies various barriers to the implementation of co-production, including poor health literacy and understanding of the concept, poor communication between professionals and service users, and service capacity and time constraints (Holland-Hart et al., 2019). Given the unprecedented disruption of services caused by the Covid-19 pandemic, it will be many years before the effectiveness of the initiative can be evaluated.

Prior, Hughes and Peckham (2012) observe that Welsh policy documents of the early 2000s, like those of Scotland, made frequent references to national identity, but in Wales's case, the policy story constructed was that of a 'small nation' that needed a fairer share of UK resources. In this policy narrative, years of underfunding needed to be addressed, and the healthcare system 'renewed' and 'repaired'. The services inherited by the Assembly were overburdened and needed fundamental change. In addition, there was inadequate system capacity, and organisational reform was vital and required joint working between NHS professionals, health and social services, and the NHS and the people of Wales. These objectives would only be achieved by 'adopting Welsh solutions to Welsh challenges' (Prior, Hughes and Peckham, 2012:10–11).

Public health

Since devolution, Scotland and Wales, like England, have created national agencies to lead on public health, working in cooperation with local NHS bodies and local government public health divisions. Both countries have seen periodic organisational changes since 2000. Scotland initially divided public health functions, such as health improvement and protection, between separate national agencies, but later shifted back to a single lead body, Public Health Scotland. Wales made periodic changes to the internal directorate structure of a single national public health organisation. Organisations in both countries have similar remits to improve and protect population health (including through health promotion programmes), to oversee disease prevention, surveillance and control of outbreaks and incidents, to reduce health inequalities and to support other agencies involved in public health work.

Public Health Scotland was established as a national health board in April 2020 in order to respond more effectively to the Covid-19 pandemic and took over the functions previously performed by Health Protection Scotland and the Information Services Division (both divisions of NHS National Services Scotland) and NHS Health Scotland (a body with a remit to reduce health inequalities). Public Health Wales is an older body, created as an NHS Trust in October 2009, and carries out similar functions to those that had been previously spilt between the Scottish organisations via its various internal divisions. The 14 Scottish regional Health Boards and seven Welsh Health Boards each have a director of public health who is supported by the national bodies. In the past decade, as in England, local government authorities in both countries have also been given greater responsibilities for public health, and the work of public health teams extends to programmes addressing health inequalities and health improvement, as well as more traditional areas, such as environmental health, sanitation and food safety (Campbell, 2018). Public Health Wales and Public Health Scotland thus each sit at the centre of a network that includes their respective devolved governments, health boards, local authorities and other agencies. In Scotland, the role of the local authorities has been given more prominence than in Wales by making the Public Health Scotland formally accountable to both the Scottish Government and the Convention of Scottish Local Authorities.

A further element in this complicated web of organisations was the replacement of Public Health England in April 2021 with the UK Health Security Agency, an executive agency of the DHSC, again as a response to the Covid-19 pandemic. The new body has certain UK-wide responsibilities, such as providing national public health science and response capabilities – not least cutting-edge analytics and genomic surveillance (Department of Health and Social Care, 2021). Exactly how these duties intersect with the work of the Scottish and Welsh agencies, given that health is a devolved matter, remains subject to negotiation at the time of writing. Commenting in June 2021 on how the network of governments and other involved agencies operates, a senior Public Health Wales source, approached as background for this chapter, said, 'governance map . . . is complicated, emerging and subject to agreements of Welsh Ministers – so it is not easy to capture all at present!'

The impact of devolved policies on finance and performance

The devolved administrations receive an annual block grant to fund public services from the UK government. Per capita public expenditure is higher in the devolved countries than in England because of the Barnet Formula that determines allocations for public expenditure from the UK Treasury. In 2019–20, Scotland received £11,604 per head, and Wales £10, 929 per head, compared with £9,604 per head for England (HM Treasury, 2020). In 2018–19, the last 'normal' year before the pandemic, the NHS spend per head was £2,396 for Scotland, compared with £2,402 for Wales and £2,269 for England, reflecting the budget allocation choices of the devolved administrations (Nicholson and Shuttleworth, 2020). The higher expenditure in Scotland and Wales partly reflects higher costs associated with geography and demography, and this must be borne in mind when assessing performance.

While comparative studies of policies concerning patient choice, patient and public involvement and health inequalities have confirmed that there are real differences in the approaches taken by the UK countries, findings on system outcomes as set out in Box 2.1 do not show that any system has a clear performance advantage. Comparisons are difficult because of different methodologies for collecting official data across the four countries. The preface to a major UK-wide comparative study by the Nuffield Trust from 2014 states:

> different policies adopted by each country appear to have made little difference to long-term national trends on most of the indicators that the authors were able to compare. Individual countries can point to marginal differences in performance in one or more areas.
>
> (Bevan et al., 2014:8)

The detailed findings suggested that, at that time, England and Scotland were doing slightly better with hospital waiting times than Wales and Northern Ireland but does not establish whether English-style market levers were necessarily better than Scottish performance management.

Box 2.1   Performance against key NHS standards at December 2019

Scotland

- 88% of attendances at accident and emergency (A&E) services were admitted, transferred or discharged within 4 hours (missed 95% standard).
- 78.9% treated within 18-week referral to treatment (RTT) standard (missed 90% standard).
- 83.3% of patients started cancer treatment within the 62 days of referral (missed 95% standard).

Wales

- 74.4% of attendances at A&E services were admitted, transferred or discharged within four hours (missed 95% standard).
- 83.5% treated within 26-week RTT standard (missed 95% standard).
- 80.6% started cancer treatment within 62 days of suspected diagnosis (missed 95% standard).

England

- 79.8% of attendances at A&E services were admitted, transferred or discharged within four hours (missed 90% standard).
- 83.7% on incomplete RTT paths waited 18 weeks or less (missed 92% standard).
- 78% of patients started cancer treatment within the 62 days of referral (missed 85% standard).

Source: Scottish Government (2022); Statistics Wales (2020); NHS England (2020).

Interestingly Scotland combined a policy emphasis on 'mutuality' with willingness to use hierarchical command and control. Guthrie and colleagues (2010) argue that there was a blend of mutuality in the form of 'control through group processes' and government 'oversight' that included performance management. From 2006, Scottish Health Boards were required to meet new HEAT (health, efficiency, access and treatment) targets, which were to become a distinctive feature of the Scottish system and more rigorous than the equivalent systems in Wales and Northern Ireland (Steel and Cylus, 2012).

Following the 2008 financial crisis, the performance of all four UK systems was affected by UK central government austerity policies. Audit Scotland reported a real-term reduction in NHS spending of about 0.7% between 2008–09 and 2014–15 (Auditor General Scotland, 2015). This was partly the result of the failure of the block grant from the UK central government to keep pace with inflation, and also because Scotland opted to share available resources across social services and other departments rather than to protect NHS budgets, as Wales had done. Reduced funding contributed to problems of rising waiting times and uneven staff recruitment. In the early years after devolution, it was suggested that the HEAT target system allowed Scotland to cope better with austerity than the other devolved administrations (see Steel and Cylus, 2012), but waiting times have continued to be a problem, and in 2015–16, HEAT targets were replaced by Local Delivery Plan Standards, which focused more on waiting-time targets.

After this relatively strong performance in earlier years, the Scottish government has faced recent criticism for failing to hit national NHS targets. Only one of the eight key national waiting-time standards was achieved in 2017–18 and two in 2018/19. In the latter year, performance declined for six out of the eight standards, with the exceptions being outpatient waits of under 12 weeks following first referral and the 31-day cancer waiting-time target (Auditor General Scotland, 2019). Any precise assessment of the relative performance of Scotland and Wales on such measures is problematic, because each country uses slightly different standards, although Box 2.1 shows that, for three high-profile targets, there is little to choose between the countries and little difference from England.

NHS Wales was widely criticised in the early 2000s for its long waiting times and its standard for referral to treatment (RTT) being set at 26 weeks compared with 18 weeks in the other home countries. As time has passed, the gap has become smaller, with performance in Scotland and England falling back. A 2015 Auditor General Wales (2015:11) report concludes:

> Overall, the NHS has improved against some public health measures and against some of its key performance measures on quality. But . . . performance against measures of waiting times – for elective care, emergency care and cancer care – have deteriorated.

Problems in managing waiting times – especially in orthopaedics and ophthalmology – meant that several health boards increased the value of activity undertaken by private providers, causing politicians to backtrack from earlier promises to end use of the private sector for NHS work.

The Covid-19 pandemic

In the early days of the pandemic, all four home countries benefited from advice from the existing UK scientific advisory structures (House of Commons, 2020). The Scientific Group for Emergencies (SAGE) reported to the UK Cabinet Office Briefing Room meetings and the Civil Contingencies Secretariat, a body within the Cabinet. SAGE brought together advice from specialist subgroups that included the Scientific Pandemic Influenza Group on Modelling, the Scientific Pandemic Influenza Group on Behavioural Science, and the New and Emerging Respiratory Virus Threats Advisory Group. The experience in setting up field hospitals, first created in London, was shared across the UK. All constituent countries began a compulsory lockdown on 23 March 2020, under powers contained in the Coronavirus Act 2020. Throughout the pandemic, personal protective equipment, diagnostics, ventilators and vaccines were procured centrally on an all-UK basis. It was only in May 2020 when the UK Government announced a phased relaxation of restrictions, guided by a newly established Joint Biosecurity Centre, that the devolved administrations complained about a lack of consultation and began to diverge from a shared UK-wide approach (Anderson et al., 2021). Scotland established the Scottish Government Covid-19 Advisory Group, while the Welsh Government created a 'technical advisory cell', both to adapt SAGE guidance for their territorial contexts.

The UK's speedy roll-out of vaccinations compared with European neighbours helped shield the government from criticism for high death rates in 2020, but even here, Wales and Scotland followed different approaches. In June 2021, Audit Wales reported that Covid-19 vaccination rates in Wales were the highest of the four UK countries and among the highest in the world (Auditor General Wales, 2021). Wales adopted UK prioritisation guidance from the Joint Committee on Vaccination and Immunisation, and messaging from the UK and Welsh governments has generally been consistent. After criticism for a slow start in February 2021, the pace of vaccination rollout quickly improved. Initially, immunisers were all registered NHS professionals, but this was extended to include general practice staff and then trained non-registered immunisers, including military personnel. An assessment by the military of sites and operating procedures for mass vaccination centres is said to have aided the pace of rollout. It has been suggested that a key factor in Wales' high vaccination rate was that the Welsh Government was prepared to use a higher proportion of available stocks soon after receipt, taking the gamble that further supplies would arrive in time for second vaccinations (Ferris, 2021). Wales also opted to move through the age cohorts more quickly than other parts of the UK, while tolerating lower uptake in top priority groups.

In mid-2021, Scotland's vaccination rate was lower than that of both Wales and England. There was a slower progression through the cohorts but greater uptake within high-risk groups than in Wales. Critics suggest that

Scotland suffered because it was slow in opening mass vaccination centres, while vaccine supplies to GPs were affected by the complexity of Scottish supply chains. They contend that the Scottish Government was slow to cooperate from the UK central government, with Scotland only negotiating the deployment of military personnel in mass vaccination centres many weeks after Wales (Rossiter, 2021). There have also been suggestions that Scotland's concern with 'mutuality' and equitable shares to health boards according to population share and geography slowed distribution (Maishman, 2021). Generally, the rules and timetable of public health measures introduced in Scotland were further from the English approach than was the case for Wales.

However, as the pandemic progressed, it was not clear that Wales' impressive vaccine roll-out had translated into a clear advantage in terms of lower infection and death rates. In the period before 25 May 2022 when Public Health Wales ceased to update data for its 'Covid-19 dashboard', the rate of estimated daily infections in Scotland was mostly lower than that in Wales, although the relative positions of the two countries fluctuated week by week. For example, in the week ending 13 May, one in 45 people in Scotland were estimated to be infected with Covid-19 compared with one in 40 in Wales. Yet in the week ending 21 May, the pattern had reversed so that one in 40 were estimated to be positive in Scotland, while the Welsh figure was one in 55 (ONS, 2022). By 25 May 2022, deaths in which Covid-19 was recorded as a factor on the death certificate stood at 12,344 in Scotland and 10,308 in Wales (Public Health Wales, 2022; Public Health Scotland, 2022), which indicates a lower mortality rate in Scotland, given a Scottish population of about 5.46 million compared with under 3.3 million living in Wales. Of course, a range of geographic, demographic and social factors, apart from differences in public policy, are likely to have affected these outcomes.

Sustainability

NHS-type systems throughout Europe are facing a squeeze arising from a combination of constrained budgets and increased demand that raises questions about sustainability. While the NHS across the UK saw a modest rise in budgets in the years after the millennium, the global financial crisis of 2008 heralded a period of austerity in which real-term government funding barely rose. Against a background of tightening budgets, Scotland and Wales must both cope with increasing levels of service utilisation arising from ageing populations and high rates of chronic illness. Compared with England, the sparsely populated geography of the two Celtic countries also means that they must support the higher costs of providing services in rural and remote areas.

Across the UK home countries, Wales has the oldest population, with Scotland in second place. Thus 21% of the population in Wales is aged 65 and over, compared with 19.1% in Scotland, and 18.4% in the more populous England. Against this, however, the proportion of over 65s in Scotland is rising faster than that in England and significantly faster than in Wales (Public Health England, 2020). A recent study by Public Health England (2020) found that the burden of disease, as measured by the Global Burden of Disease methodology, is higher in both Scotland and Wales than in England. A Welsh study published by the Health Foundation (Watt and Roberts, 2016) determined that about 58% of total inpatient spend goes on treating patients with at least one of 12 chronic conditions, and that this rises to 72% of expenditure for patients aged 50 and over. The highest costs come from admissions of patients with coronary heart disease or heart failure, chronic obstructive pulmonary disease, asthma and cancer. A Scottish study by Barnett and colleagues (2012) found a similar pattern of chronic disease and noted that over 23% of persons registered with 314 general medical practices suffered from multimorbidity (two or more chronic conditions). This was a particular problem for older people but affected those suffering socio-economic deprivation 10–15 years earlier than the most affluent.

In Wales, around 30% of the population lives in rural areas (Gartner, Gibbon and Riley, 2007), while, in Scotland, the figure is about 20% (MacVicar and Nicoll, 2013). Providing equitable healthcare provision in sparsely populated areas presents logistical and economic challenges. While there is a perception that health is generally better in rural as opposed to urban locations, the picture appears uneven so that there are pockets of deprivation. Rural populations are generally older than urban populations, compounded by outward migration of young people and inward migration of older people, and more likely to face challenges in accessing services.

While ageing populations and the rising incidence of long-term illness and multimorbidity are important drivers for rising demand for healthcare services, there may be other factors that contribute to increased utilisation. Wider socio-economic factors, such as housing, employment, and changes to benefits and universal credit, have also been noted as contributing factors to demand (Watt and Roberts, 2016).

In both Scotland and Wales, there are questions about how well NHS organisations with severely constrained budgets can cope with rising demand. Problems are similar to those of NHS England and include financial distress because of current or cumulative deficits, lower than planned income, overspending on commissioning of specialised services, year-on-year transfers of capital allocations to revenue, rising provider costs and problems in staff recruitment and retention (House of Commons, 2019). Although deficits in Wales have been smaller than in England, four of the seven health boards had significant historic debt in July 2020 when the health minister announced that the Welsh Government would write off £480 million owed by the Boards for strategic cash support (Donovan, 2020). At the time of writing, three Welsh Health Boards were operating with significant year-on-year deficits. A number of Scotland's 14 Health Boards had been reliant on similar Government 'brokerage' loans to cope with ongoing financial problems, and these debts were written off in 2019 as part of a 'new deal' associated with the introduction of three-year, rolling budgetary balance requirement (Auditor General Scotland, 2019). In 2021, four Health Boards were reported to be experiencing ongoing financial distress, and required to repay loans accrued since 2019 once the Covid-19 crisis ended (Auditor General Scotland, 2021).

Questions about the financial sustainability of the NHS are as old as the service itself, and the positive assessment contained in the Guillebaud Report (House of Commons, 1956) was an important watershed in overcoming early political opposition to public healthcare. A recent House of Lords (2017) report on the future of the NHS across the UK stated: 'Our conclusion could not be clearer. Is the NHS and adult social care system sustainable? Yes, it is. Is it sustainable as it is today? No, it is not. Things need to change.' Recent reports from Wales and Scotland echo the view that the NHS can survive but will need radical transformation. Since the Wanless Review (Welsh Assembly Government, 2003), the general strategy in Wales has been to focus more on prevention and early intervention and reconfigure services so as to develop primary and community care and relieve pressure on the acute sector. Watt and Roberts (2016) map out a 'path to sustainability' for Wales that depends on additional funding in line with General Domestic Product (GDP) increases and a continuation of the present trend of efficiency savings. They see Wales' prudent healthcare principles of improving care and doing 'only what is needed' as key mechanisms for increasing value for money. The Welsh NHS Confederation (2017) suggests that this approach is widely supported by NHS managers. It reports that NHS bodies are 'seeking to manage their financial pressures by driving out inefficiencies, while at the same time looking to derive greater value from their resources through innovative ways of working and practicing Prudent Healthcare' (Welsh NHS Confederation, 2017:1). Funding and demand pressures that threaten sustainability have also been a recurrent theme of recent Scottish Auditor General reports, and again the message has been that the service can survive by adapting to changing conditions.

A recent systematic assessment of the future of the NHS by the LSE-Lancet Commission concludes that the service is sustainable to 2030 and beyond providing that policymakers commit to sufficient investment and improvements in resource management, workforce recruitment and retention, disease prevention, health protection, clinical diagnostics, organisational learning and integration of health and social care services (Anderson et al., 2021). The Commission notes that market-based reforms have not shown evidence of benefit to date and advocates the continuation of a 'publicly funded NHS for all'. It advocates improved coordination in managing the healthcare systems of the four UK countries, a move towards greater data standardisation to facilitate comparative research and more emphasis on mutual learning.

Political commitment to the NHS remains strong in both Wales and Scotland. Both have their founding stories of early mutual or public healthcare initiatives that foreshadowed a NHS. Welsh politicians can point the Tredegar Workmen's Medical Aid Society and the inspiration it provided to Aneurin

Bevan, the minister of health who oversaw the foundation of the NHS in 1948 (Launer, 2019). Scots recall the state-funded Highlands and Islands Medical Service that provided low-cost healthcare to those living in much of remote and rural Scotland between 1913 and 1948 (McCrae, 2003). The majority parties in both countries, Welsh Labour and the Scottish Nationalist Party, have alleged that the UK Conservative government is intent on creeping privatisation of an NHS that they promise to protect. Recent opinion polls suggest that the NHS enjoys continuing strong support from the general publics in both countries.

Are the systems still faithful to the founding principles?

The establishment of the NHS in 1948 was viewed by its architects as an emphatic rejection of the healthcare market; health was to be a public good that would be both publicly financed and publicly delivered to the UK population. There would be a long period of post-war consensus in which the public NHS enjoyed wide support, including from right-wing Conservative ministers such as Enoch Powell who delivered a huge state-funded capital programme in the 1962 Hospital Plan. It was only in the 1980s that the political tide turned to favour markets and private sector methods with the Griffiths general management reforms, the growth of contracting out of hospital support services, greater use of private hospitals to reduce NHS waiting lists and the various iterations of the NHS internal market.

Market-oriented reforms and the opposition they provoked in Scotland and Wales have created schisms in the NHS and substantially re-shaped the UK healthcare landscape. However, a vision of a market-style English NHS existing in uneasy tension with alternative Celtic versions that remain truer to the original Beveridge vision oversimplifies what is a complicated and changing picture. Three elements that must be taken into account are: first, recent changes in NHS England that move it back in the direction of a planned, mainly publicly delivered service; second, the leakage of certain neo-liberal instruments in the Scottish and Welsh systems; and third, the many commonalities that these three NHS systems still share.

Since the enactment of the Health and Social Care Act 2012, the English NHS has witnessed a remarkable policy U-turn, so that legislation that appeared to open the way for privatisation and competition has been largely subverted by the creation of new entities that have no legal foundation in the Act. In outline, a system that had seemed to be about competition in a provider market unexpectedly turned back to cooperation and 'place-based planning'. As a self-protective reaction to austerity, front-line NHS bodies – the Clinical Commissioning Groups, NHS providers and NHS England's area teams – acted in concert to create new, non-legally sanctioned organisational structures to provide integrated services in local areas and maximise what could be achieved with limited budgets. The story of sustainability and transformation plans, accountable care organisations, integrated care systems and area-based local health economies or 'footprints' lies outside the scope of this chapter (see Moran et al., 2021; Paton, 2021), but in outline mean that changes introduced on the ground in recent years have narrowed the gap between England and the other UK countries.

Moving to the second point, the greater scale and central resources of NHS England result in many policy spill-overs and leakages from that system into the Scottish and Welsh NHS systems, especially the latter. For example, NHS Wales has a service-level agreement with the National Institute for Health and Care Excellence (NICE) to utilise its technology appraisals, clinical guidelines and interventional procedure guidance, as well as public health and social care guidance and the NICE Quality Standards and Clinical Pathways. The Welsh 1000 Lives Improvement Patient Flow Programme was inspired by the Health Foundation's Flow Cost Quality programme that had been successfully rolled out in several English hospitals, and the Principality's 'expert patient programme' was heavily influenced by development work undertaken by the equivalent English programme. Both Wales and Scotland make tertiary care referrals to English providers, and must pay for this activity using standard prices based on English 'Payment by Results' tariffs, albeit with smaller patient flows coming from Scotland that are largely restricted to 'highly specialised services'. More generally, there are mutual influences and a degree of convergence in several areas of health policy (Wallace, 2019).

Like England, Scotland and Wales continue to make use of independent providers to treat NHS patients, and indeed spending on this has risen in recent years (Auditor General Scotland, 2015; Smith, 2018). SNP campaigning in the run-up to the 2015 Scotland independence referendum had claimed that the ongoing English NHS reforms were a prelude to privatisation, yet spending on private treatments by the NHS in Scotland rose by about 18% in real terms in the five years to 2015 (Auditor General Scotland, 2015). This was mainly to meet waiting-time targets by increasing short-term capacity but also to provide some specialist services not available in public hospitals. Stubbornly, rising waiting lists led the Welsh Government to shelve the promise in the *One Wales* document to end use of private sector treatments by 2012. Welsh Health Board expenditure on private providers rose from £13.8 million in 2010–11 to £61 million in 2019–20 (Auditor General Wales, 2020).

Finding funds for major capital projects was difficult in a period of austerity, when the value of block grants under the Barnet formula has fallen in real terms. As a means of accessing funds, both devolved countries have used private finance initiative (PFI) type contracts to build and run health and social care facilities, with numbers of projects lower than in England but not wildly out of line with relative populations. Scotland has used private capital more than Wales, and the high cost of the PFI and its successor the 'non-profit distribution' model was heavily criticised in a report from Audit Scotland and the Accounts Commission in January 2020. In 2019, the Scottish government announced that it would be adopting Mutual Investment Model used in Wales, an alternative 'off book' system of harnessing private capital to build public-sector infrastructure that remains controversial.

The third point to consider is that Scottish and Welsh systems still bear a strong family resemblance to the English NHS, despite the emerging differences. The degree of divergence is limited by shared organisational histories and continued commitment to the founding principles of the 1948 service. All the UK NHS systems continue to be funded from general taxation, with health spending being the largest item in the budgets of the devolved administrations. Although there are differences in eligibility for free drug prescriptions and eye tests and NHS dentistry charges, medical treatments remain free at the point of need. All the systems are subject to a high degree of political direction from the national or devolved governments, with politicians generally held accountable for any shortcomings in service provision and delivery. The terms and conditions of employment and pay of staff in the various health professions are essentially the same. In all four countries, almost all GPs, NHS dentists and NHS pharmacists are contractors rather than direct employees. Moreover, the training pathways for the workforce are similar across the UK and subject to the same framework of regulation; professionals trained in Scottish medical schools or university nursing departments can work in England and Wales and vice versa. Devolution has transformed NHS governance arrangements, but it could be argued that the approaches and instruments deployed across all the UK countries was anyway moving on from the old-style central control structures of the 1948 model.

Even when market policies were in vogue, the governance of public services in the UK could be best characterised as 'centralised decentralisation', involving combinations of continued hierarchical control as well as delegation and devolution (Vincent-Jones, 2006). In England, with the purchaser/provider split still in place, decentralisation has taken the form of the delegation of service contracting and other responsibilities to local purchasers and agencies, while in Wales and Scotland, the emphasis has been more on initiatives intended to increase engagement with local communities.

The devolved administrations have given a fresh twist to command and control by portraying this as control by government departments located close to the populations they serve. Both Wales and Scotland position themselves as small countries within a system of multi-level governance, albeit in different ways. At the time of the original devolution settlements, Labour Party-led coalitions in both countries worked within the framework of reserved and devolved powers granted by the Westminster Parliament and so implicitly accepted a place in a truly UK-wide model. NHS policies could be tailored to the needs of Welsh and Scottish populations but still looked towards important elements of a shared NHS. Wales' vision of small country governance involves centrally organised health and social services that achieve greater citizen responsiveness by improved centre–periphery 'connections' and better coordination at both departmental and local levels (see Hughes, Mullen and Vincent-Jones, 2009). Interestingly Wales, like England, has used the idea of networks as an alternative to hierarchical management structures in its policy document, using the words 'a new Welsh public service based on flexible networks of diverse pathways involving a range of organisations, all working to a common citizen-centred model' (Welsh Assembly Government, 2006: para 2.24). Scottish policy documents also emphasise the importance of citizen engagement, partnerships and integrated services. But in a sparsely populated country of highlands and islands, they put less emphasis on close centre–periphery connections and more on the viability of the nation. Thus the SNP, the ruling Party in the Scottish Parliament since 2011, has long argued that sustainable independence for Scotland depends on membership of a larger economic entity in the form of the European Union (EU) (Ichijo, 2004).

Conclusion: an uncertain future?

At present, Scotland and Wales have each adopted an NHS system tailored to their own political preferences, but it is uncertain whether these arrangements will endure in the long term because of the divergent dynamics of devolved Governments and nationalist movements. In the 2021 Senedd elections, the Welsh Labour Party was returned to government with an increased majority over its nationalist rival, Plaid Cymru, and remained strongly committed to continued union with the other UK countries, albeit within an enhanced devolution settlement. By contrast, the corresponding elections for the Scottish Parliament left the SNP in a dominant position, heading a coalition with the Green Party strongly committed to an independence referendum and an application to re-join the European Union. There would be many obstacles to be overcome and many years would pass before that aspiration could be achieved, but if it came to pass, Scotland would join the minority of European nations that retain the NHS model, rather than the social health insurance (SHI) model favoured by the EU's most powerful member states.

The future of the Scottish healthcare system might then be shaped by the same forces affecting other European NHS-type healthcare systems considered in this volume. The EU regards healthcare as a non-economic 'service of general interest' (SGI), a service that public authorities must provide either through market or through non-market mechanisms in order to satisfy their public service obligations. Article 14 of the Treaty on the Functioning of the EU allows considerable flexibility in the mode of provision when it states that SGIs must 'operate on the basis of principles and conditions, particularly economic and financial conditions, which enable them to fulfil their missions'. In the healthcare field, this allows national government's freedom to determine the organisation and funding of services as long as they conform to general EU principles, but it is not certain whether this degree of policy subsidiarity will continue into the future, given the trend towards convergence in many areas of economic and social policies. If a more uniform European approach to healthcare begins to emerge, there seems a high probability that this would involve convergence towards SHI rather than the NHS model. Exactly what would emerge remains uncertain because of blurring of the boundaries that separated the classic Beveridge and Bismarck systems. In some countries, such as France, contribution-based funding has been supplemented by funding through taxation. However, any hybrid system would probably involve the widespread use of private-sector providers and co-payment characteristic of current SHI systems. Even if NHS-type systems survive, there are questions about their resilience in the face of the current trend of European economic and financial policies, which, for Eurozone countries, include the rules of the Growth and Stability Pact and 'Six Pack' and appear to have contributed to the austerity that has impacted negatively on the healthcare systems of the Mediterranean sub-region, not least on that of Greece. The idea that Scottish independence is compatible with the conferral of powers that EU membership entails remains controversial, and critics have questioned whether an escape to Europe would merely replace UK neo-liberalism with the neo-liberalism of the EU's economic policy framework (Paterson, 2015).

It seems clear that Wales will remain committed to the NHS model for the foreseeable future, and if, as an EU member in its own right, Scotland did over time shift towards the SHI model, that would put the two systems on different paths. Most Western European countries deliver high-quality healthcare with commendable efficiency, albeit at generally higher cost in terms of percentage of GDP spent. However, implementing SHI would almost certainly involve changing from access to services based on residency to more strictly defined conditional eligibility, greater use of co-payments and increased purchaser pluralism. In a recent international ranking exercise, these are among the factors that resulted in France and Germany achieving lower scores for equity, access and continuity of care compared with the British NHS (Davis et al., 2014). Interestingly, the only territory previously to break away from the UK, the Republic of Ireland, provides free public healthcare only to around a third of its population, pushing many others towards voluntary health insurance as an alternative to user charges in the state system. Ireland has the highest uptake of private insurance in the EU with around 45% of the population covered in this way.

References

Anderson, M., Pitchforth, E., Asaria, M., et al. (2021) 'LSE-Lancet Commission on the future of the NHS: Re-laying the foundations for an equitable and efficient health and care service after COVID-19', *Lancet Commissions* 397(10288): 1915–78.

Auditor General Scotland (2015) *NHS in Scotland 2015*, Edinburgh: Audit Scotland. Available at: www.audit-scotland.gov.uk/publications/nhs-in-scotland-2015

Auditor General Scotland (2019) *NHS in Scotland 2019*, Edinburgh: Audit Scotland. Available at: www.audit-scotland.gov.uk/report/nhs-in-scotland-2019#&gid=1&pid=1

Auditor General Scotland (2021) *NHS in Scotland 2020*, Edinburgh: Audit Scotland. Available at: www.audit-scotland.gov.uk/uploads/docs/report/2021/n. r_210117_nhs_overview.pdf

Auditor General Wales (2020) *NHS Wales 2019–20: Key Facts (Infographic)*, Cardiff: Audit Wales. Available at: https://audit.wales/infographics/nhs-wales-summarised-account

Auditor General Wales (2021) *Rollout of the COVID-19 Vaccination Programme in Wales*, Cardiff: Audit Wales. Available at: https://audit.wales/publication/rollout-covid-19-vaccination-programme-wales

Barnett, K., Mercer, S. W., Norbury, M., Watt, G., Wyke, S. and Gurthrie, B. (2012) 'Epidemiology of multimorbidity and implications for health care, research, and medical education: A cross-sectional study', *The Lancet* 380(9836): 37–43.

Bevan Commission (2013) *Simply Prudent Healthcare: Achieving Better Care and Value for Money in Wales*. Available at: www.bevancommission.org/sitesplus/documents/1101/Bevan%20Commission%20Simply%20Prudent%20Healthcare%20v1%2004122013.pdf.

Bevan, G., Karanikolos, M., Exley, J., Nolte, E., Connolly, S. and Mays, N. (2014) *The Four Health Systems of the United Kingdom: How Do They Compare?* London: Nuffield Trust and The Health Foundation.

Campbell, F. (2018) *A Matter of Justice: Local Government's Role in Tackling Health Inequalities*, London: Local Government Association.

Davis, K., Stremikis, K., Squires, D. and Schoen, C. (2014) *Mirror, Mirror on the Wall: How the Performance of the U.S. Health Care System Compares Internationally*, New York: The Commonwealth Fund. Available at: www.commonwealthfund.org/sites/default/files/documents/media_files_publications_fund_report_2014_jun_1755_davis_mirror_mirror_2014.pdf

Department of Health and Social Care (2021) *Transforming the Public Health System: Reforming the Public Health System for the Challenges of Our Times*. London: HMSO. Available at: www.gov.uk/government/publications/transforming-the-public-health-system/transforming-the-public-health-system-reforming-the-public-health-system-for-the-challenges-of-our-times

Donovan, O. (2020) 'Senedd roundup: Government writes off £470 million of NHS debt', *Nation Cymru*, 7 July. Available at: https://nation.cymru/news/senedd-roundup-government-writes-off-470-million-of-nhs-debt/

Ferris, N. (2021) 'How Wales leads the world in the Covid-19 vaccine race', *New Statesman*, 1 June. Available at: www.newstatesman.com/science-tech/2021/06/how-wales-leads-world-covid-19-vaccine-race

Forbes, T. and Evans, D. (2008) 'Health and social care partnerships in Scotland', *Scottish Affairs* 65(1): 87–106.

Gartner, A., Gibbon, R. and Riley, N. (2007) *A Profile of Rural Health in Wales*. Available at: https://ruralhealthandcare.wales/wp-content/uploads/2017/08/remote-and-rural-healthcare-updated.pdf

Greer, S. L. (2004) *Territorial Politics and Health Policy: UK Health Policy in Comparative Perspective*, Manchester: Manchester University Press.

Guthrie, B., Davies, H., Greig, G., et al. (2010) *Delivering Health Care Through Managed Clinical Networks (MCNS): Lessons From the North*, Report for NIHR SDO Programme, London: HMSO.

HM Treasury (2020) *National Statistics. Country and Regional Analysis*, London: HM Treasury. Available at: www.gov.uk/government/statistics/country-and-regional-analysis-2020/country-and-regional-analysis-november-2020

Holland-Hart, D., Addis, S., Edwards, A., Kenkre, J. and Wood, J. (2019) 'Coproduction and health: Public and clinicians' perceptions of the barriers and facilitators', *Health Expectations* 22: 93–101.

House of Commons (1956) *Report of the Committee of Enquiry Into the Cost of the National Health Service* (The Guillebaud Report), London: HMSO.

House of Commons (2019) *NHS Financial Sustainability: Progress Review*, Committee of Public Accounts, Ninety-First Report of Session 2017–19. Available at: https://publications.parliament.uk/pa/cm201719/cmselect/cmpubacc/1743/1743.pdf

House of Commons (2020) *The UK Response to Covid-19: Use of Scientific Advice*, House of Commons Science and Technology Committee, First Report of Session 2019–21.

House of Lords (2017) *The Long-Term Sustainability of the NHS and Adult Social Care, Select Committee on the Long-Term Sustainability of the NHS*, Report Session 2016–17, HL Paper 151. Available at: https://publications.parliament.uk/pa/ld201617/ldselect/ldnhssus/151/151.pdf

Hughes, D., Mullen, C. and Vincent-Jones, P. (2009) 'Choice versus voice? PPI policies and the re-positioning of the state in England and Wales', *Health Expectations* 12(3): 237–50.

Hughes, D. and Vincent-Jones, P. (2008) 'Schisms in the church: NHS systems and institutional divergence in England and Wales', *Journal of Health and Social Behavior* 49(4): 400–16.

Ichijo, A. (2004) *Scottish Nationalism and the Idea of Europe*, London: Routledge.

Launer, J. (2019) 'A tribute to Tredegar', *Postgraduate Medical Journal* 95: 407–8.

MacVicar, R. and Nicoll, P. (2013) 'NHS education for Scotland: Supporting remote and rural healthcare', *NES Board Paper*, August. Available at: https://rural-healthandcare.wales/wp-content/uploads/2017/08/remote-and-rural-healthcare-updated.pdf

Maishman, E. (2021) 'Covid in Scotland: Why are vaccination rates so different between health boards?', *The Scotsman*, 11 May. Available at: www.scotsman.com/health/covid-in-scotland-why-are-vaccination-rates-so-different-between-health-boards-3231620

McCrae, M. (2003) *The National Health Service in Scotland: Origins and Ideals, 1900–1950*, East Linton: Tuckwell Press.

Moran, V., Allen, P., Sanderson, M., McDermott, I. and Osipovic, D. (2021) 'Challenges of maintaining accountability in networks of health and care organisations: A study of developing sustainability and transformation partnerships in the English National Health Service', *Social Science and Medicine* 268: 113512.

NHS England (2020) *NHS Performance Statistics*, January/February. Available at: www.england.nhs.uk/statistics/wp-content/uploads/sites/2/2020/01/Combined-Performance-Summary-January-November-December-data-2020-c7d3g.pdf; www.england.nhs.uk/statistics/wp-content/uploads/sites/2/2020/02/Combined-Performance-Summary-February-December-January-data-2020-oi2U9.pdf

Nicholson, E. and Shuttleworth, K. (2020) *Devolution and the NHS*, London: Institute for Government. Available at: www.instituteforgovernment.org.uk/explainers/devolution-nhs.

Office of National Statistics (ONS) (2022) *Coronavirus (COVID-19) Infection Survey*, UK, 20 May 2022. Available at: www.ons.gov.uk/peoplepopulationandcommunity/healthandsocialcare/conditionsanddiseases/bulletins/coronaviruscovid19infectionsurveypilot/20may2022

Paterson, B. (2015) 'Questioning the "common sense": Was Scottish independence really an alternative to UK neoliberalisation?', *Capital and Class* 39(3): 493–514.

Paton, C. (2021) '"There's the end of an auld sang": Farewell to the NHS market', *International Journal of Health Planning and Management* 36(5): 1392–96. Available at: https://doi.org/10.1002/hpm.3173.

Pearson, C. and Watkins, N. (2018) 'Implementing health and social care integration in Scotland: Renegotiating new partnerships in changing cultures of care', *Health and Social Care in the Community* 26(3): e396–403.

Prior, L., Hughes, D. and Peckham, S. (2012) 'The discursive turn in policy analysis and the validation of policy stories', *Journal of Social Policy* 41(2): 271–89.

Public Health England (2020) *The Burden of Disease in England Compared With 22 Peer Countries: A Report for NHS England*, London: PHE. Available at: https://assets.publishing.service.gov.uk/government/uploads/system/uploads/attachment_data/file/856938/GBD_NHS_England_report.pdf

Public Health Scotland (2022) *COVID-19 Daily Dashboard*. Available at: https://public.tableau.com/app/profile/phs.covid.19/viz/COVID-19DailyDashboard_15960160643010/Dailyupdate

Public Health Wales (2022) *ONS Mortality Data for Wales*. Available at: https://public.tableau.com/app/profile/public.health.wales.health.protection/viz/CovidDashboard_ONSmortality/ONSdeaths

Riley, C. (2016) 'The challenge of creating a "Welsh NHS"', *Journal of Health Service Research Policy* 21: 40–2.

Robson, K. (2011) *The National Health Service in Scotland: Subject Profile*, Edinburgh: Scottish Parliament.

Rossiter, J. (2021) 'What's holding up Scotland's vaccine rollout?', *The Spectator*, 4 February. Available at: www.spectator.co.uk/article/what-s-holding-up-scotland-s-vaccine-rollout-#

Saks, M. (2010) 'Analyzing the professions: The case for the neo-Weberian approach', *Comparative Sociology* 9(6): 887–915.

Scottish Government (2022) *NHS Scotland Performance Against LDP Standards*. Available at: www.gov.scot/publications/nhsscotland-performance-against-ldp-standards/pages/accident-and-emergency-waiting-times/; www.gov.scot/publications/nhsscotland-performance-against-ldp-standards/pages/18-weeks-referral-to-treatment/; www.gov.scot/publications/nhsscotland-performance-against-ldp-standards/pages/cancer-waiting-times/

Smith, M. (2018) 'The eye-watering amounts of money the Welsh NHS is spending on private companies to treat patients for them', *Wales Online*, 30 November. Available at: www.walesonline.co.uk/news/health/eye-watering-amounts-money-welsh-15473532

Statistics Wales (2020) *NHS Activity and Performance Summary*, December 2019/January 2020. Available at: www.slideshare.net/StatisticsWales/nhs-activity-and-performance-summary-december-2019-and-january-2020

Steel, D. and Cylus, J. (2012) 'United Kingdom (Scotland) health system review', *Health Systems in Transition* 14(9): 1–150.

Taylor, A. (2015) 'New act, new opportunity for integration in Scotland', *Journal of Integrated Care* 23(1): 3–9.

Vincent-Jones, P. (2006) *The New Public Contracting: Regulation, Responsiveness, Relationality*, Oxford: Oxford University Press.

Wallace, J. (2019) 'Understanding wellbeing and devolution in Scotland, Wales and Northern Ireland', in Wallace, J. (ed) *Wellbeing and Devolution: Reframing the Role of Government in Scotland, Wales and Northern Ireland*, Basel: Springer International Publishing.

Watt, T. and Roberts, A. (2016) *The Path to Sustainability Funding Projections for the NHS in Wales to 2019/20 and 2030/31*, London: Health Foundation. Available at:

www.health.org.uk/sites/default/files/PathToSustainability_0.pdf#:~:text=Our%20
projections%20suggest%20that%20longterm%20fiscal%20sustainability%20
of,rate%20for%20efficiency%20growth%20of%201%25%20a%20year

Welsh Assembly Government (2003) *The Review of Health and Social Care in Wales: The Report of the Project Team Advised by Derek Wanless*, Cardiff: WAG. Available at: www.wales.nhs.uk/documents/wanless-review-e.pdf

Welsh Assembly Government (2006) *Beyond Boundaries: Citizen-Centred Local Services for Wales* (Beecham Review Report), Cardiff: Welsh Assembly Government.

Welsh NHS Confederation (2017) *Finance and the NHS in Wales*. Available at: www.nhsconfed.org/-/media/Confederation/Files/public-access/Welsh-NHS-Confederation-Finance-Briefing.pdf

The Scandinavian macro-region

3   Sweden

Paula Blomqvist and Ulrika Winblad

Introduction

The Swedish healthcare system has a long history of state involvement, while market dynamics have been rare and underdeveloped. When the modern system was constructed after 1945, it came to reflect the dominant political ideology of social democracy and the Swedish social democratic party's preference for a system where both financing and care delivery was public, in line with the British National Health Service (NHS) model. Following the heritage of independent local and regional government, the system became strongly decentralised, with counties, later renamed regions, as the main providers of care.

In the 1980s, the system became exposed to strong financial pressure while at the same time being criticised for inefficiency and poor responsiveness to patient demands. As a result, a series of reforms was initiated, which aimed to introduce market elements such as competition and patient choice. This neoliberal reform trend continued in the following decades, leading to a gradual increase of private care providers in the outpatient sector. At the same time, regional political planning and steering continued to shape the system, for instance through reforms rationalising hospital care. Neither of these reform trends affected the system's financing structure, which meant that it retained its character of decentralised, Scandinavian-type NHS system.

At the same time, the universalistic principles on which the system is founded have become challenged by social developments. Disparities in income and living conditions increased in Sweden during the last decades – a development which has also led to reduced health equality, despite general improvements in public health. The low-educated and foreign-born are groups which stand out as having higher mortality and lower health status than the rest of the population. Such disparities in health were exposed during the Covid-19 pandemic, where the foreign-born in low- and middle-income countries were reported to have a substantially higher risk of infection and death than the general population.

In this chapter, we provide an overview of developments in the Swedish healthcare system loosely in a neo-Weberian and neo-institutionalist frame of reference since the early 1980s, including marketisation, privatisation,

DOI: 10.4324/9781003139799-7

structural reforms and new measures to monitor care quality. The changes which have taken place during the last four decades concern foremost the delivery of care services and modes of governance within the system. Taken together, these changes have made the system not only more pluralistic and responsive to patients' demands but also more fragmented and, in some ways, less egalitarian.

A short history of the Swedish healthcare system

The long legacy of statism in the Swedish healthcare system can be explained by the early establishment of a unitary state in the sixteenth century and the weak role of the church after the county's reformation in 1590s, when the Crown seized most of its property. The first hospitals were enacted through royal decree in the sixteenth century, and, in 1862, the main responsibility for managing hospitals was transferred to the regional level (Gustafsson, 1987). Outpatient care became organised in 1671 through a national system of state-employed doctors catering to the needs of the largely rural population – a system that remained in place until the 1960s. The private market for health providers was small and mainly limited to the few larger cities.

The Swedish state also became involved early on the financing of healthcare. The first public, voluntary, health insurance was created in 1891, but in contrast to health insurance in most other countries at the time, the Swedish insurance scheme was funded mainly by the state. Private health insurance remained a marginal feature – a fact that can be attributed to the low availability of commercial health services and poor market conditions (Ito, 1980). In 1947, health insurance was made compulsory, and, in 1955, a tax-funded universal health insurance which also covered medical drugs was enacted.

In the following decades, an expansion of the organisation for providing health services at the regional level followed, guided by ideals of public planning and public health promotion (Anell and Claesson, 1995). An important step towards a more coherent and integrated public healthcare system was taken in the early 1960s when the responsibility of regions for inpatient care was extended to outpatient health services. A system of district-based health centres employing medical teams of foremost general practitioners and nurses was created a few years later with the aim of offering basic health services to local populations within geographically defined areas. The new health centres (*vårdcentraler*), which replaced the old system of district-based doctors, were given responsibility not only for providing services to those who requested them but also for investigating health needs within their districts and working pro-actively to erase health inequalities. The creation of a national system of public health centres meant that not only hospital care but also primary care came under regional political control.

In 1970, a final step towards a completely public system was taken through a reform which severely limited opportunities for doctors to engage in private practice. The so-called Seven-Crowns reform, stipulating that doctors could only charge seven Swedish crowns (less than one euro) for patient visits, led to a further reduction of privately employed doctors. The reform, which was strongly opposed by the political right and the medical profession, was motivated by the goal of social equality, as it eliminated the last remaining financial barriers to healthcare for low-income groups (Serner, 1980; Immergut, 1991). The reforms from 1950 to 1970 and their new direction towards working proactively to address the medical needs of the population were codified in the 1982 Health Services Act, which also formalised the relatively independent role of the regions in financing and providing care to all residents. To summarise, the stepwise creation of the modern Swedish healthcare system between 1945 and 1982 resulted in a system that was uniquely public, with even primary care physicians being public employees, and regionally elected politicians directly controlling all resource allocation. Private practice was rare, and private health insurance was virtually non-existent. This organisation implied a healthcare system that was strongly egalitarian in terms of access to care but where patients had little opportunity to choose health providers freely or seek care outside their geographic area of residence.

During the 1980s, the Swedish economic situation deteriorated as the growth levels of previous decades declined while inflation and unemployment rose. During the same period, political attitudes towards the welfare state began to change, particularly in relation to public services, which were criticised as being inefficient, bureaucratic and user-unfriendly (Blomqvist and Rothstein, 2000; Mellbourn, 1986). The criticism came to include the healthcare system, which was described as wasteful, irresponsive to patient demands and with notoriously long waiting lines for care by right-wing groups. Some of these criticisms were acknowledged by the governing social democratic party, particularly the system's lack of cost-efficiency and value of choice as a means to empower patients. At this time, the Swedish healthcare debate was strongly influenced by the New Public Management (NPM) doctrine, particularly ideas about performance-related payments, quasi-markets and consumer choice (Garpenby, 1992; Blomqvist, 2004). Over the following decades, these concepts would provide inspiration for a series of reforms undertaken within the system, initiated by both left-wing and right-wing governments.

Reforms from the 1980s to 2020

The search for economic efficiency

The increasing financial pressure of the healthcare system during the 1980s was added to by a growing share of elderly in the population. Increased demands for care were also generated by new technological innovations enabling more invasive procedures. The increased waiting times for care during the period contributed further to criticisms of the system's inefficiency and low productivity. A particular problem was that hospital beds often were occupied by elderly patients awaiting discharge, so-called bed block-ers (Styrborn and Thorslund, 1993). Towards the late 1980s, many health-care regions experienced severe financial strains, enhanced by reduced state grants and 'tax freezes' where the state prohibited the raising of regional income taxes. As a result, a general search for new means to reduce costs and to increase economic efficiency started, led by the central organisation, the Swedish Association for Local Authorities and Regions (SALAR). This paved the way for a wave of regional experimenting with new, market-oriented, organisational models, such as decentralised budgeting, purchaser–provider splits and performance-based payments in the following decade (Anell, 1996; Garpenby, 1992). Another response to the strained financial situation in the regions towards the end of the 1980s was attempts to rationalise the hospital sector. Compared to most other European countries at the time, the Swed-ish system had a heavy bias towards inpatient care. Rationalisation reforms came to include hospital specialisation, mergers of hospitals and the closing of smaller hospitals. This led to a marked reduction in total hospital beds. During the period 1985–95, the number of beds decreased by 67%, from 15 to 5 per 1,000 inhabitants (Gralén, Hjalte and Persson, 2019).

The search for cost containment and economic efficiency in the health-care system in the late 1980s and early 1990s also manifested itself in two reforms which transferred the main responsibility for nursing home care and long-term care for the mentally ill from the regions to the municipalities. Reforms, enacted in 1992 and 1994, led to institutions for long-term care for the elderly and psychiatric clinics for the mentally challenged being closed or transferred to municipal ownership. Apart from economic motives such as reducing the number of costly hospital beds and freeing them up for acute care patients, the reforms aimed at improving life quality through de-insti-tutionalisation and more independent living (Szebehely, 1998; Markström, 2003). To summarise, the efficiency-enhancing reforms carried out during the late 1980s and early 1990s contained a dual logic of marketisation and planned rationalisation.

Privatisation and market orientation

In 1991, a new centre-right government took office in Sweden, declaring that they would reform the public welfare system by introducing more mar-ket elements along with consumer choice. In the following years, reforms were enacted in both the primary care and hospital sector which re-opened the doors to private care providers and offered patients the opportunity to choose these as an alternative to public providers. This re-orientation had already been initiated by Social Democratic governments during the 1980s when they began to reform the public social service sector by improving financial conditions for non-profit organisations, allowing service users more choice between different service providers. After 1991, more radical steps were taken through a series of reforms encouraging the establishment also of for-profit providers in the healthcare sector. An important part of the political shift was new legislation of public procurement in 1992 which allowed county councils and municipalities to contract out healthcare provision and other public welfare services to private actors. A year later, the same government introduced the General Practitioner Reform (*Husläkarreformen*), which gave general practitioners the right to freely establish themselves within the county councils and receive county council funding on the basis of the number of listed patients. Soon thereafter, in 1994, a similar right was extended to private specialists, which were to be reimbursed on a fee-for-service basis. These reforms constituted a radical policy break in that their main objective was to end the virtual public monopoly on healthcare provision which had characterised the system since the 1970s.

On the regional level, many policymakers continued to experiment with NPM-inspired reforms, such as purchaser/provider splits, performance-based payments and various forms of internal markets. In a few cases, hospitals were sold or put out to tender. Attempts to market-oriented care delivery at this time also included transforming hospitals into public enterprises which meant that they were managed as independent entities. Regional marketisation reforms were most common in, but not confined to, regions led by right-wing parties (Saltman and Bergman, 2005).

In the end, many of the marketisation reforms introduced during the first half of the 1990s were later modified or reversed, as it was discovered that they did not, in most cases, reduce costs even though they increased administration (Harrison and Calltorp, 2000). Even so, the NPM-inspired reforms of the late 1980s and early 1990s came to have a lasting effect on the Swedish system in that they raised cost-awareness, opened the gates to private establishment in the outpatient sector and introduced new management systems on the clinical level. During the late 1990s and 2000s, the share of private health providers gradually increased in the system, particularly in the bigger cities. In the hospital sector, privatisation efforts in practice subsided after the 1990s, partly because of the unwillingness of many of the regions, partly because of lack of interest from the market itself (Anell, 2011). In 2019, specialised somatic care (both inpatient and outpatient care) from private healthcare providers amounted to 8% of the total costs for specialised somatic care – a figure that has remained constant since the early 2000s (Anell, 2011; SALAR, 2021a).

After 2006, when a parliamentary election returned a centre-right coalition to government, a second wave of privatisation reform was enacted. The Primary Care Choice Reform (PCCR) (*Primärvårdsreformen*), enacted in 2009, stipulated that all regions must introduce so-called choice systems whereby private care providers would be free to establish themselves if they fulfilled certain basic criteria and thereafter be financially reimbursed by the region on the basis of how many listed patients they attracted. The PCCR had many similarities with the 1993 General Practitioner Reform but was more open to regional adaption. The political motives behind the reform were to increase opportunities for choice on the part of patients, stimulate private entrepreneurship and improve access to care (Fredriksson, 2013). Evaluations have shown that the PCCR led to a 20% increase in the share of private primary care providers in the years after its implementation, albeit with great local variation. In 2019, primary care purchased from private healthcare providers amounted to 40% of the total costs for primary care (SALAR, 2021a). The vast majority of the new private providers have been for-profit, in many cases part of large international venture capital corporations (Angelis, Häger Glenngård and Jordahl, 2016). The reform also led to an increase in primary care patient visits, indicating that it did improve access to care for many (Andersson, Janlöv and Rehnberg, 2014). A persistent critique of the PCCR has been that the improvement in access has been confined foremost to patient groups in urban settings, as the new private health centres have established foremost in such areas (Swedish National Audit Office, 2014). It has also been shown that establishment of private care providers has been more common in areas with higher-income levels and fewer unemployed (Isaksson, Blomqvist and Winblad, 2015). These establishment patterns indicate a growing dispersion in access to care between regions, as well as between different socio-economic groups within regions.

A year prior to the PCCR, similar legislation on choice systems was created through the 2008 Act on System of Choice in the Public Sector. The 2008 reform, which, in contrast to the PCCR, was voluntary to implement on part of regional and municipal authorities, provided a legal framework for introducing choice systems to a range of social care services including nursing home care, home-based care for the elderly and disabled and specialist healthcare. In 2020, choice systems had been introduced within nursing home care in approximately half of the municipalities, leading to about 20% of all beds in the sector being provided by private providers in 2019 (NBHW, 2021a). Within healthcare, nine out of 21 regions had choice systems for specialised somatic and/or psychiatric care in 2020 (SALAR, 2020b). 'Choice systems' (*valfrihetssystem*), based on the principles of free establishment for private actors and consumer choice, thus became the new terminology for privatisation of social service delivery in Sweden in the 2000s.

The privatisation reforms after 1991 also led to an increased establishment of private specialist care providers outside the hospitals, particularly in the larger cities. The majority of these are funded by the regions on a fee-for-service basis and has led to increased opportunities for patients to seek care freely without remittances, which is typically required for specialist care at the hospitals. Together with increased opportunities for patient choice, this has led to a more *consumerist* healthcare sector, where providers advertise for customers and patients shop around for care. Alongside the publicly financed healthcare market, there has also been a development towards a private health service market, financed by private health insurance. In 2020, the number of private insurance holders had increased by several hundreds of percent since the mid-1990s but was still only about 800,000, corresponding to about 10% of the population of working age (Kullberg, Blomqvist and Winblad, 2019). The private insurance market that developed during this period was primarily for complementary health services, that is, services that are already provided through the public healthcare system. A large majority of all private insurance holders obtained insurance through employment, in most cases in the private sector. Several studies indicate that an important motive for obtaining private health insurance in Sweden is that it guarantees faster access to and more coordinated care (Kullberg, Blomqvist and Winblad, 2019; Lapidus, 2017).

Patient responsiveness

The impact of NPM ideas in the Swedish healthcare debate in the 1980s and 1990s led to concerns regarding the role of patients which was shared by right- and left-wing groups, becoming formulated as a lack of patient *choice*. As a result, a string of reforms was initiated with the aim of creating more opportunities for patients to choose care provider. For the right-wing parties, choice was intimately linked to privatisation and market competition, while left-wing actors like the Social Democratic Party initially tried to create choice opportunities within the public healthcare sector (Blomqvist, 2004). The first choice reform was the so-called patient choice recommendation in 1989, a voluntary commitment on part of the regions to secure the right to a free choice of care provider for patients. In the early 1990s, the 1993 General Practitioner Reform mandated the regions to provide a free choice of provider and let capitation payments follow the choices of patients. In 2010, Primary Care Choice Reform mandated the regions to introduce so-called choice systems, giving all individuals the right to choose a public or a private primary healthcare provider not only within the region but also anywhere in the country.

Another type of reform which concerned the role of patients was the waiting-time guarantees. Long waiting times for certain treatments had long been a concern in the system; in some regions, patients could wait 1–2 years for hip or knee replacements. The first waiting-time guarantee was introduced as a recommendation by SALAR in 1992 and stated that patients had the right to treatment within three months for 12 specific diagnosis groups. This was initially effective in reducing waiting times but had the side effect of crowding-out other patient groups. In 2005, the government and SALAR reached another agreement, resulting in three-month waiting-time guarantee combined with economic bonuses to regions which managed to honour the guarantee. This voluntary agreement was turned into binding law in 2010, either obliging the regions to offer specialist treatment to all patients within three months of receiving their diagnosis or being obliged to assist them in seeking care elsewhere at the expense of the home region (or, in some cases, the referring clinic) (Winblad and Hanning, 2013; Winblad, Vrangbæk and Östergren, 2010). Despite this law, waiting lines for care grew in several regions again after 2010 (SALAR, 2020a).

A third way in which Swedish policymakers sought to strengthen the role of patients in the healthcare system over the last decades is the adoption of the Patient Rights' Act in 2015. The Act stipulates that patients shall have the right to full information regarding treatment alternatives, co-determination in treatment decisions and – in cases of serious medical illness – a so-called second opinion. The act also states that patients shall have free choice of ambulatory care in the whole country. It has been criticised, however, for poor implementation and containing only 'soft', or non-legally enforceable, rights (SAHCSA, 2017).

Improved quality control

NPM ideas also influenced Swedish healthcare in that they led to an increased focus on measuring performance and improving quality within the system. New tools of quality management were introduced in the heath sector at both the national and regional levels. One of the first new methods for quality control was *national guidelines*, the first of which were introduced in 1996. Formally non-binding, national guidelines are developed by the National Board of Health and Welfare (NBHW) in collaboration with medical expertise. Their goal is to ensure that diagnosis-setting and treatment methods are evidence-based and uniform across the country. In contrast to national guidelines in most other countries, part of the guidelines are directed to regional politicians, providing guidance on prioritising (Fredriksson, Blomqvist and Winblad, 2014). In 2019, treatment guidelines were produced in 18 different areas, including mental health, diabetes, cardiovascular disease and dementia.

Another quality-enhancing reform has been national collection and publication of clinical outcome data through so-called *medical quality registries*. In the mid-1990s, the NBHW and SALAR became involved in the funding and management of quality registers previously established by medical professionals, transforming them into a steering tool used to monitor medical quality outcomes in the regions (Levay and Waks, 2009; Örnerheim, 2018). The registers contain individualised patient data concerning diagnoses, medical interventions and treatment outcomes which are reported by medical personnel. In 2019, there were 108 national quality registries within the system, covering all of the most common medical diagnoses. The development of the medical quality registers led to another policy development to strengthen medical quality within the system, the so-called *Open Comparisons*. The Swedish NBHW started, in 2006, to publish comparative data from regions and care providers of a range of indicators of quality and efficiency from the medical quality registers. The purpose of the Open Comparisons is to enhance quality within the system by making performance and outcomes in the healthcare system more transparent, to facilitate comparisons between regions and individual care providers and to create stronger incentives for quality improvement through benchmarking. Just like the national guidelines and medical quality registers, the Open

Comparisons came to constitute a steering tool for national authorities in that it created considerable pressure on regions with poor results to improve their performance (Fredriksson et al., 2014). The striving for enhanced performance monitoring on part of national authorities was also manifested in the establishment of new audit agencies at the national level, such as the Health and Social Care Inspectorate in 2013 and the Swedish Agency for Health and Care Services Analysis (SAHCSA) in 2014. Since 2018, the national quality management has been intensified through SALAR's initiative to create a more comprehensive infrastructure called the National System for Knowledge-based Management. This system evolves around 26 diagnostic groups, for which quality information is developed and shared (SALAR, 2021b).

Re-scaling the system

When the modern Swedish health system was developed in the post-war era, it became strongly decentralised, with a complex and somewhat fluid division of labour between the national, regional and local levels. Parallel to the NPM-influenced reforms regarding marketisation, patient choice and quality control, there has been an ongoing discussion about the system's structure and the division of responsibilities between the geographical levels within it. The most salient issues have been the number and size of the regions, the role of the central government in relation to them and the problems regarding coordination between the regions and the municipalities, responsible for provision of social and long-term care.

Several reforms have been initiated during the 1990–2020 period to reduce the numbers and size of the regions, but most have been unsuccessful due to political divisions and resistance from the regions. During the 1990s, several regional mergers took place, creating the larger regions of Västra Götaland and Skåne (Blomqvist and Bergman, 2010). In the mid-2000s, a public commission proposed that the remaining 21 units merge into 6–10 regions with an estimated 1–2 million inhabitants. The proposal was, however, never implemented. A social democratic government in 2014 made another attempt at mergers, but this proposal too failed to win parliamentary support. The main argument in favour of larger regions has been that many of the existing regions are too small to provide care services effectively.

A second reform trend relating to the multi-level governance structure of the system has been attempts to re-centralise governing power within it by enhancing the role of the national authorities. One example is the enhancement of performance monitoring through audit and data-collection. Another is the increased use of binding regulation, although the tradition of soft governance, for instance in the form of agreements with the regions or non-binding recommendations, is still very much alive (Blomqvist and Winblad, 2021). A further example of the re-centralisation within the system is that the efforts steer and standardise the medical practice through the introduction of national guidelines. It should be noted, however, that the re-centralisation tendency only refers to the *regulation* of the system, as the regions have retained their financial autonomy. The re-centralisation trend was further reinforced during the Covid-19 pandemic, as it became clear that the decentralised system hindered an effective and coordinated response to the pandemic. This led to the government mandating its national authorities, principally the NBHW and Health and Social Care Inspectorate, to take a more active role in coordination activities between the regions – for instance regarding the distribution of medical equipment, transfer of patients between them, and securing the delivery of vaccines and other supplies through procurement on the international market (Pierre, 2020; Winblad, Swenning and Spangler, 2022).

A third example of reforms aimed at altering relations between different levels in the system in recent decades concerns the coordination between the regional healthcare and municipal social care systems. The fact that the regions are the main providers of healthcare services while municipalities provide home care, home-based assistance and, in most cases, home-based healthcare, creates a need for collaboration, as for instance when patients are discharged from hospitals. Another area of collaboration concerns nursing home residents, as the municipalities are not permitted to employ physicians and therefore must secure medical services through contracts with the regions or private care providers. The Covid-19 pandemic placed the coordination issue, particularly regarding elderly patients, in focus. By the end of April 2020, 50% of all who lived in nursing homes died from Covid-19 infection in Sweden, while 26% had home-based assistance (NBHW, 2020b). The pandemic also exposed the lack of adequate medical care and medical equipment in many nursing homes (Diderichsen, 2021; Pierre, 2020). Coordination problems between different actors in the system, which have been enhanced by the increased plurality of providers, also include incompatible information systems, a lack of cost incentives for collaboration and differing organisational and professional cultures (SAHCSA, 2020). In 2018, the Coordination Act (*Samverkanslagen*) was passed, making primary care providers mainly responsible for coordinating regional health authorities and municipal social care authorities during patient discharge. So far, however, most evaluations point to the Act having had limited effect on care coordination (SAHCSA, 2020; NBHW, 2021b). The Coordination Act can be seen as part of a larger reform trend under way in Swedish healthcare which attempts to, yet again, shift resources from the hospital sector towards primary care. In summary, it is clear not only that the multi-level character of the Swedish healthcare system has undergone several revisions in previous decades but also that it has proved hard to change. A clear trend is nevertheless the strengthening of the role of the national government in regulating and overseeing the system.

Developments in public health

Public health in Sweden is good by international comparison and has improved further during the last decades – life expectancy increased from 80 years for women and 75 years for men in 1990 to 84 and 80 years, respectively, in 2019. Infant mortality decreased during the same period from 5.9 in 1990 to 2.1 per 1,000 in 2019 (Statistics Sweden, 2021). Smoking decreased markedly during the same period, as did mortality from several diseases, including cardiovascular and tumour issues (PHA, 2019). The positive developments in public health during recent decades are believed to be the result of increased living standards, reduced smoking and improvements in the medical treatment of deadly diseases like cancer, heart failure and stroke (PHA, 2019). There were also some negative public health trends since the 1990s, foremost increased obesity and higher incidences of self-reported poor mental health, particularly among young women (PHA, 2019; Löfstedt et al., 2017).

Behind the figures, showing a general improvement in population health during the last decades in Sweden is, however, a pattern, where differences in health and mortality between different socio-economic groups in Sweden persist and in some cases even widen (Månsdotter and Lindeskog, 2014). Individuals with pre-secondary education have been reported to have higher mortality in many diseases and also run a higher risk of violence and injury, compared to those with post-secondary education. Life expectancy in this group is also markedly lower, particularly for women, and has not increased as much as for those with post-secondary education during recent decades (PHA, 2021a). The Public Health Authority (PHA) lists three prime reasons behind these differences: the general improvement in standard of living has not included all social groups; the persisting differences in health-related behaviour such as smoking and dietary habits; and the fact that unemployment, which is a known risk factor for poor health, is considerably more common among the low-educated (PHA, 2021a).

Another social development in Sweden affecting public health is the increase in the share of foreign-born, which increased from 9.2% in 1990 to 19.6% in 2020 (Statistics Sweden, 2021). This marked increase reflects, above all, immigration by refugees from the Balkans, Africa and the Middle East. Foreign-born populations from low- and middle-income countries in Sweden have been known to run higher health risks, as they tend to have lower education, higher rates of unemployment and lower health literacy, referring to knowledge about and motivation to improve individual health, than the native population (Mårtensson et al., 2020). Poor health among immigrants can thus to some extent be seen as the result of failed integration, while it can also serve as a hindrance for integration.

The Covid-19 pandemic sadly exposed social inequalities in health in Sweden, revealing how they also manifest themselves in communicable diseases. The risk of Covid infection and related death has been shown to be more than twice as high among those born in low- and middle-income countries as compared to the native Swedish population (OECD, 2020). This was attributed to factors such as poorer initial health status, more crowded living arrangements (including inter-generational living) and higher employment in sectors where working from home has not been possible (Diderichsen, 2021;

Valeriani et al., 2020). During the vaccinations against Covid-19 in the spring of 2021, uptake has also been reported to be lower among the foreign-born, a pattern that has been explained by both language barriers and lower trust in public authorities (PHA, 2021b). In this sense, the Covid-19 pandemic has highlighted the fact that health inequalities in Sweden today follow not only class-based but also ethnic cleavages in Swedish society.

The impact of reforms on the system

The reforms undertaken in Swedish healthcare during the last three decades have transformed the system in several ways. Most notably, care delivery has been restructured and marketised; national monitoring and quality measurement enhanced; and new modes of governance introduced on all levels. To assess the impact of all the different types of reforms which have taken place during the period is a daunting task, not least in light of the fact that the functioning of healthcare systems is also affected by other, external, factors such as economic and social change, technological developments or migration. Still, a few remarks can be made regarding developments in relation to central dimensions like efficiency, access to care, care quality and system governability.

When it comes to *economic efficiency*, most observers seem to agree that substantive improvements have been made, particularly during the 1990s and early 2000s (Anell, 2005, 2011; SALAR, 2010). These are attributed foremost to rationalisations in the hospital sector, which, as described earlier, led to a marked decrease in hospital beds and increased specialisation among hospitals. In 2019, Sweden had the lowest number of hospital beds per inhabitant in the European Union with 2.1 hospital beds per 1,000 inhabitants (OECD, 2021). Critics have argued that the bed reductions have gone too far and that there is now a shortage of beds in several hospitals, particularly in the bigger cities (Swedish Medical Association, 2021). The impact of the rationalisations in the hospital sector is also evident in the reduction of staff in the sector, which has been estimated to have been diminished by 20% during the 1990s alone (SALAR, 2010). The rationalisation of care in the hospital sector during this period is evident too in the shortening of treatment periods for somatic care. Between 1992 and 2007, the average hospital length of stay decreased from 8 days to 5 days, and in 2019, it had decreased further to 3.9 days (NBHW, 2020a; SALAR, 2010).

The 1990s also witnessed a reduction of total costs in the system, a development which can be explained by the long-term care reforms, shifting patients to the municipal sector, and budget cuts. After the 1990s, spending levels within the system increased again. Between 2000 and 2017, the health share of Gross Domestic Product went from 8% to 11% – a faster increase than in most other European countries during the same period (Gralén, Hjalte and Persson, 2019). During the same period, costs per patient visit grew as well, indicating reduced productivity. Real prices of healthcare costs such as doctors' wages have also increased markedly after 2000 (SALAR, 2018; Gralén, Hjalte and Persson, 2019). The privatisation reforms during the 1990s, which increased the supply of care in terms of both the number of care providers and patient visits, are not believed to have contributed much to cost increases in the system however, as regional budgets are still capped (Andersson, Janlöv and Rehnberg, 2014). Summarising these developments, it appears that economic efficiency did increase in the Swedish healthcare system following the rationalisations in the inpatient sector during the 1990s but that these gains have been at least partly offset by cost increases in the system during the 2000s and 2010s. In 2016, a public commission concluded that the healthcare system suffered from inefficiencies and that productivity in the Swedish hospital sector was lower than that in the neighbouring Nordic countries. Several reasons were listed, the most important of which was a lack of capacity in the primary care sector, which was seen as leading to patients being treated in hospitals when their needs could have been met at a lower level of care (Swedish Public Commission, 2016).

In the case of access to care, the picture is mixed as well. As noted previously in the chapter, the PCCR reform led to a substantive increase in the share of private providers leading to access being improved in the primary care sector after 2010 (Beckman and Anell, 2013; Dietrichson, Ellegård and Kjellsson, 2020; Glenngård and Anell, 2016). At the same time, concerns have been expressed that the PCCR reform had negative effects on equity in access (Burström et al., 2017; Isaksson, Blomqvist and Winblad, 2015). In addition to improved access to primary care, access to care can also be seen as being enhanced by choice reforms and reforms strengthening the right to co-determination and a second opinion on the part of patients. A less positive development can be noted when it comes to waiting times for care, which decreased during the 1990s and early 2000s but grew again after 2014. The problems with access to care in the inpatient sector are also manifested in overcrowding and bed-spacing (that is, the patient being placed in another clinic than where he/she is enrolled) in hospitals, which has become a growing problem in Sweden since 2010. Taken together, these developments demonstrate that, despite decades of reforms, the healthcare system is still not able to meet the demands of the population. Waiting lines have been described as the Achilles heel of the Swedish healthcare system, and it is clear that it continues to be a significant problem.

When it comes to the impact of reforms on the quality of care, the picture is rosier. Sweden has performed very well in international evaluations of medical quality in recent years, and most observers agree that there has been a notable improvement. There is general agreement that the improvement can be related at least in part to quality management reforms like the quality registers, evidence-based guidelines and the publication of quality indicators, making it possible to compare performance between regions and care givers. These reforms are seen as having contributed not only to a general quality improvement but also to an equalisation of quality within the system, as regions and care givers with lower performance have been given strong incentives to catch up (Fredriksson et al., 2014; SAHCA, 2017). When it comes to the impact of privatisation reforms, there is no evidence that these reforms have either improved or reduced care quality within the system (Anell, 2011; Andersson, Janlöv and Rehnberg, 2014).

Regarding the impact of reforms on patient satisfaction, which can be seen as another quality dimension, the evidence is less conclusive. National surveys show that patient satisfaction has decreased slightly during the last decades, along with a lowered confidence in the healthcare system from just under 70% in 2011 to just over 60% in 2019 (SALAR, 2020a). However, when patients who have recently used health services are asked, the picture is more positive, particularly among those being treated in hospital, among which almost 90% have a high or very high satisfaction level (SALAR, 2020a). When it comes to indicators such as patient participation and coordination of care, both domestic and international surveys indicate that patients are still dissatisfied (SAHCSA, 2017, 2021). These findings indicate that reforms aimed at increasing patient empowerment since the 1990s have not been particularly successful, even if rising expectations in the population regarding participation and co-determination are likely to have played a role too.

Finally, it can be asked what the effects of reforms undertaken in the 1990–2020 period have had on the *governability* of the system. A first observation is that the system's governability has probably been enhanced because of improved information about costs, resource allocation and performance in the system. Compared to the late 1980s, policymakers today have considerably more information regarding all such matters. This is, in large measure, not only due to the collection and publication of data through the Open Comparisons but also due to increased competence and specialisation on part of the regional purchasing units. Second, governability within the system has increased also at the central state level, which has obtained more tools for steering and monitoring the system. Of particular importance in this regard are evidence-based guidelines, but national steering has also been reinforced through direct coordination and binding regulation.

Furthermore, it could also be argued that governability has increased at the clinical level within the system, reflecting developments such as through the professionalisation of managers and the introduction of new management techniques (Bejerot and Hasselblad, 2011; Elg et al., 2011). At the same time, there is evidence of growing discontent with working condition among healthcare staff in the Swedish system. Complaints about working conditions, particularly in the hospital sector, are commonplace, and there is clearly a lack of confidence in the regions in employers (Anell, 2020). The dissatisfaction with working conditions in the system can be seen as a result of both rationalisation and management reforms, forcing the staff to spend more time on data reporting and documentation and less time with patients (Andersson, Janlöv and Rehnberg, 2014).

Is the Swedish healthcare system sustainable?

The future sustainability of the Swedish healthcare sector, which can be seen in terms of its financial viability, public legitimacy and its ability to meet the medical needs of the population, appears quite good in some respects. The relatively strong performance of the Swedish economy during the last decade has led to the system being reasonably well funded, with resources available for the planned expansion of the primary care sector. The pandemic years, where the government resources were transferred from the state to the regions on an unprecedented scale, demonstrated that this is possible and easily implemented if there is a need. At the same time, it is clear that the cost expansion that has taken place within the Swedish system during the last two decades cannot continue at the same pace. Considering expected demographic developments, where the oldest group in the population (over 85 years) is expected to more than double before 2050, it is apparent that further rationalisation and efficiency gains within the system are called for. This has also been the conclusion of several public committees over the last years (Swedish Public Commission, 2016). The main strategy for increasing efficiency in the system at present concerns a further shift of resources to the primary care sector, improved coordination between health and social care authorities to prevent avoidable hospitalisation and further digitalisation of care. When it comes to digital care, Sweden is far ahead compared to most other countries; this was evident not least during the pandemic, where a large share of all patient visits could be conducted online (Pierre, 2020).

Regarding the sustainability of the system's legitimacy and public support, conditions also seem fairly promising even if challenges exist here too. There has long been a strong public support for the fundamental principles of the system – that it is publicly financed and that care is offered to all permanent residents on the same conditions, regardless of income or occupation. This support has not declined during the last decades (Blomqvist, 2016). At the same time, there are clear signs of public discontent with some parts of the system, such as (continued) waiting lines for specialist care, particularly in some regions, and the low level of responsiveness to patient demands for information, participation and continuity of care. As long as these short-comings remain, there is a risk that increasing numbers will turn to the private market for care, which is now available for those with complementary health insurance. In such a scenario, the system's solidaristic character will be undermined even if the tax-based funding structure remains.

The future sustainability of the Swedish healthcare system also depends on its ability to address the growing health inequalities in the population, concerning both social class and ethnicity. This implies that it must improve its ability to reach low-educated groups with preventive care measures such as pre-natal and infant care as well as life-style changes to reduce health risks. A particular challenge in this regard, which became visible not least during the pandemic, is the lower level of trust in public health authorities among immigrants, which leads to a reduced tendency to seek timely care as well as to accept vaccinations (Valeriani et al., 2020). Overall, it seems that the Swedish healthcare system should be fairly well equipped to address this challenge, given that social equity both in access and, what is more difficult, in health outcomes has long been a central goal within the system. What is problematic is that, so far, preventive care has not been prioritised among the regions, despite national policy proclamations in this regard (Swedish Public Commission, 2017). Moreover, the current, performance-based reimbursement systems that dominate in the primary care sector do not create incentives to invest in preventive care. A more fundamental problem is that the PCCR reform in effect removed the previous system of district-based areas of responsibility for population health which were created in the 1960s. The (partial) privatisation of the primary care sector has led to a more fragmented system of competing health centres and single providers, where patients shop around freely. This fragmentation implies that preventive care services have tended to become individualised, while programmes aimed at whole patient groups, or geographic districts, have become harder to organise.

Conclusion

In this chapter, we have described reforms undertaken in the Swedish healthcare reforms during the last four decades, from the late 1980s to 2020. At the beginning of this period, the Swedish system could be described as almost completely public in both financing and provision. In fact, there were probably few systems in the world at the time that were as completely dominated by the public sector as the Swedish system was at this time (Immergut, 1991). Since then, a significant element of marketisation has taken place within the system, particularly in the primary care sector, where private providers now compete with those in the public sector, creating a mixed delivery system with public funding. In the hospital sector, marketisation reforms were initiated during the 1990s but largely faded out in the 2000s, leading to the vast majority of hospitals remaining public. In terms of funding as well, there has been a return to global budgets, rather than performance-related payments. Reform in the hospital sector has instead followed a different track, where restructuring and rationalisation in the form of hospital mergers and closures dominated, leading to a stark reduction of hospital beds. Taken together, the market-oriented reforms undertaken in Swedish healthcare between the years 1990 and 2020 had a profound but not radical impact on the Swedish healthcare system. None of the reforms implemented concerned the financing side of the system or its basic organisation of decentralised, democratic governance. What they did was to alter the provision structure in the primary care sector, which went from a virtual public monopoly to a mixed system of public and private providers. They also transformed governance in the hospital sector, as hospitals, even though the great majority remained public, became governed more independently and with stronger elements of managerialist internal steering systems.

Parallel to reforms in the delivery of healthcare services, the 1980–2020 period has also seen a string of reforms aimed at improving quality within the system. Such reforms focused on increasing the transparency of the system in terms of its performance as well as its costs. Innovations such as medical quality registers, evidence-based national guidelines and benchmarking have led to quality levels being raised and differences in performance between regions and providers being reduced. The increased availability of information about resource allocation and performance has also improved governability within the system, at both the regional and national levels. A downside of the increased transparency is the rise of administrative burdens for healthcare staff.

Given the fact that the reforms in Sweden during the studied period concerned the provision side of the system, rather than its financing, the system remains a solid NHS system of the Scandinavian, decentralised type. The tax-based financing structure has not been called into question, even by political right-wing groups, and the solidaristic principle of care resources being distributed on basis of need, rather than ability to pay, still underpins the system. At the same time, the egalitarian ethos of the system has been challenged by several developments during the period, including the increase in private health insurance uptake, a tendency of care providers to establish disproportionally in more prosperous areas, and increased disparities in health outcomes among different socio-economic groups. Taken together, these developments imply that the system has become less egalitarian and that, even if access to healthcare is still formally equal for all citizens, circumstances like residence location, socio-economic status and individual initiative have come to play a bigger role in the distribution of health services.

References

Andersson, F., Janlöv, N. and Rehnberg, C. (2014) *Konkurrens, kontrakt och kvalitet – hälso-och sjukvård i privat regi* (Rapport till Expertgruppen för studier i offentlig ekonomi och Myndigheten för vårdanalys 2014:5), Stockholm: Frizes.

Anell, A. (1996) 'The monopolistic integrated model and health care reform: The Swedish experience', *Health Policy* 37(1): 19–33.

Anell, A. (2005) 'Swedish healthcare under pressure', *Health Economics* 14(S1): S237–54.

Anell, A. (2011) 'Choice and privatisation in Swedish primary care', *Health Economics, Policy and Law* 6(4): 549–69.

Anell, A. (2020) *Vården är värd en bättre styrning*, Stockholm: SNS förslag.

Anell, A. and Claesson, R. (1995) *Svenska sjukhus förr och nu – Ekonomiska aspekter på struktur, politik och framtida förutsättningar*, Lund: IHE, Institutet för hälso-och sjukvårdsekonomi.

Angelis, J., Häger Glenngård, A. and Jordahl, H. (2016) *Att styra och leda en vårdcentral: Hur går det till och vad kan förbättras?* Stockholm: SNS förlag.

Beckman, A. and Anell, A. (2013) 'Changes in health care utilisation following a reform involving choice and privatisation in Swedish primary care: A five-year follow-up of GP-visits', *BMC Health Services Research* 13(1): 1–9.

Bejerot, E. and Hasselbladh, H. (2011) 'Professional autonomy and pastoral power: The transformation of quality registers in Swedish health care', *Public Administration* 89(4): 1604–21.

Blomqvist, P. (2004) 'The choice revolution: Privatization of Swedish welfare services in the 1990s', *Social Policy and Administration* 38(2): 39–155.

Blomqvist, P. (2016) 'NPM i välfärdsstaten: Hotas universalismen?', *Statsvetenskaplig tidskrift* 118(1): 39–67.

Blomqvist, P. and Bergman, P. (2010) 'Regionalisation Nordic style: Will regions in Sweden threaten local democracy?', *Local Government Studies* 36(1): 43–74.

Blomqvist, P. and Rothstein, B. (2000) *Välfärdsstatens nya ansikte: Demokrati och marknadsstyrning inom den offentliga sektorn*, Stockholm: Agora.

Blomqvist, P. and Winblad, U. (2021) 'Sweden', in Immergut, E. M., Anderson, K. M., Devitt, C. and Popic, T. (eds) *Health Politics in Europe: A Handbook*, Oxford: Oxford University Press.

Burström, B., Burström, K., Nilsson, G., Tomson, G., Whitehead, M. and Winblad, U. (2017) 'Equity aspects of the primary health care choice reform in Sweden – A scoping review', *International Journal for Equity in Health* 16(1): 1–10.

Diderichsen, F. (2021) 'How did Sweden fail the pandemic?', *International Journal of Health Services* 51(4): 417–22.

Dietrichson, J., Ellegård, L. M. and Kjellsson, G. (2020) 'Patient choice, entry, and the quality of primary care: Evidence from Swedish reforms', *Health Economics* 29(6): 716–30.

Elg, M., Stenberg, J., Kammerlind, P., Tullberg, S. and Olsson, J. (2011) 'Swedish healthcare management practices and quality improvement work: Development trends', *International Journal of Health Care Quality Assurance* 24(2): 101–23.

Fredriksson, M. (2013) 'Is patient choice democratizing Swedish primary care?', *Health Policy* 111(1): 95–8.

Fredriksson, M., Blomqvist, P. and Winblad, U. (2014) 'Recentralizing healthcare through evidence-based guidelines-striving for national equity in Sweden', *BMC Health Services Research* 14(1): 1–9.

Fredriksson, M., Eldh, A. C., Vengberg, S., Dahlström, T., Halford, C., Wallin, L. and Winblad, U. (2014) 'Local politico-administrative perspectives on quality improvement based on national registry data in Sweden: A qualitative study using the consolidated framework for implementation research', *Implementation Science* 9(1): 1–11.

Garpenby, P. (1992) 'The transformation of the Swedish health care system, or the hasty rejection of the rational planning model', *Journal of European Social Policy* 2(1): 17–31.

Glenngård, A. H. and Anell, A. (2016) 'Introducing quasi-markets in primary care: The Swedish experience', in Lapsley, I. and Knutsson, H. (eds) *Modernizing the Public Sector*, Abingdon: Routledge.

Gralén, K., Hjalte, F. and Persson, U. (2019) *Hälso- och sjukvårdsutgifternas utveckling i Sverige* (IHE Rapport 5), Lund: IHE.

Gustafsson, R. A. (1987) *Traditionernas ok: den svenska hälso-och sjukvårdens organisering i historie-sociologiskt perspektiv*, Doctoral thesis, University of Gothenburg.

Harrison, M. I. and Calltorp, J. (2000) 'The reorientation of market-oriented reforms in Swedish health-care', *Health Policy* 50(3): 219–40.

Immergut, E. M. (1991) *Medical Markets and Professional Power: The Economic and Political Logic of Government Health Programs* (Volume 24). Centro de

Estudios Avanzados en Ciencias Sociales, Instituto Juan March de Estudios e Investigaciones, Madrid.

Isaksson, D., Blomqvist, P. and Winblad, U. (2015) 'Free establishment of primary health care providers: Effects on geographical equity', *BMC Health Services Research* 16(1): 1–10.

Ito, H. (1980) 'Health insurance and medical services in Sweden and Denmark 1850–1950', in Heidenheimer, A. J. and Elvander, N. (eds) *The Shaping of the Swedish Health System*, London: Croom Helm.

Kullberg, L., Blomqvist, P. and Winblad, U. (2019) 'Health insurance for the healthy? Voluntary health insurance in Sweden', *Health Policy* 123(8): 737–46.

Lapidus, J. (2017) 'Private health insurance in Sweden: Fast-track lanes and the alleged attempts to stop them', *Health Policy* 121(4): 442–9.

Levay, C. and Waks, C. (2009) 'Professions and the pursuit of transparency in healthcare: Two cases of soft autonomy', *Organization Studies* 30(5): 509–27.

Löfstedt, P., Wiklander, L., Bremberg, S., et al. (2017) 'Why are psychosomatic symptoms in young people increasing in Sweden?', *European Journal of Public Health* 27(Supplement 3).

Månsdotter, A. and Lindeskog, P. (2014) 'Sociala investeringar för jämlikhet i hälsa – Vad är nytt ur folkhälsoperspektivet?', *Socialmedicinsk tidskrift* 91(3): 232–44.

Markström, U. (2003. *Den svenska psykiatrireformen: bland brukare, eldsjälar och byråkrater*, Doctoral dissertation, Umeå University.

Mårtensson, L., Lytsy, P., Westerling, R. and Wångdahl, J. (2020) 'Experiences and needs concerning health related information for newly arrived refugees in Sweden', *BMC Public Health* 20(1): 1–10.

Mellbourn, A. (1986) *Bortom det starka samhället: socialdemokratisk förvaltningspolitik 1982–1985*, Stockholm: Carlsson.

NBHW (2020a) *DRG-statistik 2019. En beskrivning av vårdproduktion och vårdkonsumtion i Sverige* (Socialstyrelsen Report 2020–11–7042).

NBHW (2020b) *Statistik om smittade och avlidna med Covid-19 bland äldre efter boendeform* (Socialstyrelsen Dnr. 6.7–15552/2020).

NBHW (2021a) *Statistik om socialtjänstinsatser till äldre och personer med funktionsnedsättning efter regiform 2020* (Socialstyrelsen Art.nr: 2021–3–7266).

NBHW (2021b) *Återinskrivningar av sköra och multisjuka äldre* (Socailstyrelsen Report 2021–2–7195).

Organisation for Economic Cooperation and Development (2020) *What Is the Impact of the COVID-19 Pandemic on Immigrants and Their Children?* Paris: OECD Publishing.

Organisation for Economic Cooperation and Development (2021) *Hospital Beds (Indicator)*, Paris: OECD.

Örnerheim, M. (2018) 'Policymaking through healthcare registries in Sweden', *Health Promotion International* 33(2): 356–65.

PHA (2019) *Folkhälsans utveckling* (Årsrapport 2019). Folkhälsomyndigheten. Available at: www.folkhalsomyndigheten.se/contentassets/d162673edec94e5f8d-1da1f78e54dac4/folkhalsans-utveckling-arsrapport-2019.pdf

PHA (2021a) *Folkhälsans utveckling* (Årsrapport 2021). Folkhälsomyndigheten. Available at: www.folkhalsomyndigheten.se/contentassets/39ef6af33177445bb6d2ad88829cc5ce/folkhalsans-utveckling-arsrapport-2021.pdf

PHA (2021b) *Utrikesfödda och covid-19. Konstaterade fall, IVA-vård och avlidna bland utrikesfödda i Sverige 13 mars 2020–15 februari 2021.* Folkhälsomyndigheten. Available at: www.folkhalsomyndigheten.se/contentassets/2dddee08a4e c4c25a0a59aac7aca14f0/utrikesfodda-och-covid-19.pdf

Pierre, J. (2020) 'Nudges against pandemics: Sweden's COVID-19 containment strategy in perspective', *Policy and Society* 39(3): 478–93.

SAHCSA (2017) *Lag utan genomslag. Utvärdering av patientlagen 2014–2017* (Vårdanalys Report 2017:2), Stockholm: Myndigheten för vård- och omsorgsanalys.

SAHCSA (2020) *Laga efter läge. Uppföljning av lagen om samverkan vid utskrivning från slutenvården* (Vårdanalys Report 2020:4), Stockholm: Myndigheten för vård- och omsorgsanalys.

SAHCSA (2021) *En lag som kräver omtag. Uppföljning av patientlagens genomslag, med en fördjupning om valfrihet* (Vårdanalys Report 2021:10), Stockholm: Myndigheten för vård- och omsorgsanalys.

SALAR (2010) *Statistik om hälso- och sjukvård samt regional utveckling 2009* (SKL Report June 2010), Stockholm: Sveriges Kommuner och Landsting.

SALAR (2018) *Ekonomirapporten, december 2018. Om kommunernas och landstingens ekonomi* (SKL Report December 2018), Linköping: Sveriges Kommuner och Landsting.

SALAR (2020a) *Hälso- och sjukvårdsrapporten 2020. Öppna Jämförelser* (SKR Report 2020), Stockholm: Sveriges Kommuner och Landsting.

SALAR (2020b) *Valfrihetssystem i regionerna – beslutsläge* (SKR PM 2020), Stockholm: Sveriges Kommuner och Landsting.

SALAR (2021a) *Regionernas köp av verksamhet.* Available at: https://skr.se/skr/ ekonomijuridik/ekonomi/sektornisiffror/kopavverksamhet.35817.html

SALAR (2021b) *National System for Knowledge-Driven Management within Swedish Healthcare.* Available at: https://kunskapsstyrningvard.se/kunskapsstyrningvard/ omkunskapsstyrning/nationalsystemforknowledgedrivenmanagementwithinswedish healthcare.56857.html

Saltman, R. B. and Bergman, S. E. (2005) 'Renovating the commons: Swedish health care reforms in perspective', *Journal of Health Politics, Policy and Law* 30(1–2): 253–76.

Serner, U. (1980) 'Swedish health legislation: Milestones in reorganisation since 1945', in Heidenheimer, A. J. and Elvander, N. (eds) *The Shaping of the Swedish Health System*, London: Croom Helm.

Statistics Sweden (2021) *SCB, Befolkningsstatistik i sammandrag.* Available at: www.scb.se/hitta-statistik/statistik-efter-amne/befolkning/befolkningens-sam-mansattning/befolkningsstatistik/pong/tabell-och-diagram/helarsstatistik – riket/ befolkningsstatistik-i-sammandrag/

Styrborn, K. and Thorslund, M. (1993) '"Bed-blockers": Delayed discharge of hospital patients in a nationwide perspective in Sweden', *Health Policy* 26(2): 155–70.

Swedish Medical Association (2021) *Vårdplatser. Dags att möta behovet av vårdplatser och minska "vårdskulden".* Available at: https://slf.se/var-politik/vardplatser/

Swedish National Audit Office (2014) *Primärvårdens styrning: behov eller efterfrågan?* (RiR 2014:22), Stockholm: Riksrevisionen.

Swedish Public Commission (2016) *Effektiv vård – Slutbetänkande av En nationell samordnare för effektivare resursutnyttjande inom hälso- och sjukvården* (SOU 2016:1), Stockholm: Wolters Kluwers.

Swedish Public Commission (2017) *Nästa steg på vägen mot en mer jämlik hälsa* (SOU 2017:47), Stockholm: Wolters Kluwers.

Szebehely, M. (ed) (1998) *Äldreomsorgsforskning i Norden: en kunskapsöversikt,* Copenhagen: Nordic Council of Ministers.

Valeriani, G., Sarajlic Vukovic, I., Lindegaard, T., Felizia, R., Mollica, R. and Andersson, G. (2020) 'Addressing healthcare gaps in Sweden during the COVID-19 outbreak: On community outreach and empowering ethnic minority groups in a digitalized context', *Healthcare* 8(4): 445.

Winblad, U. and Hanning, M. (2013) 'Sweden', in Siciliani, L., Borowitz, M. and Moran, V. (eds) *Waiting Time Policies in the Health Sector: What Works?*, Paris: OECD Publications.

Winblad, U., Swenning, A. and Spangler, D. (2022) 'Soft law and individual responsibility: A review of the Swedish policy response to COVID-19', *Health Economics, Policy and Law* 17(1): 48–61.

Winblad, U., Vrangbæk, K. and Östergren, K. (2010) 'Do the waiting-time guarantees in the Scandinavian countries empower patients?', *International Journal of Public Sector Management* 23(4): 353–63.

4 Denmark

Karsten Vrangbæk

Introduction

This chapter utilises the neo-Weberian/neo-institutionalist framework to analyse developments in the Danish health system. Developments will be presented and discussed with reference to the main stakeholder groups in the health sector and particularly healthcare professionals, state, regional and local governments, patients and the medical–industrial complex. Since healthcare is an integrated part of the Danish welfare state, there will also be reference to broader institutional developments of the welfare state.

The chapter shows that historical ambitions and political compromises have gradually created a system that is state regulated, largely funded by taxation and dominated by public ownership of hospitals. However, the system also has significant private components in terms of voluntary supplementary insurance to cover co-payments, and reliance on outpatient general and specialist practices that are privately owned and managed, but tightly integrated into public planning and regulation and largely funded by public means. These features are rooted in political responses to specific historical conditions and provide a specific hybrid flavour to the Danish version of the Nordic National Health Service (NHS). The role of private actors, and most importantly, the private general practitioners (GPs) and practising specialist doctors has been maintained over time for functional reasons *and* due to the interests and power of the medical profession. The private GPs have thus maintained a level of autonomy and a relatively strong bargaining position for economic resources. In return, they have accepted to serve important roles as gatekeepers and coordinators and are seen as key contributors to maintaining a cost-efficient healthcare system.

The hybrid institutional position of the GP sector is one of the reasons for the misclassification of the Danish system in the efforts by Reibling, Ariaans and Wendt (2019) to develop a new typology of health systems with multiple subtypes of the NHS variant. The Danish healthcare system is 'regulation oriented' in the sense that state politicians and agencies play a significant role, but due to the strong role of general practice and municipal health-care, it comes closer to the performance- and primary-care-oriented public

DOI: 10.4324/9781003139799-8

systems along with the other Nordic countries. The primary care orientation is clear in the emphasis on critical role of GP services (Pedersen, Andersen and Søndergaard, 2012) and the expansion of municipal/local health services with a strong focus on prevention, rehabilitation and long-term care over the past decades (Olejaz et al., 2012). Another reason for misclassifications by Reibling and colleagues is the inclusion of performance dimensions in the typology. Performance data are backward looking and often not truly comparable. They are therefore a much weaker basis for empirically based typologies than careful comparison of systemic features. Nevertheless, the general ambition to update typologies is commendable, and as this chapter shows, there is good reason to consider how New Public Management (NPM) and other governance developments, as well as the governance of Covid-19, can be reflected in the terminology of 'neo-Beveridgian' NHS-type systems.

Origins of the National Health Service in Denmark

The NHS is a central part of the Danish welfare state which originates from rudimentary institutions to care for the poor and disabled in the eighteenth century. The first large-scale public hospital was established in 1757 in Copenhagen by King Frederik V with inspiration from similar institutions in Berlin (1710) and London (1719 and 1722). The hospital was initially for the poor, as wealthier citizens mostly used private doctors providing services at home (Vallgårda, 1989). During the nineteenth century, several additional hospitals were built in Copenhagen along with a number of local hospitals established by Danish towns and counties. The local hospitals were financed with property taxes and, to a lesser extent, charity and user charges. These hospitals were also initially intended for the poor, but this gradually changed at the end of the nineteenth century. From the 1930s onwards, the national government subsidised hospitals to an increasing degree, while counties maintained the responsibility for delivering hospital services (Vallgårda and Krasnik, 2014).

The establishment of hospitals coincided with a process of establishing the medical profession more firmly as part of the state-backed authority structures for medical practice (Jørgensen, 2007; Larsen, 2008). The medical profession successfully built alliances with the state, which is reflected in the growing number of laws to regulate the medical field. The profession also gained positions in various committees and authoritative agencies to develop legislation and regulate medical practices and sale of pharmaceuticals. Competing actors in the field were gradually excluded and their methods were de-legitimised. This is institutionalised in the 'quack regulation' from 1794 (Jørgensen, 2007). Internally, the medical profession was consolidated and strengthened, as the surgical and the medical specialties were united in 1834 following scientific advances in both fields (Larsen, 2008). The medical profession has continued to play a strong role in the scientific development and clinical governance of healthcare in Denmark. Medical societies are represented in policy committees coordinated by national- and regional-level governments and have a role in developing guidelines and standards for medical practice (Olejaz et al., 2012). However, this integration in the state and regional governance structure and the fact that health professionals working in hospitals are salaried employees also mean that their power has been constrained and that professional autonomy has been balanced with economic constraints and broader prioritisation decisions (Vrangbæk, 2021).

Health insurance developed during the second half of the nineteenth century. The conservative government introduced state subsidies to voluntary insurance schemes offered by mutual societies in 1892. This happened in response to the formation of other political movements and the organisation of labourers and farmers into unions, associations and cooperatives. These developments are often considered to be prerequisites for the development of the extensive Nordic welfare state (Korpi, 1983; Esping-Andersen, 1990). However, the initial development of the Danish healthcare can be characterised as a combination of state-supported corporatist and liberal welfare components in terms of health insurance funds (until 1973) and continued reliance on privately owned practices for primary care. In this sense, we can characterise Denmark as an early example of a hybrid NHS-based system where the institutional structures have been adjusted over time in response to specific policy problems and constellations of interests (Schmid et al., 2010).

Insurance schemes initially covered user charges associated with hospital admissions and paid for care provided by GPs, thus enabling a high number and equal distribution of GPs in Denmark. Initially, health insurance membership was exclusively comprised of the lower-income population. In 1900, insurance schemes only covered 20% of the population; by 1925, they covered 42%. In 1973, however, when insurance schemes were replaced by the universal public scheme and contributions could be considered an earmarked tax, coverage was 90%.

The period from 1945 to the 1980s represents an expansion of the welfare state and the comprehensive public healthcare system. The initial step was the first Danish Hospital Law in 1946. This was a framework law whereby Parliament left much of the detailed planning to county politicians, health professionals, bureaucrats and sickness funds. Politically, there was broad agreement about the principles of equity in access and public funding of hospitals (Vallgårda and Krasnik, 2014). This can be explained by the post-World War II political commitment to build societal welfare institutions.

During the 1950s and 1960s, the expansion of the health system was mainly led by the counties and municipalities and often involved a combination of public and private actors. However, by the late 1960s, Social Democrats were gaining ground and pushing for further development of public welfare state institutions. At the same time, there was a growing confidence in the ability to engineer the welfare state by comprehensive central planning schemes. The Social Democrats were not just at the centre of this development, but they also solicited support from a broad spectrum of political parties, thus illustrating the well-established Danish political norm to base major societal reforms on broad-based agreements. This is rooted in a parliamentary system with many small parties and frequent minority and coalition governments (Jensen, 2014; Vrangbæk, 2021).

Since the 1940s, there has been agreement among the political parties that access to healthcare should be independent of where one lives and of economic resources (Vallgårda, 1989). The principle of universality has been combined with a strong reliance on decentralised political initiatives and a high level of trust in medical expertise, particularly in the expansion period from 1945 to the 1980s. This has led to a technical and pragmatic policy style underpinned by a tradition of broad political compromises on welfare reforms at the national level. The parliamentary setup of many small parties and shifting coalition and minority governments has contributed to this dynamic. Furthermore, there is a long tradition of pragmatic collaboration at the regional and municipal levels, due to the institutional structure with broad-based committees. Overall, it can be concluded that the development of the Danish health system was formed at the national level, while most of the activities aimed at providing health and social care were established by towns and counties. This division of labour between the central state and decentralised political authorities characterises Danish healthcare even today with a strong role for regions and municipalities in the governance of health systems within a national-level framework. Indeed, it can be argued that technical governance issues between the central state and the decentralised authorities have become increasingly important while traditional left/right debates have played a minor role (except in occasional discussions about the marginal role of the private sector in Danish healthcare).

Main health reform policies since the 1970s

The tax-based universal health system was established in a major reform in 1971, designating counties as the political and administrative entities responsible for hospital ownership and services. The 1970–73 reform also gave municipalities extensive responsibilities for a number of health-related welfare services including social services, care for the elderly, non-clinical long-term care, and child and maternity care. Part of the municipality reform was updating the financing scheme by abolishing sickness funds and establishing county and state taxation as the primary funding vehicle for healthcare. Healthcare and welfare services thus became organised by democratically elected councils at the county (now region) and municipal levels and funded by county/municipal taxation and general block grants from the state. Thus, the municipality reform of 1970–73 was a major milestone, as it streamlined the governance of hospitals with the counties as owners and managers within a framework of state regulation (Vallgårda and Krasnik, 2014). The amalgamation of municipalities and counties and the streamlining of decentralised political governance consolidated the institutional path that is still followed today, as illustrated by the subsequent Structural Reform in 2007, which replaced the 13 counties with five larger regions and reduced the number of municipalities from 271 to 98 (Christiansen and Vrangbæk, 2018).

The period since the 1980s has been characterised by various challenges to the welfare- and profession-centred consensus. Core issues relate to concerns about the economic sustainability of the previous growth rates. Health systems are also subject to general societal development trends entailing demands for choice and participation rather than simply accepting decisions of medical and bureaucratic authorities. While the majority of voters maintain their support for the public healthcare system and accept being taxed to pay for healthcare, the past three decades have also seen stronger demands for general tax cuts from voters and economic-liberal interest organisations. These demands have met positive responses – particularly from liberal-conservative coalition governments. This has led to conflicting pressures on politicians to accommodate growing demands and needs for healthcare, while at the same time facing constrained resources. The solution has been an ongoing effort to improve efficiency through a combination of regulation, economic incentives and softer governance measures. However, efforts to increase efficiency have also created tension, such as between the national government that carries the responsibility for overall economic coordination and the decentralised authorities that are responsible for the actual delivery of services, as well as between public decision makers and healthcare professionals. Tensions have also been fuelled by a tendency for national-level politicians to intervene more directly in specific areas of healthcare through regulation, targets and economic incentives. Institutionalised budget negotiations between the state and the regions/municipalities have become an important arena for discussing economic- and governance-related issues, although, in recent years, they have been circumscribed by a national-level 'budget law' that imposes hard budget constraints and automatic sanctions for overspending (OECD, 2019).

A major reform of the political and administrative structure in 2007 created larger municipalities and regions (replacing the counties) and reshuffled responsibilities. The reform was based on concerns for the long-term sustainability of the county and municipal welfare governance and on a desire to take on more control from the national level. In spite of the comprehensive nature of the reform, however, it is notable that the basic institutional principles of decentralised political management, universal coverage and public funding were maintained. As such, the reform can be seen as an extension of the historical path of Danish health policy rather than a fundamental shift (Vrangbæk, 2021). Further changes to the overall structure for healthcare governance have been proposed as part of the election campaigns in 2011 and 2019 by the liberal party and supported by other major right-of-centre parties. Key elements were to replace the five regions with larger and more autonomous health regions and to establish a set of 'health clusters' for integration of hospitals, GPs and municipal healthcare. However, in both cases, these parties were voted out of government, and the Social Democratic-led governments have decided to maintain the structure with five democratic regions as the main governance units for hospitals and specialised care, while also investing in local 'health houses' and announcing a reform initiative in 2022 based on some variant of health clusters. A number of additional incremental changes are described later.

Impact on system architecture

The current health system is a multi-level governance structure consisting of the national state level, the five regions and 98 municipalities. Political councils are in charge of regions and municipalities. The councils are supported by administrations and are represented in joint interest organisations called Danish Regions and Local Government Denmark. These organisations negotiate annual agreements with the state on economic conditions and general policy directions. Danish Regions also negotiate collective agreements with health professionals to determine salaries for hospital doctors and fees for GPS and practising specialists. Furthermore, regions and municipalities negotiate health agreements every four years to coordinate activities and facilitate integrated care solutions. These agreements are subject to approval by national authorities (Olejaz et al., 2012).

National authorities are responsible for framework legislation and coordination of the general public-sector economy. The main institutional actors include Parliament, the Ministry of Health, the Danish Health Authority, the Danish Medicines Agency and the Danish Patient Safety Authority. National health authorities also have responsibilities related to the general supervision of health personnel and overall quality management based on national clinical guidelines and standards. These national authorities also develop plans that determine the location of highly specialised services, while the regions are in charge of operational planning and determine the location of regular hospital services. The regions also supervise and pay medical practitioners, while municipalities are in charge of health promotion and long-term care services (Olejaz et al., 2012; European Commission, 2021).

The five regions provide tax-financed hospital and outpatient medical care, as well as mental health and long-term care services for all legal residents of Denmark, as well as dental services for children under the age of 18. The regions subsidise prescription drugs, adult dental care, physiotherapy and optometry services. There is no defined benefit package for healthcare services, but, in general, the regions provide comprehensive care, as long as treatments are evidence-based and clinically proven. In principle, the regions have autonomy to make decisions about service levels and new medical treatments. In practice, this takes place in coordinated processes, where the regions coordinate decisions, while adhering to a framework of national laws, state-municipal agreements, guidelines and standards.

Since the Structural Reform in 2007, public health expenditures are financed by state and municipal taxes, which are redistributed to the regions that are not allowed to levy taxes. General block grants from the national government finance 77% of regional activities. Grants are allocated according to a formula based on demographic and socio-economic characteristics. A minor portion of state funding for regional and municipal services is activity-based or tied to specific priority areas. The remaining 20% of financing for regional services comes from municipal co-payments. Municipal expenditures are financed through a combination of local taxes and block grants. There are no out-of-pocket payments for regional hospitals or GPs (Olejaz et al., 2012; European Commission, 2021).

Almost two million Danes are covered by supplementary private health insurance that gives access to private treatment facilities. Most of the insurance policies are paid for by employers as part of collective agreements and/ or as a relatively minor addition to pension plans (Sagan and Thomson, 2016). According to the business association for insurance and pension companies, the number of Danes holding supplementary voluntary health insurance (VHI) has increased from 1.5 million to 2.3 million from 2009 to 2020 (Forsikring og Pension, 2021). This can be compared to a total population of 5.8 million Danes.

Centralisation and efficiency of hospitals

One of the aims of the 2007 reform was to strengthen the capacity to do integrated planning and modernisation of hospital capacity. Several governance initiatives were taken to secure this. First, the 13 counties were amalgamated into five regions to create more efficient and stronger administrative units. Second, the government launched a major investment plan in the wake of the reform, making the allocation of national funding for new hospitals conditional upon regional plans adhering to centralisation guidelines from the state. Third, the reform increased the power of the Danish Health Authority (DHA) and centralised the economic power to the national level, as the regions were no longer able to issue taxes. All in all, this meant that the pursuit of the general aims of the reform became strongly influenced by national authorities. While the DHA issued general guidelines with respect to specialty planning, an important task for the democratically elected politicians in each regional board was to initiate local specialty planning to comply with national guidelines. The specialty planning by the DHA included a definition of which specialties should be present at the regional level, and which should be available at a smaller number of hospitals to serve patients across regions. In this process, it was decided which specialties should be present in regions at which hospitals that remained open were to have changed functions. Compliance with the guidelines was a prerequisite to receive funding for the renewal of hospitals, and this gave the regions an incentive to comply. The process took place over several years and involved negotiations between each region and the DHA before a final plan was issued by the DHA. The clinical community was involved in the process by participating in a dialogue with each region and also at the national level by guiding the DHA with respect to what was feasible for a country like Denmark (OECD, 2013; Christiansen and Vrangbæk, 2018).

In the end, the number of acute hospitals was reduced from about 40 to 21 major hospitals with joint acute facilities. Many of these hospitals include two or more physical locations. The restructuring and geographical placement of acute hospitals took place in a democratic process subject to central guidelines and requirements. Since the reform, hospital productivity has increased by more than 2% per year and costs have been stable. Productivity increases are simply measured by comparing the total number of DRG points (activities) produced to the regional expenditure for hospitals (Sundhedsdatastyrelsen, 2021). In addition to the specialised hospitals, most municipalities have established 'health houses' – sometimes in collaboration with the regions. These institutions vary in terms of structure and function but generally aim to provide services to chronic care and elderly patients within the local community. Some also provide co-location of GPs, private specialist doctors and other service providers, such as physiotherapists and podiatrists. The 'health houses' are part of a conscious and ongoing effort to move patients, who do not require highly specialised care, to either GPs or municipal-/local-level care. This is further supported by economic incentives such as the municipal co-payment for hospital care, changes in the DRG payment scheme and the so-called 'proximity financing' scheme, which incentivises regional/municipal efforts to avoid unnecessary (re)admissions and to accelerate the use of telemedicine. Treatment guidelines for chronic care also support these efforts and typically include triaging guidelines, emphasising that most chronic care patients should be treated in primary care facilities. This policy of moving care out of hospitals is highly dependent on strengthening the coordination of care in networks of local, primary and specialised care providers. In this sense, much of the current policy thinking is closer to ideas of New Public Governance (NPG), networks and multi-level neo-Weberianism. The multi-level aspect requires democratic entities at state, region and municipal levels to collaborate in spite of institutional differences and diverging interests. Key venues for such negotiations are the annual negotiations about the economic framework and negotiations between regions and municipalities about formal 'health agreements'. The regular negotiation of national-level agreements between GPs and the regions is another important institutional forum for policy development.

Impact on population health

The health of the Danish population is relatively good; patients are generally satisfied with the health system – 89% express satisfaction compared to 71% in countries in the Organisation for Economic Cooperation and Development (OECD, 2021) – and overall levels of happiness are among the highest in the world (Helliwell et al., 2021). Life expectancy has been increasing over the past decades, and Denmark is slowly catching up with its Nordic neighbours. A Danish female born in 2020 can expect to live 83.6 years, while the figure in 2000 was 79.2. Comparable figures for the other Nordic countries are Sweden is 84.2 and 82, Norway 84.9 and 81.5 and Finland 85 and 81.2 (www.nordicstatistics.org/statistics/). A legacy of poor lifestyle choices, and particularly the high prevalence of female smokers in the past, is considered the main reason for poorer performance than Sweden and Norway. The consumption of alcohol among adolescents is also among the highest in Europe. All of these are reflected in the difference between preventable and treatable mortality, which illustrates that the main causes of poor health performance should be found outside the health system, in the culture and lifestyle choices of Danes as highlighted in Figure 4.1.

From 2019 to the pandemic year 2020, the life expectancy for Denmark increased by 0.1 years, and for Finland and Norway, it increased by 0.2 years, while for Iceland it decreased by 0.1 years. For Sweden, the life expectancy decreased by as much as 0.7 years, mostly due to a relatively high level of Covid-19-related deaths among older persons in Sweden. Figures 4.2–4.4 show improvements in life expectancy and an important reduction in mortality due to heart disease and cancer. This reflects a focused effort in these areas which have seen the introduction of successive 'packages' of increased funding combined with detailed, structured descriptions of standard pathways and aggressive monitoring of process performance indicators.

Disease management programs have also been introduced for chronic diseases, including chronic obstructive pulmonary disease (COPD) and diabetes, and the health status in those areas is slowly improving, although social inequities remain. The Danish Health Authority published a comprehensive report about inequality in health in 2020 (Udesen et al., 2020). The report provides details about developments from 2010 to 2017 differentiating between high, medium and low levels of social inequality. It shows persistently high social inequality in self-rated health, which is otherwise high in comparison to other countries. Social inequality is also high in dental health for children and adults and a number of health risk factors, such as smoking, obesity, working life conditions, stress and loneliness. This is further reflected in high levels of social inequality in life-style-related diseases, such as diabetes, COPD, lung cancer and musculo-skeletal diseases. Many of these findings are related to lifestyle rather than the health system as such, and the report shows that there are low levels of inequality in access to treatment on all dimensions except dental care for adults, where co-payments are applied.

The Danish health system has performed well during the Covid-19 pandemic. The number of Covid-19 deaths was lower than that in most other European Union (EU) countries. This was partly due to quick upscaling of testing capacity at the beginning of the pandemic, which enabled effective detection, tracing and isolation of confirmed cases early on. The Danish response was also characterised by a high level of flexibility in scaling up intensive care capacity which was never endangered during the epidemic. Rapid implementation

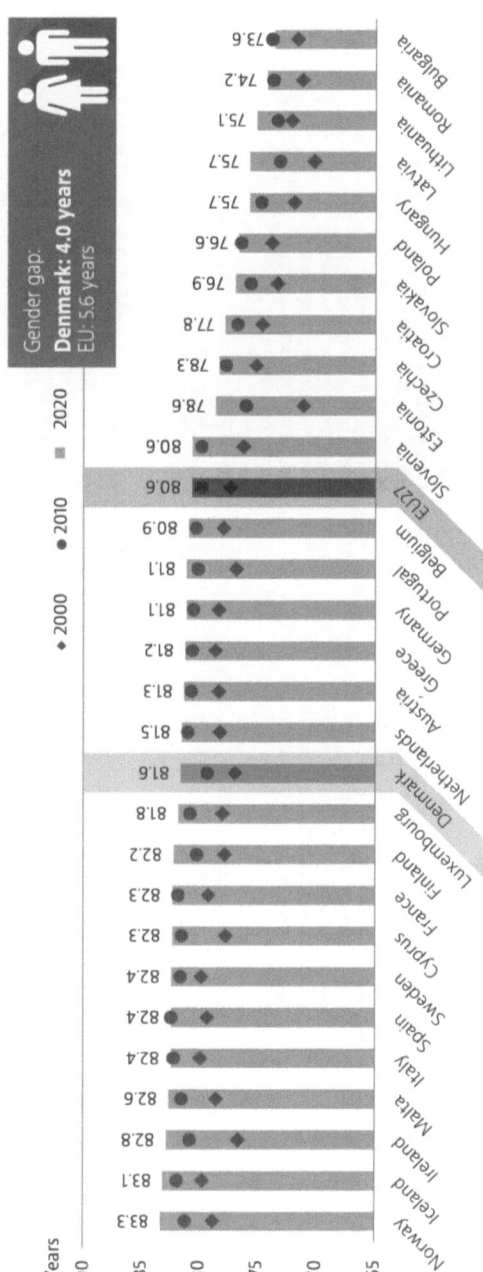

Figure 4.1 Mortality in European societies

Source: European Commission (2021).

Reproduced with permission from the OECD/European Observatory on Health Systems and Policies

Note: The EU average is weighted. Data for Ireland refer to 2019.
Source: Eurostat Database.

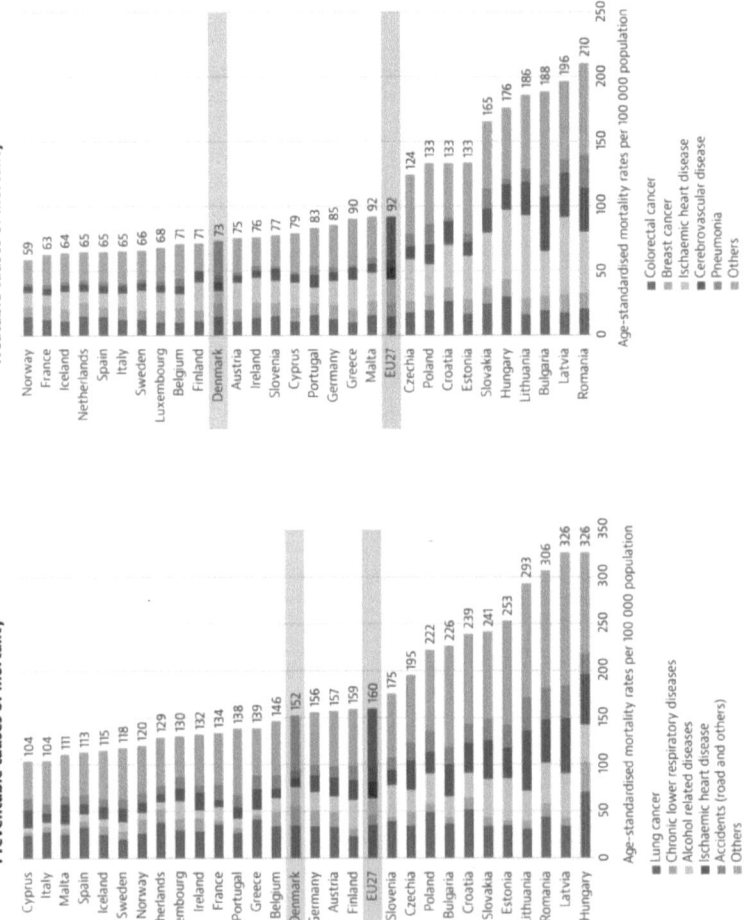

Preventable causes of mortality

Cyprus	104
Italy	104
Malta	111
Spain	113
Iceland	115
Sweden	118
Norway	120
Netherlands	129
Luxembourg	130
Ireland	132
France	134
Portugal	138
Greece	139
Belgium	146
Denmark	152
Germany	156
Austria	157
Finland	159
EU27	160
Slovenia	175
Czechia	195
Poland	222
Bulgaria	226
Croatia	239
Slovakia	241
Estonia	253
Lithuania	293
Romania	306
Latvia	326
Hungary	326

Age-standardised mortality rates per 100 000 population

■ Lung cancer
■ Chronic lower respiratory diseases
■ Alcohol related diseases
■ Ischaemic heart disease
■ Accidents (road and others)
■ Others

Treatable causes of mortality

Norway	59
France	63
Iceland	64
Netherlands	65
Spain	65
Italy	65
Sweden	66
Luxembourg	68
Belgium	71
Finland	71
Denmark	73
Austria	75
Ireland	76
Slovenia	77
Cyprus	79
Portugal	83
Germany	85
Greece	90
Malta	92
EU27	92
Czechia	124
Poland	133
Croatia	133
Estonia	133
Slovakia	165
Hungary	176
Lithuania	186
Bulgaria	188
Latvia	196
Romania	210

Age-standardised mortality rates per 100 000 population

■ Colorectal cancer
■ Breast cancer
■ Ischaemic heart disease
■ Cerebrovascular disease
■ Pneumonia
■ Others

*Note: Preventable mortality is defined as death that can be mainly avoided through public health and primary prevention interventions. Treatable mortality is defined as death that can be mainly avoided through health care interventions, including screening and treatment. Half of all deaths for some diseases (e.g. ischaemic heart disease and cerebrovascular disease) are attributed to preventable mortality; the other half are attributed to treatable causes. Both indicators refer to premature mortality (under age 75). The data are based on the revised OECD/Eurostat lists.
Source: Eurostat Database (data refer to 2018, except for France 2016).*

Figure 4.2 Comparative life expectancy in EU countries

Source: European Commission (2021).
Reproduced with permission from the OECD/European Observatory on Health Systems and Policies

Any cardiovscular diseases: 1-year all-cause mortality
(ages 35+)

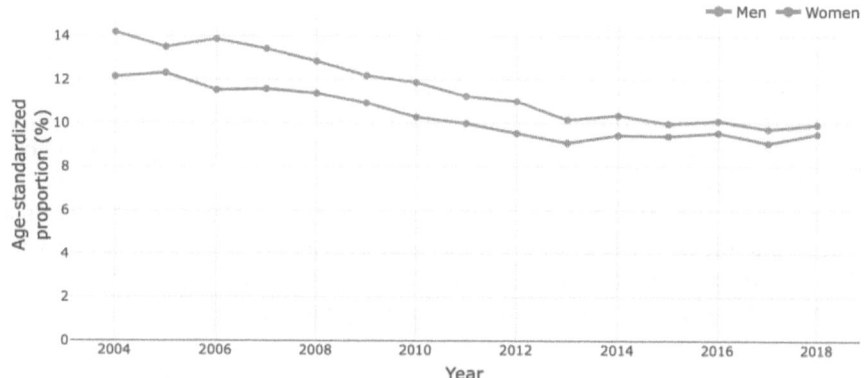

Figure 4.3 Cardiovascular diseases in Denmark
Source: Danish Heart Association (2018).

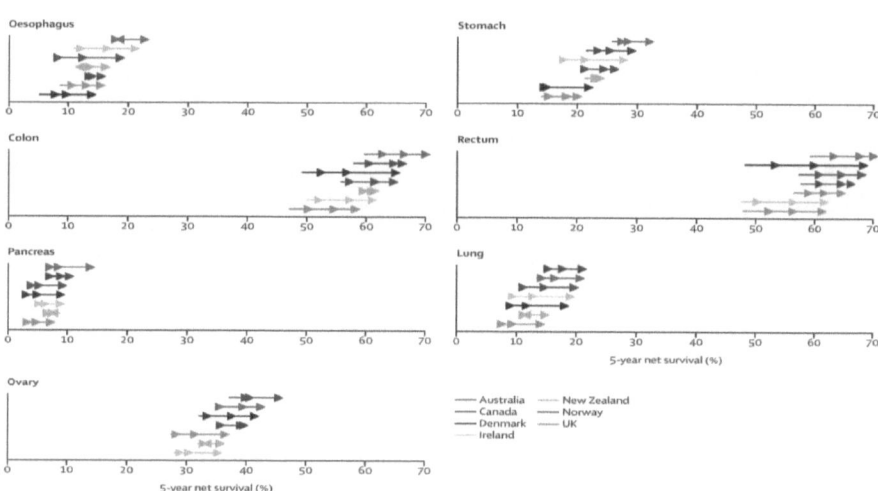

Figure 4.4 Cancer five-year mortality in selected countries
Source: Arnold, Rutherford, Bardot et al. (2019).

of teleconsultations alleviated pressure on primary care services (European Commission, 2021). The institutional structure of the governance structure in Denmark allowed for a high level of coordination of efforts. State, regional and municipal authorities held daily coordination meetings, and a national-level crisis response unit had the task of coordinating across different areas of society. A fast revision of the 'epidemic law' allowed the national parliament to make swift decisions on pandemic responses and apply restrictions that have largely been accepted by the population (Seing et al., 2021). The high degree of acceptance can be explained by a generally high level of trust in government institutions (OECD, 2021) and by the fact that, for example, mobility restrictions were less severe than in many other countries. Danes were never confined to stay in their homes when not infected or 'close-contacts', and there were no restrictions on travel within the country. From an institutional governance perspective, we can interpret the successful response to the pandemic as the result of a well-functioning neo-Weberian model with tight coordination of efforts orchestrated by a strengthening of power at the national apex of government and associated agencies.

Evaluation of future sustainability

The Danish health system is performing relatively well and has demonstrated a remarkable ability to adjust to new contingencies such as the economic crisis in the 1980s and the changing needs and expectations in the population (Christiansen and Vrangbæk, 2018; OECD, 2013). The successful response to Covid-19 is another illustration of the resilience of the system (European Commission, 2021).

Yet several challenges must be addressed in the future. The ageing of the population means that the prevalence of chronic diseases and co-morbidities will increase in the future. This puts pressure on resources and the capacity to coordinate services across hospitals, GPs and local care in an efficient manner. While future generations of over 60-year-olds appear to be healthier than previously, they will still incur health problems requiring treatment and driving expenditures. Furthermore, future generations of elderly are accustomed to high standards and are likely to demand more individualised and extensive service than previous generations. At the same time, health technologies are developing rapidly, and some of the technologies are very costly such as advanced cancer treatments and drugs for neuro-degenerative diseases. Hospital-administered pharmaceuticals are a major cost driver today, and this is likely to be even more important in future as more and more customised treatments become available.

It is evident that the system must strive to continuously develop solutions to optimise service delivery across care levels and to improve prevention and rehabilitation at the municipal level and to address the social biases and relatively poorer health in some parts of the population as explained earlier (Sundhedsdastyrelsen, 2021). Telemedicine and other digitally based solutions may reduce expenditures in the long run, but extant experience mostly point to improved quality, not cost reductions. This may change if some of the ongoing pilot projects are rolled out on a larger scale.

An ageing population also means fewer people of working age and more competition for human resources. Already today we see challenges in recruiting and retaining skilled nurses. Similarly, it is increasingly difficult to attract medical doctors to positions in rural areas and areas with social problems. Attracting foreign healthcare professionals has relieved some of the problems, but this strategy is not ethically sustainable as the countries of origin also need healthcare professionals in the future. The difficulties in recruiting and retaining nurses were exacerbated during the Covid crisis, which also fuelled a major conflict about salaries and working conditions in the summer of 2021. The conflict ended with a government intervention, which has soured the relations and led to further loss of personnel. The issue is critical in some hospitals and more broadly indicates the ongoing need to negotiate new compromises between the professions and the state.

A broader challenge for the public health system is the political willingness to uphold a collective solution. While support has remained strong for the universal health system, it is also evident from the high number of persons purchasing VHI that Danes are willing to seek private solutions, if the public service level is perceived to fall behind. However, as this is most relevant for affluent persons in the workforce, this may introduce further social bias in access to healthcare. Maintaining a satisfactory service and quality standard in the public sector is thus a critical challenge for the future as expectations, needs and technological possibilities are likely to challenge the costs of the system. So far, Danes have a high level of satisfaction with the health services (OECD, 2021). Part of the reason is perhaps that it has been possible to incorporate and adjust NPM ideas of increased choice of provider and performance-based payments within the system in ways that are largely seen as service increases. Key examples include the free choice of public hospitals and the diagnosis and treatment guarantee, which opens for choice of private providers in case the regions are unable to provide a diagnosis within 30 days. The potential for public participation in democratic governance at the regional and local levels may also contribute to the support for the system. Even though the regions and municipalities increased in size with the reform in 2007, there is still a relatively high level of participation in elections, and politicians are generally relatively easy to approach in Denmark.

Danes also have a high level of trust in public institutions – 72% compared to 51% in the rest of the OECD countries (OECD, 2021). This is likely to be a main reason behind the relatively high level of support for Covid-19 policies including recommendations for vaccination (Helliwell et al., 2021) and the low level of mortality from the pandemic.

Neo-liberal health reforms?

Radical neo-liberal health reforms have not been introduced in the Danish health system, which has largely maintained its status as a public, tax-financed scheme with services that are largely free at the point of delivery. Figure 4.5 shows that public healthcare expenditures remain high, while out-of-pocket payments and voluntary insurance payments are limited compared to most other European countries.

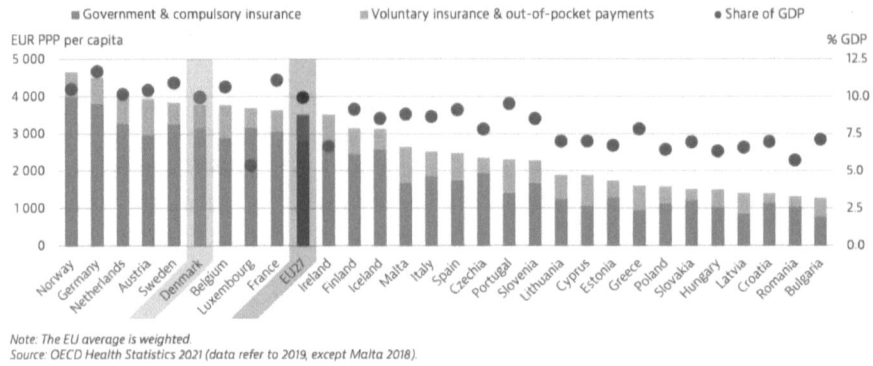

Note: The EU average is weighted.
Source: OECD Health Statistics 2021 (data refer to 2019, except Malta 2018).

Figure 4.5 Healthcare expenditure in European countries

Source: Organisation for Economic Cooperation and Development (2019) Heath Statistics.

While there have not been 'big bang' NPM reforms, the Danish system has incorporated a number of governance ideas associated with the NPM (Hood, 1991). The NPM ideas have generally been adapted as instruments to achieve specific purposes in the health system. For instance, market principles have been introduced in the form of 'free choice of hospitals' upon referral from the 1990s and 'extended free choice' from 2002 which essentially allows for access to private hospitals and clinics if waiting times exceed a predefined level of one month. Liberal-conservative governments have also supported a private sector alternative by providing tax breaks for employees who receive VHI as part of their benefit package. While this incentive has now been dismantled by the Social Democratic government, there continues to be a growth in the number of citizens with VHI coverage, although the actual contribution to health expenditures remains marginal (Sagan and Thomson, 2016). The gross income associated with these policies was 2.5 billion DKK in 2020, while the gross payments were slightly more than 2 billion DKK (Forsikring og Pension, 2021). This can be compared to about 190 billion DKK in public healthcare expenditure.

The past three decades have also seen a significant increase in the use of performance measures, which are often published in a way that allows for comparisons and benchmarking over time. While these measures are generally not tightly related to economic incentives, they are indirectly part of the governance structure as they provide the basis for choice (with money following patients to other regions or private hospitals) and more importantly for various types of administrative interventions if suboptimal performance is identified.

While it is possible to find examples of NPM-inspired governance initiatives, the Danish health system has also been affected by two other types of governance trends. The first is broadly described as 'digital era governance'

(DEG) (Dunleavy et al., 2005) and the second is a bundle of instruments, known by the broad headline of NPG.

According to Dunleavy and colleagues (2005), DEG consists of three main elements: 1) integration of service through digital solutions; 2) need-based holistic service based on 'real time' matching of citizen needs and service offers; and 3) digitalisation of contact points and administrative processes. The Danish health system has often described as one of the most digitalised in Europe. Information Technology (IT) is used at all levels of the health system as part of a national strategy supported by the National Agency for Health IT. Each of the five regions uses electronic health record (EHR) systems for hospitals, with adherence to national standards for compatibility. All citizens in Denmark have a unique electronic personal identifier that is used in all public registries, including health databases. The government has implemented an electronic medical card, storing encoded information about each patient's prescriptions and medication use; this information is accessible by the patient and all relevant health professionals (Gjødsbøl et al., 2021).

GPs also have access to an online medical handbook with updated information on diagnosis and treatment recommendations. Two regions are currently implementing a comprehensive new EHR and data capture system developed by the American IT firm called EPIC. While the initial implementation has been problematic due to a poor fit with Danish system conditions and massive critique from healthcare professionals about excessive levels of detail and illogical workflows (Røhl and Nielsen, 2019), it is expected to provide benefits in the long run. The three other regions are using a system developed by Systematic. Shared standards facilitate communication between the two IT systems at the general level, but with a number of challenges at the detailed clinical level.

The national health information portal, Sundhed.dk, offers differentiated access for health staff and the wider public. It provides general information on health and treatment options and access to individuals' own medical records and history. For professionals, the site serves as an entry to medical handbooks, scientific articles, treatment guidelines, hospital waiting times, treatments offered and patients' laboratory test results. The portal also serves as a communication platform for referral, discharge and prescription information among primary care providers, regions, hospitals and pharmacies (Vrangbæk, 2020; Vrangbæk et al., 2021). NPG emphasises network structures, co-creation and joined-up service delivery structures (Osborne, 2009).

Such ideas have also been critical in health policy debates in Denmark, particularly since the 1990s where seamless and efficient care across sectoral boundaries was formulated as a key issue. The ambition of eliminating ambiguity and strengthening coordination was also at the heart of the 2007 structural reform in Denmark and has been reinforced by governance mechanisms such as the mandatory health agreements between regions and municipalities, the municipal co-financing of hospital care and the introduction of disease management programs to structure the complexity of care for chronic patients. More recently, the government changed part of the funding scheme for the regions from activity-based incentives for hospitals to a 'proximity payment scheme' that rewards performance in regard to prevention of unnecessary hospital admissions and faster introduction of telemedicine to facilitate patient co-creation and involvement of local care delivery structures. A new government policy initiative from 2022 further emphasises the importance of networks between hospitals, GPs and municipal healthcare organisations for the future of healthcare governance (Sundhedsministeriet, 2022).

Conclusion

The Danish NHS system is characterised by a high degree of continuity or path dependence in terms of the overall structures (public funding and public ownership of hospitals, public funding and mixed private/public delivery in primary care) but with gradual adaptation and inclusion of NPM, NPG and DEG governance dimensions. This means that the current system is perhaps best characterised as a multi-level 'neo-Beveridgian' hybrid system. The Danish system resembles the other Nordic healthcare systems on many dimensions but also with some special features in terms of a more radical structural reform in 2007, stronger growth in VHI and continued reliance on privately owned GP practices.

The general path dependency of the Danish healthcare system can be explained by 'blame avoidance' strategies and a broad political consensus behind the overall aims of equity, quality and efficiency in the health policy arena. This can be interpreted in light of ideas in the seminal book by Pierson (1994) about welfare reforms and institutional path dependency. Following his core argument, it can be observed that Danish governments since the late 1970s have been caught between the need for cost containment and high expectations about healthcare in the voting population. The solution has been to focus much of the internal governance attention on developing instruments to control costs while at the same time securing a sufficiently high level of service and quality to avoid blame for failures or claim credit for advances. This has led to the policy consensus behind a controlled growth in expenditure levels and fewer 'hidden retrenchments' than in other parts of the welfare state. Reforms have been incremental and designed to maintain public governance control, while avoiding blame or claiming credit from voters and avoiding conflicts with the major stakeholder interests among health professionals, patients and medical industry. The latter has largely been achieved, although a few major conflicts with GPs and nurses have occurred – most recently in 2020, where a major strike among nurses was ended with a government decree.

The major structural reform in 2007 was presented as a way to improve quality, while streamlining the capacity to deliver highly specialised services in fewer and larger hospitals. The challenging part of the reform was that it presupposed a significant increase in capacity at the local and primary care levels and a stronger coordination across sectors. This has proven harder to achieve, although many policies in the past decades have taken inspiration from NPG and DEG to move towards these aims. The NPG and DEG reform elements have also attempted to place a different emphasis on patient involvement than the previous choice-oriented policies, which have been maintained and adapted to the Danish context, and the general democratic involvement mechanisms of voting and participating in local, regional and state assemblies (Vrangbæk, 2018). Examples of new types of patient involvement can be seen in the extensive efforts to develop and utilise patient-reported outcome measures and to use telemedicine and digital tools for communication and management, particularly of chronic diseases. Such developments require changes in the roles of healthcare professionals and new compromises with the state, which can be difficult to achieve in a period with many other new requirements and challenges in retaining staff in some parts of the system. Many patients benefit from the extensive digitalisation of healthcare in Denmark, as it provides opportunities to be treated at home and to engage in a more informed dialogue with the healthcare professionals. However, there also remains a group of digitally 'illiterate' citizens for whom the migration to digital solutions remains challenging. Overall, this may exacerbate some of the inequality that remains in the system, despite a long-standing emphasis on reducing the social gradients in access and health outcomes.

The Covid-19 response has been relatively successful in Denmark. It has also illustrated the capacity of the national state to assert its power within the multilevel governance structure of state, regions and local governments (Seing et al., 2021). However, the decentralised government levels continue to play a strong role in the implementation and ongoing governance of healthcare delivery.

References

Arnold, M., Rutherford, M. J., Bardot, A., et al. (2019) 'Progress in cancer survival, mortality, and incidence in seven high-income countries 1995–2014: A population-based study', *The Lancet Oncology* 20(11): 1493–505.

Christiansen, T. and Vrangbæk, K. (2018) 'Hospital centralization and performance in Denmark – Ten years on', *Health Policy* 122(4): 321–8. Available at: https://doi.org/10.1016/j.healthpol.2017.12.009

Danish Heart Association (2018) Available at: https://hjerteforeningen.shinyapps.io/HjerteTal-en/?_inputs_&agCVD=%22national%22&varCVD=%22v12%22&oCVD=%22d1%22&bar=%22cvd%22&year=%222018%22

Dunleavy, P., Margetts, H., Bastow, S. and Tinkler, J. (2005) 'New public management is dead – long live digital-era governance', *Journal of Public Administration Research and Theory* 16: 467–94.

Esping-Andersen, G. (1990) *The Three Worlds of Welfare Capitalism*, Cambridge: Cambridge University Press.

European Commission (2021) *State of Health in the EU. Denmark. Country Health Profile*. Available at: https://ec.europa.eu/health/system/files/2021-12/2021_chp_da_english.pdf

Forsikring og Pension (2021) Available at: www.forsikringogpension.dk/statistik/
sundhedsforsikringer/

Gjødsbøl, I. M., Høyer, K., Langstrup, H., Kayser, L. and Vrangbæk, K. (2021) 'Digitalisering i det danske sundhedsvæsen?', *Samfundsoekonomen*, nr. 1. Available at: www.djoef-forlag.dk/openaccess/samf/samfdocs/2021/2021_1/Samf_4_1_2021.pdf

Helliwell, J. F., Layard, R., Sachs, J. and De Neve, J. (eds) (2021) *World Happiness Report 2021*, New York: Sustainable Development Solutions Network.

Hood, C. (1991) 'A public management for all seasons?', *Public Administration* 69(1): 3–19.

Jensen, C. (2014) *Velfærdsstaten – en introduktion. 2. udgave*, København: Hans Reitzels Forlag.

Jørgensen, E. B. (2007) 'Genese og struktur af klinisk medicin og klinisk sygepleje – om hvordan medicin og sygepleje som moderne fag, erhverv og uddannelser har konstitueret sig i Danmark samt forbindelsen mellem dem. For lægeerhvervet er perioden 1736–1937 og for sygeplejeerhvervet er perioden 1863–1957', *Forlaget Hexis*. Available at: http://www2.viauc.dk/bibliotekerne/holstebro/Documents/Projekter%20Undervisere/emmysafhandling.pdf

Korpi, W. (1983) *The Democratic Class Struggle*, London: Routledge.

Larsen, K. (2008) 'Brydningstid i dansk medicin 1750–1850: Om positioner, kampe, videnskab og praksis i medicinsk felt. Forskningsnoter DPU, forskningsnoter K. Larsen', *Working Paper*, Aalborg Universitet.

Olejaz, M., Nielsen, J. A., Rudkjøbing, A., Okkels, B. H., Krasnik, A. and Hernández-Quevedo, C. (2012) 'Denmark: Health system review', *Health Systems in Transition* 14(2): 1–192.

Organisation for Economic Cooperation and Development (2013) *Reviews of Health Care Quality: Denmark 2013. Rising Standards*, Paris: OECD. Available at: www.oecd-ilibrary.org/social-issues-migration-health/oecd-reviews-of-health-care-quality-denmark-2013_9789264191136-en

Organisation for Economic Cooperation and Development (2019) *Budgeting and Public Expenditures in OECD Countries 2019*, Paris: OECD. Available at: https://doi.org/10.1787/9789264307957-en

Organisation for Economic Cooperation and Development (2021) *Government at a Glance*, Paris: OECD.

Osborne, S. (ed) (2009) *The New Public Governance? Emerging Perspectives on the Theory and Practice of Public Governance*, Abingdon: Routledge.

Pedersen, K. M., Andersen, J. S. and Søndergaard, J. (2012) 'General practice and primary health care in Denmark', *Journal of the American Board of Family Medicine* (Supplement 1): S34–S38. Available at: https://doi.org/10.3122/jabfm.2012.02.110216

Pierson, P. (1994) *Dismantling the Welfare State?: Reagan, Thatcher and the Politics of Retrenchment*, Cambridge: Cambridge University Press.

Reibling, N., Ariaans, M. and Wendt, C. (2019) 'Worlds of healthcare: A healthcare system typology of OECD countries', *Health Policy* 123(7): 611–20.

Røhl, U. and Nielsen, J. (2019) 'Sundhedsplatformen i modvind: En analyse af aktørernes teknologiforståelser i danske medier', *Samfundslederskab i Skandinavien* 34. Available at: https://doi.org/10.22439/sis.v34i3.5810

Sagan, A. and Thomson, S. (2016) *Voluntary Health Insurance in Europe. Role and Regulation*, Copenhagen: World Health Organization.

Schmid, A., Cacace, M., Götze, R. and Rothgang, H. (2010) 'Explaining health care system change: Problem pressure and the emergence of "hybrid" health care systems', *Journal of Health Politics, Policy and Law* 35(4): 455–86. Available at: https://doi.org/10.1215/03616878-2010-013

Seing, I., Thórný Stefánsdóttir, N., Wassar, K. J., et al. (2021) 'Social distancing policies in the coronavirus battle: A comparison of Denmark and Sweden', *International Journal of Environmental Research and Public Health* 18(20). Available at: https://doi.org/10.3390/ijerph182010990

Sundhedsdatastyrelsen (2021) *Løbende offentliggørelse af produktivitet i sygehussektoren*, København: Sundhedsdatastyresen. Available at: https://sundheds-datastyrelsen.dk/da/tal-og-analyser/analyser-og-rapporter/sundhedsvaesenet/produktivitet-i-sygehussektoren

Sundhedsministeriet (2022) *Sundhedsreformen. Gør Danmark Sundere*, København: Sundhedsministeriet (Ministry of Health).

Udesen, C. H., Skaarup, C., Schmidt Petersen, M. N. and Ersbøll, A. K. (2020) 'Social ulighed i sundhed og sygdom Udviklingen i Danmark i perioden 2010–2017', *Statens Institut for Folkesundhed*, København: Sundhedsstyrelsen. Available at: www.sst.dk/-/media/Udgivelser/2020/Ulighed-i-sundhed/Social-ulighed-i-sundhed-og-sygdom-tilgaengelig.ashx?la=da&hash=CB63CAD067D942FE54B99034085E78BE9F486A92

Vallgårda, S. (1989) 'Læger, sundhedsvæsen og befolkning i det 19. århundrede', *Ugeskrift for læger* 4(maj): s.16–28.

Vallgårda, S. and Krasnik, A. (2014) *Sundhedsvæsen og sundhedspolitik*, 4th edition, København: Munksgård.

Vrangbæk, K. (2018) 'The regulation of health care in Scandinavia: Professionals, the public interest and trust', in Chamberlain, J. M., Dent, M. and Saks, M. (eds) *Professional Health Regulation in the Public Interest: International Perspectives*, Bristol: Policy Press.

Vrangbæk, K. (2020) *International Health Care System Profiles. Denmark*, New York: The Commonwealth Fund. Available at: www.commonwealthfund.org/international-health-policy-center/countries/denmark

Vrangbæk, K. (2021) 'Denmark', in Immergut, E., Anderson, K., Dewitt, C. and Popic, T. (eds) *Health Politics in Europe: A Handbook*, Oxford: Oxford University Press. Available at: https://global.oup.com/academic/product/health-politics-in-europe-9780198860525?q=Immergut&lang=en&cc=de

Vrangbæk, K., Høyer, K., Langstrup, H., Kayser, L. and Gjødsbøl, I. M. (2021) 'Digitalisering i det danske sundhedsvæsen', *Samfundsøkonomen*, Copenhagen: DJØF.

5 Norway

Pål E. Martinussen and Jon Magnussen

Introduction

'I'd like to have a healthcare system in Norway adapted to the customer, offering the treatment you require. . . . Obviously, there's a difference between people and cars. But it's about the mindset'. These were the words of the Norwegian Labour Party health minister upon visiting the Toyota factory in Japan on 9 January 2009. Seven years earlier, on 1 January 2002, a Labour Party government initiated a 'big bang' hospital reform in Norway almost overnight. The reform transferred hospital ownership from the locally elected county councils to the central government and introduced new management principles for the hospitals based on a decentralised enterprise model. The reform involved 100,000 employees and 40 billion NOK (almost $5 billion) and is thus one of the most encompassing Norwegian public-sector reforms ever. The introduction of the enterprise model came five years after the implementation of activity-based financing (ABF) in hospitals. This reform, too, was initiated by a Labour government. In between, patient rights had been strengthened and expanded through the introduction of free choice of hospitals.

All these reforms were a part of a larger shift in the Norwegian public administration system and can partly be seen as an ideological change in Norwegian political parties, including the Labour Party, towards New Public Management (NPM) and private sector models (Lægreid, Opedal and Stigen, 2005). Norwegian public management research has mainly built on a broad institutional perspective, combining conventional organisational research and neo-institutionalism (Christensen and Lægreid, 2001). The introduction of performance management has thus been interpreted in terms of the historical-institutional context of national style of governance and modes of institutional regulation, based on specific identities, histories and dynamics (Olsen, 1997). As put forward by Per Lægreid (2020:585), one of the leading researchers on Norwegian public management: '[I]t is a story of the complex interplay between competing logics, loyalties and influences, demanding more elaborate models of decision-making and change than assumed by the Weberian ideal model'. While the hospital reform was most visibly inspired

DOI: 10.4324/9781003139799-9

by NPM thinking, a central point to be made here is that business management principles and market ideology had also been introduced into Norwegian healthcare both through ABF and a free choice of hospitals: the hospital
reform was simply a natural culmination of this trend. Today, the major
political debate in neo-Weberian and neo-institutionalist terms is again about
how the healthcare system should be organised, and in particular whether to
keep the enterprise model for hospitals or not.

Origins of the National Health Service

The Norwegian healthcare system found its form in the years following
World War II. Strongly inspired by the Beveridge plan, the foundations for
the welfare state were laid in the joint political programme prepared by the
political parties in the summer of 1945. With the Labour Party governing
alone with a majority in parliament in the period 1945–65, the modern welfare state emerged as a clear social democratic project, although there was a
multiparty agreement about the need for social security and redistribution.
The period therefore saw a rapid expansion of hospitals, institutions and
eventually primary health services, often little subjected to political debates
despite the need for large investments in other sectors (Larsen, 1996; Larsen,
Berg and Hodne, 1986; Schiøtz, 2003). This period saw the establishment
of the key financial, political and administrative actors in the health system:
While the configuration of these has varied somewhat, the main structures
have been stable and today these actors are: The Ministry of Health and
Care Services, the National Insurance Scheme, the Directorate of Health,
the National Institute of Public Health and the Board of Health Supervision.
Helped by the discovery of the petroleum resources in the North Sea, the
period after 1970 was characterised by large investments in the health sector, with growing provision of specialised services and an increasing role of
hospitals (Saunes, Karanikolos and Sagan, 2020).

Norway is a good example of the oscillation between political/administra-
tive centralisation and decentralisation in healthcare. During the first decades
after World War II, healthcare evolved as the result of mostly uncoordinated
efforts by counties, municipalities, private non-profit organisations and sometimes the state. The Hospital Act that was passed by Parliament in 1969 was
therefore an attempt to better coordinate and put a national emphasis on the
planning and operating of a sector that previously had been subjected to few
centralised decisions. The Hospital Act formally placed the responsibility for
planning, building and managing the hospitals with the 19 counties. This set
the stage for a gradual evolution of a three-level system of healthcare governance. Regionalisation was established as a structural principle in 1974 when
counties were grouped in five healthcare regions. Although these had neither
a political nor administrative responsibility, the small population of several
counties combined with large geographical distances provided opportunities
for economies of scale through centralisation. The municipalities were given

the responsibility for primary healthcare in 1980 (Parliamentary Proposition no. 36, 1980–81), and the responsibility for the nursing homes was transferred from the counties to the municipalities in 1988.

This decentralised model was challenged and modified in terms of both centralised policy initiatives and a higher degree of centralised funding in the period up to the hospital reform in 2002. While the country was divided into five health regions in 1974, recognising that counties would not cooperate voluntarily, regional cooperation was made mandatory in 1999. When, in addition, the introduction of ABF in 1997 meant more central funding, there was in essence little left of the original decentralised model upon entering the 2000s. The hospital reform can, therefore, be seen as the final and formal stage of a re-centralisation of the hospital sector (Martinussen and Magnussen, 2009).

Main health reform trends

In the period following the Hospital Law in 1969, the Norwegian healthcare system has been almost continuously under reform. Initially, hospitals were funded based on the number of bed-days. From 1980, however, the system changed to global budgeting. The counties would first be given fixed sector-specific budgets, but from 1986, this was changed to a need-adjusted per capita financing of counties. They would then be free to allocate resources between the services they were responsible for. This lasted until 1997, when a system of partly activity-based financing was introduced. The hospital payment reform was the first of several NPM-inspired reforms and was followed by the family doctor reform in 2001, free choice of hospitals in 2001 (extended to include private hospitals in 2015), the hospital reform of 2002 and the coordination reform of 2012 (Byrkjeflot and Neby, 2008; Nyseter, 2015; Rommetvedt et al., 2014). Common to all these reforms is that they have targeted organisational structures and ownership forms, political governance, patient rights, quality and economy. Thus, the changes in the system from the 1970s and up till today have been quite radical. Whereas the hospital reform is the reform that most explicitly built on NPM ideas, it only came as a conclusion of several NPM-inspired changes. In addition, the major reforms in this period was also characterised by increased focus on performance indicators and comparable data between hospitals, focus on management roles, and laws and regulations on unified leadership that links responsibility to manager positions rather than to professions.

Activity-based financing

As noted, between 1980 and 1997, Norwegian hospitals were reimbursed through a system of global budgeting. Hospitals would receive a fixed budget from the county at the beginning of each year, mainly based on historical costs. Counties, on the other hand, would get their income from a capitation model similar to the capitation models found in other tax-based countries, such as the other Nordic countries and the United Kingdom (UK).

With the introduction of ABF in the hospital sector from 1 July 1997, a fraction of the block grant from the state to the county councils was replaced by a matching grant depending on the number and composition of hospital treatments. The reimbursement from the state was given as a percentage of the diagnostic related group-based cost of a treatment: 30% the first year, before increasing gradually to 60% in 2003. Between 2004 and 2006, the share fluctuated between 40% and 60%, but from 2006 to 2013, the ABF share remained at 40%, before increasing to 50% from 2014. The introduction of ABF followed a period of relatively low growth in hospital budgets, resulting in high waiting lists and waiting time for elective treatment (Martinussen and Hagen, 2009). One argument for ABF was therefore to increase the number of elective treatments, which was needed in order to fulfil the waiting-list guarantee that had been adopted by the parliament. Whereas an increase in the block grant to the county councils was assumed to spill over to other county sectors such as secondary schools and transportation, the introduction of ABF was assumed to shift the county councils' priorities in the direction of hospitals (Biørn et al., 2003).

Free choice of hospitals

The debate over patient rights began in the 1980s and early 1990s, following a situation with long waiting lists for elective treatment. The minority Labour Party governments during the 1990s had generally been sceptical towards free-choice reforms, but after pressure from the opposition parties, the first Patient Rights Act was finally passed in 1999 (Parliamentary Proposition no. 12, 1998–99). The Act both simplified and consolidated already existing legislation and implemented new rights, thus covering a broad package of rights that extended far beyond the free choice of hospitals, such as evaluation within 30 days, second opinion, participation and information, access to medical records, special rights relating to children and complaints and assistance from the Patients' Ombudsman. Several amendments were made to the Patient Rights Act in 2003 and 2004, including an extension of free choice of hospital to private hospitals with a tender agreement with the regional health authorities (Parliamentary Proposition no. 63, 2002–2003).

In 2014, the choice of hospital was extended from being limited to public hospitals, or hospitals with a tender agreement, to all public and private hospitals. Prior to the election of 2013, the Conservative Party had campaigned in favour of extending patients' choice of hospital (Ringard, Saunes and Sagan, 2016). The inclusion of private non-contracted providers into the choice scheme and allowing a larger role for providers with tender agreements functioned as an important driver of change for the supply side of the system (Saunes, Karanikolos and Sagan, 2020).

The family doctor reform

Important reforms have also taken place in the primary healthcare sector. In 2001, the Family Doctor reform implemented a list system, which implied that the general practitioners (GPs) were essentially privatised (Parliamentary Proposition no. 99, 1998–99). Whereas GPs were mostly municipally employed before the reform, the new system meant that the majority of GPs became self-employed, acting as family doctors serving a specific patient list. GPs must now be contracted with a municipality to receive public payment, and each municipality will have a number of GP contracts based on the size and composition of the population, from which the inhabitants can choose between. It is mandatory for each inhabitant to be on the list of one GP, and the average list size is around 1,500.

The main argument for organising primary care as a list system/family doctor scheme was partly the need for continuity for frail elderly persons with chronic conditions and other vulnerable groups, which could be obtained through a regular GP contract. Another argument was that a regular GP contract would simplify cooperation on patients with the need for coordinated services (Veggeland, 2018). Particularly in the urban cities, there was a need to avoid doctor-shopping in order to increase control over the prescription of addictive drugs (Bay and Hellevik, 2002). The Family Doctor scheme builds on the purchaser–provider model as well as ABF, in line with the NPM principles. Since the gatekeeper system means that all referrals to hospitals and specialists have to go via a GP, the list system seemingly creates a market where free choice of hospital can be realised (Veggeland, 2018).

The hospital reform

The Norwegian hospital reform differed significantly from similar reforms in other countries, with its central and rapid implementation. The parliamentary process behind the reform took only one year from initial proposal in parliament to a decision, which stands in sharp contrast to the incremental and locally initiated changes in the neighbouring countries of Denmark, Sweden and Finland (Vrangbæk, 2009). The intention of the reform was to fulfil a number of specific aims, particularly to improve management, to increase equality in service accessibility, to improve the medical quality of the services and to increase hospital productivity (Parliamentary Proposition no. 66, 2000–01). Central features of the reform were increased delegation of authority to the hospitals, increased use of contracts for governing providers, professional rather than interest-based boards, clearer division between health policy and service production and increased freedom of choice for patients, thus reflecting the main principles of NPM.

The reform was based on two main elements. The first was the transfer of hospital ownership from the locally elected county councils to central government, and the delegation of the responsibility for providing hospital services to five (later reduced to four) autonomous regional health authorities. The main argument for state ownership was to give the state the complete responsibility for the specialised health services, by gathering sector responsibility, financing responsibility and ownership on one hand. This should ensure that there is no doubt among the population and health sector actors that the state holds both the formal and genuine responsibility for the hospital sector, thus preventing gaming on who are in charge. The other main element of the reform was to organise the hospitals into enterprises instead of public administration entities, thus making the hospitals separate legal entities and not an integral part of the central government administration. The introduction of enterprise organisation signified a clear break with Norwegian public administrative tradition, since it represents a new management philosophy: organisation as enterprises marks a clear organisational distinction between the operative activities and the executive political body.

The coordination reform

The final reform to be presented here is the Coordination Reform, which came into effect on 1 January 2012 (Parliamentary Proposition no. 47, 2008–09). The reform was born from the same problems and challenges that face most modern healthcare systems today: how to handle the increasing number of patients, and particularly the elderly and chronically ill who move between primary and specialised care. The reform thus attempted to create more coherent pathways for patients in a sector that is characterised by fragmentation and specialisation. The other Nordic countries, and also England and the Netherlands, have implemented similar reforms as the Norwegian, and a common feature is the decentralisation of tasks and responsibilities. The Danish '*Sundheds-og strukturreform*' of 2007 was a particular inspiration for the Norwegian reform, with the introduction of, for instance, municipal co-financing and contracts between municipalities and hospitals. There were first and foremost three challenges that the reform attempted to solve: (1) dealing with the challenges related to patients' needs for coordinated services, especially across the primary and secondary level; (2) increasing the focus on health prevention and public health in the health services; and (3) dealing with the ageing population and changing range of illnesses among the population.

One key element of the reform was to give the municipalities full responsibility for patients ready to be discharged from hospital treatment by providing intermediate care units; that is, local emergency beds for patients with the need for pre- or post-hospital services. The municipalities were also made responsible for co-financing of hospital care, but this was later abandoned in order to reduce the municipalities' financial risk (Saunes, Karanikolos and Sagan, 2020). The second key element was to give the municipalities more responsibility for health prevention and public health work, with the intention of reducing the number of hospital admissions.

Public health

As mentioned earlier, the local authorities play an important role in public health in Norway. One of the objectives of the Coordination reform was to contribute to promotion of health and the implementation of more effective preventive measures, and to take responsibility at an early stage. Through the new Public Health Act introduced on 1 January 2012, the municipalities were given greater responsibility for prevention within the health service, as well as public health work across sectors (Norwegian Ministry of Health and Care Services, 2013). The aim of the Public Health Act was to improve coordination of public health work horizontally, across various sectors and actors, and vertically, between the local, regional and national authorities. Whereas the municipalities are responsible for implementing cross-sectoral public health interventions locally, the overall responsibility rests with the Ministry of Health and Care Services, with the Directorate of Health and with the National Institute of Public Health (NIPH), also playing important roles in supporting the implementation and monitoring of public health policies (Saunes, Karanikolos and Sagan, 2020). The ambitious public health policy goals are that Norway shall rank among the top three countries with the highest life expectancy in the world and that the population shall experience more years of good health and well-being, with reduced social inequalities in health, and the promotion of good health throughout the entire population (Norwegian Ministry of Health and Care Services, 2013).

With the ongoing Covid-19 pandemic, it is of particular interest to shortly outline how the country has responded to this. In Norway, NIPH has overseen all data collection and measurements, since Covid-19 was first listed as a notifiable disease in Norway, while the municipalities are responsible for detecting, reporting and surveilling the spread of infectious diseases. The testing first took place in hospitals, but later special testing sites were established in the municipalities. All samples were analysed in hospital laboratories, and the results were submitted electronically directly to the Norwegian Surveillance System for Communicable Diseases Laboratory database (Ursin, Skjesol and Tritter, 2020).

Impact on the architecture of the system

The Norwegian healthcare reforms have first and foremost targeted organisational structures and ownership forms, political governance, patient rights, quality and economy – in other words, what we would refer to as administrative reforms. Particularly, the changes from the 1970s and up till today have been all-encompassing. From the 1990s, the principles of NPM have been guiding many of the changes. The popular engagement and debates around the healthcare system in general – and the hospitals in particular – have therefore been strong and continuous. A paradox is that even though the healthcare system has been the subject of reforms and consistent efforts to improve, the situation is often portrayed as if the sector remains in a state of constant crisis (Vaglum, 2020).

Yet the overarching health policy goals for the healthcare sector have been the same since the Hospital Act of 1969. There is a broad agreement that, in Norway, healthcare shall be accessible for everyone, of a high quality and efficiency, shall contribute to public health and shall remain mainly public. In particular, the objectives of equal access independent of socio-economic status and place of residence have remained stable and important. The many reforms have *not* challenged this picture: overall, the reforms have therefore contributed to 'do things differently' rather than 'do other things'. The main challenges and accompanying policy measures have first and foremost been administrative (Martinussen et al., 2017).

There has traditionally been a strong emphasis in the Norwegian health-care system on political governance and public participation through locally elected political bodies. This has distinguished the country from the more centralised tax-based systems such as in the UK. This practice has been challenged by the 'business orientation' reflected in the organisational forms that was introduced with healthcare reforms, described with terms such as enterprises, divisions, centre structures and unified leadership. The governance of the hospitals now emphasises scorecards, performance management and professionalised leadership. The hospital reform of 2002 was the natural end point of this development. In line with the general development in Norwegian public administration, the hospital reform represented a withdrawal of politics, by introducing delegation of authority, discretion for managers and boards and limited involvement of politicians. A main principle of the reform was to 'keep politicians at arm's length': to give hospital management full control and responsibility of the daily running of the hospitals without interference from politicians and other administrative levels. In practice, therefore, the reform removed the local democratic arena for health policymaking from the counties, thus centralising democratic decision-making and narrowing the room for direct political intervention.

At national level, health policy governance now takes place through grants, laws and regulations, and through ownership control, but in principle not through the type of direct political instructions which takes place in the traditional public administration model. This has limited the health minister's control space, both because the national parliament has increased its power and because the channels for influence are fewer. In the years following the reform, parliament has challenged the balance of political control and enterprise autonomy, which formed the basis of the reform, by being more involved than ever in hospital issues (Opedal and Rommetvedt, 2005). This has confronted the 'arm's length' principle that was so central to the reform: to let the hospital leaders lead.

The two main impacts of the last 40 years' health policy reforms on the architecture of the health system can thus be summed up in two trends: from decentralisation to centralisation and from traditional public administration to enterprise organisation.

Impact on population health

A question, then, is whether the health policy reforms have had any notable effect on population health. To answer this would require a precise understanding of the relationship between health system characteristics and population health, as well as a separation of the effects of health policy reforms from the effects of other policy changes, changes in medical technology, changes in population income, and so on. This is a formidable task well outside the scope of this chapter. Thus, we narrow this down to briefly presenting some major trends in population health.

First, we note that life expectancy at birth in Norway has increased steadily in the period after 1990 as indicated in Table 5.1. There is an established relationship between per capita healthcare expenditures and life expectancy. Linden and Ray (2017) found that, in countries with a high share of public expenditures, an *increase* in private and public spending contributes equally to increased life expectancy at birth. Norway is one of the countries with the highest share of public spending, thus policy reforms that would increase the share of private spending would not be expected to lead to a lower increase in life expectancy.

Second, there was also an increase in healthy life expectancy in the period from 1990 to 2013 (Knudsen et al., 2016). Tollånes and colleagues (2018) also observe that, adjusted for age, the burden of illness decreased in the period 2006–2016.

As noted, the degree of decentralisation has been a recurrent theme in policy reforms. One argument for centralisation is that a centralised model is better suited to achieve equity. Notably, we observe that there has been an increasing social gradient in life expectancy in the past 30 years. Figure 5.1 shows the differences in five-year average life expectancy between those with secondary level or higher education and those only with compulsory education. We note that the difference is smaller for women and that the gender difference is reduced over this period. Furthermore, while the difference has increased, it also seems to have stabilised.

Figure 5.2 shows life expectancy at birth for men and women. Steadily increasing over this period, we note that the difference between men and women is substantially lower today than it was 30 years ago.

There is also a substantial geographical variation, although this is largely explained by socio-economic differences (Tollånes et al., 2018). As described

Table 5.1 Life expectancy at birth in Norway

	1990	2000	2010	2020
Men	73.44	75.96	78.85	81.48
Women	79.81	81.38	83.15	84.89

Source: Statistics Norway (2020).

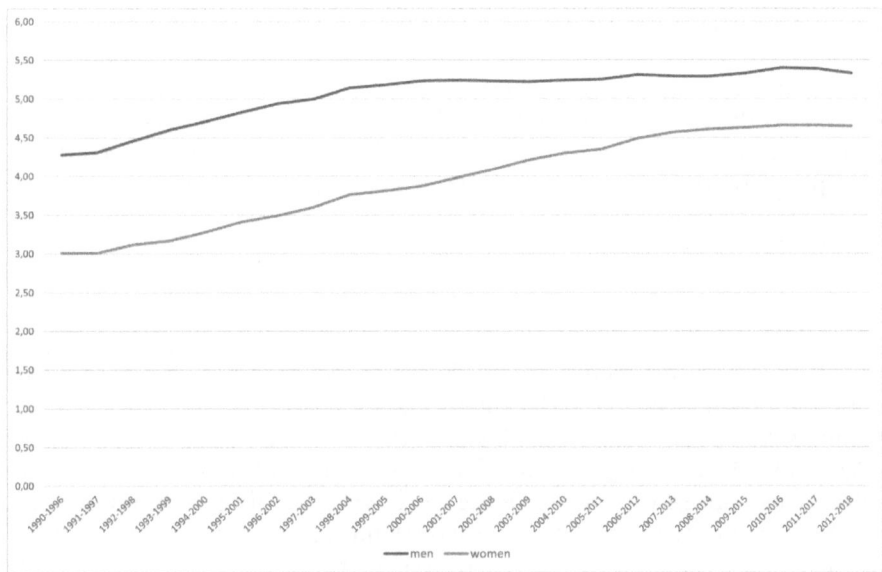

Figure 5.1 Difference in life expectancy in Norway: Secondary or higher education versus compulsory only education

Source: Norhealth (2019).

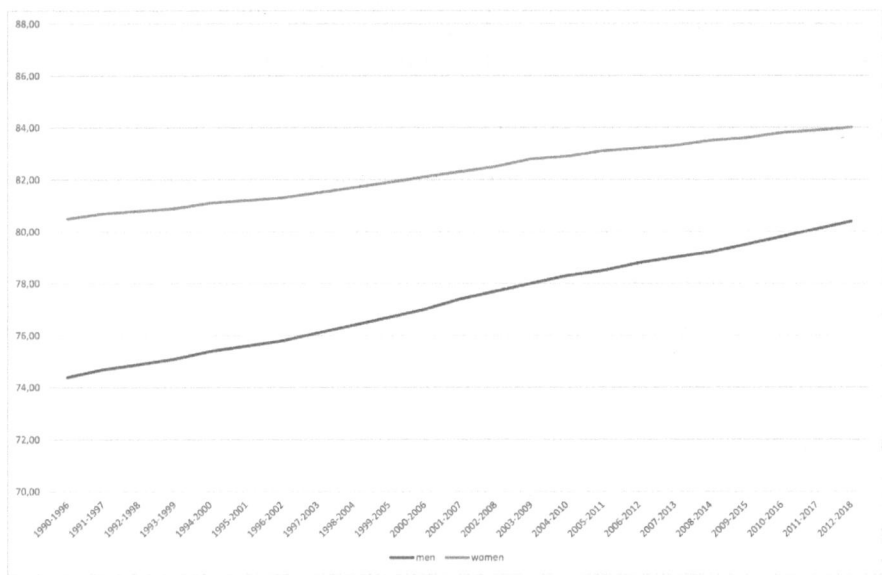

Figure 5.2 Life expectancy at birth in Norway: Men and women

Source: Norhealth (2019).

earlier, since the early 1980s, municipalities, counties and regional health authorities have been funded through a need-adjusted capitation model. Thus, in principle, the system is designed to support a goal of equal access to services. As discussed earlier, however, both municipalities and counties have a large degree of freedom in the way they allocate resources between different types of services. There are also large geographical variations in the use of services (Ingebrigtsen et al., 2020) that does not reflect the availability or resources.

Future sustainability

In 2019, healthcare expenditure in Norway accounted for 10.5% of Gross Domestic Product, which is the eighth highest among the Organisation for Economic Cooperation and Development (OECD) countries and fifth highest in the World Health Organization European region. Health expenditure per capita is also one of the highest in the world with $6,547 per capita in 2019, which is third only to the US and Switzerland. In recent years, the share of public financing in Norway has remained stable at around 85%, which is the highest in Europe. Life expectancy in Norway increased by nearly four years from 2000 and is now one of the highest in Europe at 82.2 years.

The Norwegian healthcare system faces many of the same challenges as systems in other high-income countries. An ageing population leads to a higher need for healthcare services while at the same time drawing on a lower workforce. In their White Paper *Perspektivmeldingen* (Parliamentary Proposition no. 14, 2020–2021), the government discusses future challenges for the public welfare system based on projections stating that:

- The share of 80+ in the population may increase from 4.5% in 2020 to 12% in 2060.
- The number of healthcare workers will increase from 310,000 in 2018, through 425,000 in 2030, to 570,000 in 2060.

Furthermore, the predicted growth in demand for personnel rests on assumptions of improved public health as well as productivity growth (Hjemås, Holmøy and Haugstveit, 2019). Without these, demand will be expected to increase even more. On the other hand, an increase in private (family) care and refraining from improving the standard of care will reduce the growth in future demand.

Predicting the future burden of illness is difficult, but the expectation is that there will be an increase in burden of illness from non-communicable diseases, such as cancer, diabetes and dementia. In other areas, such as cardiovascular diseases, there has been a rapid decline in the past 20 years, and this is expected to continue. While aggregate burden of illness in the population is expected to increase, a continued reduction in per capita burden-of-illness is expected (Parliamentary Proposition no. 41, 2020–21).

Broadly phrased, we would point to three challenges for future sustainability. First, aggregate demand is likely to increase, driven both by demographic changes and by demand for higher quality. Second, differences in socio-economic distribution of health and healthcare are likely to remain an issue. Third, a growth in private healthcare and individual willingness to pay for such care may lead to a two-tiered healthcare system. The White Paper describes six policy tools to secure the future sustainability of the system: first, a clear system for priority-setting; second, increased focus on prevention; third, a more knowledge-based provision of services; fourth, technological improvement; fifth, increased use of co-payment; and, sixth, dismantling some 'outdated' welfare goods.

The policy tools are a familiar mix of demand and supply side measures. Lowering demand but increasing focus on prevention is an uncontroversial strategy, although not much is known about the effects of increased prevention of future demand for services. Other tools will be more controversial; removing 'outdated' services and rationing by increasing co-payment are likely to have distributional effects, and thus might increase social inequalities. Systems for priority-setting and knowledge-based services are intended to sort and remove unnecessary demand. Again, these are expected to be less controversial due to negative distributional effects. Notably, further NPM-type reform, aimed at increasing the efficiency in the provision of services, is not suggested.

In Norway, the overall satisfaction with health services is generally high (Skudal et al., 2016) as is the support for public responsibility of healthcare (Martinussen and Magnussen, 2019). Still, while most healthcare services in Norway are publicly provided and funded, the role of the private health sector is increasing. This is reflected both in terms of the increased use of private actors in supplying publicly funded services, as well as in the provision of supplementary private insurance and the accompanying rise in the number of private providers. The emergence of a parallel private market for healthcare has caused some concern, as it is sometimes contended that an increasing use of private health services may be accompanied by a decrease in the support, and willingness to pay taxes, for the public sector. Also, private health insurance may lead to the crowding out of resources from the publicly funded part of the sector, rather than the expected increasing capacity (Propper, 2000). In Norway, the use of private health insurance has increased 12 times from 2007 to 2017 – from around barely 50,000 to over 500,000 individuals.

If a higher usage of private healthcare leads to less commitment to fund public healthcare, it could in the worst case lead to the evolution of a two-tiered healthcare system, with those well off receiving their services from the private sector and the public system ending up as a 'poor service for the poor' (Propper, 2000). While empirical evidence for Norway suggests that only moderate concern is warranted that the growth in employer-provided public health insurance would affect the support for the public healthcare system (Martinussen and Magnussen, 2019), social inequalities in healthcare are still increasing. For many years, it was generally believed that the egalitarian Norwegian welfare state, whose aim has been to provide equally high standards for all citizens, would also produce less socio-economic differences in health outcomes compared to other countries. However, somewhat unexpectedly, several studies have demonstrated that socio-economic inequalities in morbidity and mortality are high, as compared with other European regions (Mackenbach et al., 1997; Dahl, 2002; Eikemo et al., 2008).

The effects of reforms on the nature of the National Health Service

The view on markets and competition is one of the fundamental dividing lines in politics. The positions range from those who see competition as having no place in services aimed at protecting the sick to those who claim that competition is the antidote for bloated, inefficient services and even saves lives (Goddard, 2015). There is a growing body of evidence that suggests positive effects of competition in hospital markets (Cooper, Gibbons and Skellern, 2018; Croes, Krabbe-Alkemade and Mikkers, 2018; Propper, 2018), but unfortunately, there are no specific studies on the effect of hospital competition in Norway.

However, the hospital reform was evaluated in 2005 and 2006 with focus on five dimensions: accessibility, priorities, efficiency, user participation and employee participation/work environment (Norwegian Research Council, 2007). The evaluation showed that the rate of hospital activity increased more in the period following the reform than in the period before, which would imply that overall access probably improved. Waiting time was furthermore reduced, and so was also the share of patients with waiting times exceeding the recommended timeframe. Yet the assignment of priorities in practice did not improve, as differences in waiting times between high and low-priority groups diminished rather than increased. Hospital efficiency (productivity) increased more (3–4%) than in the other Nordic countries. User participation was formalised through the introduction of user councils and has been more successfully implemented at the regional level than in the municipalities. The evaluation indicated that employee participation on strategic decisions was experienced as low, while the working environment appeared to be satisfactory, with local variations.

There are also several studies on the effect of competition among GPs in Norway (Brekke et al., 2019; Godager, Iversen and Ma, 2015; Iverson and Ma, 2011; Markussen and Røed, 2017). In contrast to the largely favourable international literature on hospital competition, these studies indicate that increased competition is accompanied by increased prescription of drugs, increased use of sickness certificates and increased referral rates to radiological services. Thus, it could be argued that competition among GPs to some extent has led to an oversupply of services.

The use of incentives through payment systems

As noted, the introduction of ABF in 1997 was the first major NPM-inspired reform in the Norwegian healthcare sector. The main motivation was to increase efficiency as well as activity (Biørn et al., 2003). As noted earlier, the share of ABF has varied over the years, reflecting both the difficulties in balancing conflicting incentives in the system and ideological beliefs in the merits of prospective payment systems.

One concern with ABF is that it may affect the selection of patients to hospitals. There are several studies looking at the potential effect of ABF on cream-skimming in Norway (Anthun, Bjørngaard and Magnussen, 2017; Januleviciute et al., 2016; Martinussen and Hagen, 2009; Melberg, Olsen and Pedersen, 2016). While all studies find support for patient selection or strategic coding, the effects are generally moderate. Kjøstolfsen and colleagues (2021) also find that the share of physicians that are concerned about the potential negative selection effects is substantially higher than the share that doubts that such effects actually take place. Studies of hospital productivity find an immediate positive effect of ABF, but then there is a quite moderate subsequent productivity growth (Anthun, Bjørngaard and Magnussen, 2017; Biørn et al., 2003).

Notably, the share of ABF is higher for GP services provided by private GPs than for hospitals. Between two-thirds and three-quarters of GP income comes from out-of-pocket payments and fee-for-service reimbursements from the National Insurance Scheme. Brekke and colleagues (2019) find that the likelihood of a GP issuing sickness certificates not only increases with the degree of competition but also is higher for private fee-for-service-funded GPs than public salaried GPs.

Managerialism – the diminishing role of professions

The evaluation of the hospital reform concluded that the working environment appeared satisfactory, although there were local variations and indications that personnel experienced a low degree of participation in strategic decision-making. The health minister at the time maintained that the only thing that mattered was whether the reform had led to a better health service, with hospitals that provide good and safe services when needed. She therefore concluded that the evaluation showed that the reform had mainly fulfilled its goals (Dommerud, 2007).

However, other studies indicate that the picture may not be as straightforward. The health professions had strongly opposed the reform, expressing concerns that it would increase the emphasis on the economic aspects of healthcare on behalf of the medical principles in guiding hospital activities. A study based on a survey of a representative sample of hospital physicians four years after the reform confirmed this: as many as half of the hospital physicians were negative towards it (Martinussen and Magnussen, 2011).

Moreover, while a majority (58%) reported that the reform had increased hospital productivity, 38% reported poorer and 54% reported no change in medical quality, and 29% and 52% reported less or no change in equality of access, respectively. Not surprisingly, respondents with managerial responsibilities were found to be more positive towards the reform, which seems to support a polarisation thesis; that is, instead of managerialist values taking over the medical profession through a process of hybridisation, there is heterogeneity within the profession: some physician managers adopt management values and tools, and others remain alienated from them. Furthermore, building on the same data, Aasland, Rosta and Nylenna (2010) found that a majority (62%) of the hospital physicians reported that the reform gave incentives to prioritise 'profitable patient groups', although a somewhat lower proportion (45%) felt that such behaviour *actually* took place as a result of the reform. A later study, built on a similar survey among hospital physicians from 2016, confirmed this negative impression: it found that the physicians were still generally sceptical towards the current enterprise model and ABF (Martinussen et al., 2017). The preferences of the hospital physicians are for more locally based leadership, shorter decision paths and less incentive-based management.

On the other hand, the reform has apparently not affected the job satisfaction of the hospital physicians. Aasland, Rosta and Nylenna (2010) showed that there was a significant increase in satisfaction from 2000 to 2006, with a non-significant dip in 2002 (the year of the reform), which according to the authors suggest a robust job satisfaction based on internal values more than external changes such as comprehensive health reforms. The view that the reform has led to increased cream skimming (selection of profitable patients) also received little support in an analysis of patient data from the period 1995–2005 (Martinussen and Hagen, 2009). The analysis gives some evidence of cream skimming in the first period of ABF, in particular within the less severe orthopaedic diagnoses. However, cream skimming did not increase after the 2002 reform but was stable and, for some DRGs, even reduced.

The introduction of market mechanisms and business management principles into public healthcare systems is controversial. This stems from the lack of evidence that the stated objectives have been achieved, a general ideological resistance to markets in healthcare and – not least – the reformers' failure to consider health professionals' opinions. NPM-type health reforms challenge the role, identity and autonomy of the medical professionals, and the centrally initiated, 'big-bang' nature of the Norwegian hospital reform that was implemented almost overnight may explain why it has met with such particular strong resistance from the hospital physicians. The reform has failed to combine changes in legislation and incentives with changes in organisation and management that are well received by the medical profession in general and not only by those in managerial positions (Martinussen and Magnussen, 2011).

Conclusion

As in other countries, the Covid-19 pandemic has affected the healthcare sector. The general impression is that the present organisational and financial structures stood up well to the test of Covid-19. On a positive note, we have seen a transition to more use of 'digital' healthcare, that is, online consultations. Also, the role of the municipal primary healthcare sector, and in particular the municipal chief medical officer (most often a physician with specialisation in public health), has proved to be a strength of the system. In periods with large (expected) numbers of hospitalisations due to Covid-19, capacity had to be diverted from other patient groups. This led to a substantial reduction in activity-based income and eventually to two rounds of supplementary funding from the state. This illustrates that, although ABF provides ample risk sharing when activity exceeds its expected level, high fixed costs make it more difficult to cope when activity falls. More disturbingly a lack of capacity, most notably in Intensive Care Unit capacity, has led to stricter Covid-related restrictions in order to limit the number of hospitalisations. While overall capacity is primarily a question of the size of healthcare budgets, there has been a renewed debate about links between the lack of hospital intensive care capacity and the present model of governance and funding. A new Labour-Center government has announced an intention of a less market-oriented healthcare system and a possible White Paper reviewing the current model. Still, the political debate does not point in the direction of specific new reform initiatives. The Norwegian healthcare sector still has the highest share of public funding among the European Union/European Economic Area countries, and private care is still a marginal add-on to a predominantly publicly funded and regulated sector. If anything, we would expect to see a modest reversal of some of the features of the existing system, most notably in the direction of a stronger political participation in the governance of the healthcare sector and – perhaps – less reliance on economic incentives. Time will provide the answer.

References

Aasland, O. G., Rosta, J. and Nylenna, M. (2010) 'Healthcare reforms and job satisfaction among doctors in Norway', *Scandinavian Journal of Public Health* 38: 253–8.

Anthun, K. S., Bjørngaard, J. H. and Magnussen, J. (2017) 'Economic incentives and diagnostic coding in a public health care system', *International Journal of Health Economics and Management* 17: 83–101.

Bay, A. H. og Hellevik, T. (2002) *Kompetanse- og utdanningsbehov innenfor trygde- og arbeidsmarkedsetaten*, NOVA Rapport November.

Biørn, E., Hagen, T. P., Iversen, T. and Magnussen, J. (2003) 'The effect of activity-based financing on hospital efficiency: A panel data analysis of DEA efficiency scores 1992–2000', *Health Care Management Science* 6: 271–83.

Brekke, K. R., Holmås, T. H., Monstad, K. and Straume, O. R. (2019) 'Competition and physician behaviour: Does the competitive environment affect the propensity to issue sickness certificates?', *Journal of Health Economics* 66: 117–35.

Byrkjeflot, H. and Neby, S. (2008) 'The end of the decentralized model of healthcare governance? Comparing developments in the Scandinavian hospital sectors', *Journal of Health Organization and Management* 22: 331–49.

Christensen, T. and Lægreid, P. (eds) (2001) *New Public Management. The Transformation of Ideas and Practice*, Aldershot: Ashgate.

Cooper, Z., Gibbons, S. and Skellern, M. (2018) 'Does competition from private surgical centres improve public hospitals' performance? Evidence from the English National Health Service', *Journal of Public Economics* 166: 63–80.

Croes, R. R., Krabbe-Alkemade, Y. J. F. M. and Mikkers, M. C. (2018) 'Competition and quality indicators in the health care sector: Empirical evidence from the Dutch hospital sector', *European Journal of Health Economics* 19: 5–19.

Dahl, E. (2002) 'Health inequalities and health policy: The Norwegian case', *Norsk epidemiologi* 12: 69–75.

Dommerud, T. (2007) 'Reformen var på sin plass', *Dagensmedisin*, 21 February. Available at: www.dagensmedisin.no/artikler/2007/02/21/-reformen-var-pa-sin-plass/

Eikemo, T. A., Huisman, M., Bambra, C. and Kunst, A. E. (2008) 'Health inequalities according to educational level in different welfare regimes: A comparison of 23 European countries', *Sociology of Health and Illness* 30: 565–82.

Godager, G., Iversen, T. and Ma, C. A. (2015) 'Competition, gatekeeping, and health care access', *Journal of Health Economics* 39: 159–70.

Goddard, M. (2015) 'Competition in healthcare: Good, bad or ugly?', *International Journal of Health Policy and Management* 4: 567–9.

Hjemås, G., Holmøy, E. and Haugstveit, F. (2019) *Fremskrivninger av etterspørselen etter arbeidskraft i helse – og omsorg mot 2060*, SSB Rapport, December.

Ingebrigtsen, T., Balteskard, L., Guldhaugen, K. A., Kloster, R., Uleberg, B., Grotle, M. and Solberg, T. K. (2020) 'Behandlingsrater for ryggkirurgi i Norge og Helse Nord 2014–18', *Tidsskrift for Den norske legeforening*. Available at: https://doi.org/10.4045/tidsskr.20.0313

Iversen, T. and Ma, C. A. (2011) 'Market conditions and general practitioners' referrals', *International Journal of Health Care Finance and Economics* 11: 245.

Januleviciute, J., Askildsen, J., Kaarbøe, E. O., Siciliani, L. and Sutton, M. (2016) 'How do hospitals respond to price changes? Evidence from Norway', *Health Economics* 25: 620–36.

Kjøstolfsen, G. H., Baheerathan, J. P., Martinussen, E. and Magnussen, J. (2021) 'Financial incentives and patient selection: Hospital physicians' views on cream skimming and economic management focus in Norway', *Health Policy* 125: 98–103.

Knudsen, A. K., Kinge, J. M., Skirbekk, V. and Vollset, S. E. (2016) *Sykdomsbyrde i Norge 1990–2013. Resultater fra Global Burden of Diseases, Injuries, and Risk Factors Study*, Oslo: Norwegian Institute of Public Health.

Lægreid, P. (2020) 'Public administration research in Norway: An organizational and institutional approach to political organisations', in Werner, J. and Bouckaert, G. (eds) *European Perspectives for Public Administration*, Leuven: Leuven University Press.

Lægreid, P., Opedal, S. and Stigen, I. M. (2005) 'The Norwegian hospital reform: Balancing political control and enterprise autonomy', *Journal of Health Politics, Policy and Law* 30: 1027–64.

Larsen, Ø. (ed) (1996) *The Shaping of a Profession*, Canton, MA: Science History Publications.

Larsen, Ø., Berg, O. and Hodne, F. (1986) *Legene og samfunnet*, Oslo: Den norske lægeforening.

Linden, M. and Ray, D. (2017) 'Life expectancy effects of public and private health expenditures in OECD countries 1970–2012: Panel time series approach', *Economic Analysis and Policy* 56: 101–13.

Mackenbach, J. P., Kunst, A. E., Cavelaars, A., Groenhof, F., Geurts, J. J. M., Andersen, O., et al. (1997) 'Socioeconomic inequalities in morbidity and mortality in western Europe', *Lancet* 349: 1655–9.

Markussen, S. and Røed, K. (2017) 'The market for paid sick leave', *Journal of Health Economics* 55: 244–61.

Martinussen, P. E., Frich, J. C., Vrangbæk, K. and Magnussen, J. (2017) 'Organisatoriske forhold og løsninger i spesialisthelsetjenesten – hva mener sykehuslegene?', *Michael* 14(Supplement 19): 95–105.

Martinussen, P. E. and Hagen, T. P. (2009) 'Reimbursement systems, organisational forms and patient selection: Evidence from day surgery in Norway', *Health Economics, Policy and Law* 4: 139–58.

Martinussen, P. E. and Magnussen, J. (2009) 'Healthcare reform: The Nordic experience', in J. Magnussen, J., Saltman, R. B. and Vrangbæk, K. (eds) *Nordic Health Care Systems: Recent Reforms and Current Policy Challenges*, Berkshire: Open University Press.

Martinussen, P. E. and Magnussen, J. (2011) 'Resisting market-inspired reform in healthcare: The role of professional subcultures in medicine', *Social Science and Medicine* 73: 193–200.

Martinussen, P. E. and Magnussen, J. (2019) 'Is having private health insurance associated with less support for public healthcare? Evidence from the Norwegian NHS', *Health Policy* 123: 675–80.

Melberg, H. O., Olsen, C. B. and Pedersen, K. (2016) 'Did hospitals respond to changes in weights of Diagnosis Related Groups in Norway between 2006 and 2013?', *Health Policy* 120: 992–1000.

Norhealth (2019) Available at: www.norgeshelsa.no

Norwegian Ministry of Health and Care Services (2013) 'Report to the storting. Summary: Public health report: Good health – a common responsibility', *White Paper no. 34 (2012–2013)*, Oslo: Norwegian Ministry of Health and Care Services.

Norwegian Research Council (2007) *Resultatevaluering av sykehusreformen. Tilgjengelighet, prioritering, effektivitet, brukermedvirkning og medbestemmelse*, Oslo: Norwegian Research Council.

Nyseter, T. (2015) *Velferd på avveie. Reformer, verdier, veivalg*, Oslo: Res Publica.

Olsen, J. P. (1997) 'Civil Service in transition: Dilemmas and lessons learned', in Hesse, J. J. and Toonen, T. A. J. (eds) *The European Yearbook of Comparative Government and Public Administration*, Vol. III, Baden-Baden: Nomos.

Opedal, S. and Rommetvedt, H. (2005) 'Sykehus på Løvebakken. Stortingets engasjement og innflytelse før o getter sykehusreformen', *Tidsskrift for Samfunnsforskning* 46: 99–132.

Parliamentary Proposition no. 12 (1998–99) *Lov om pasientrettigheter (pasientrettighetsloven)*, Oslo: Ministry of Health and Care Services.

Parliamentary Proposition no. 14 (2020–21) *Perspektivmeldingen*, Oslo: Ministry of Finance.

Parliamentary Proposition no. 36 (1980–81) *Om lov om helsetjeneste i kommunene*, Oslo: Ministry of Social Services.

Parliamentary Proposition no. 47 (2008–09) *Samhandlingsreformen – Rett behandling – på rett sted – til rett tid*, Oslo: Ministry of Health and Care Services.

Parliamentary Proposition no. 63 (2002–03) *Om lov om endringer i lov 2. juli 1999 nr. 63 om pasientrettigheter (pasientrettighetsloven) m.m*, Oslo: Ministry of Health and Care Services.

Parliamentary Proposition no. 66 (2000–01) *Om loven om helseforetak m.m. (Helseforetaksloven)*, The Health Enterprise Law, Oslo: Ministry of Health and Care Services.

Parliamentary Proposition no. 99 (1998–99) *Om lov om endringer i lov 19. november 1982 nr. 66 om helsetjenesten i kommunene og i visse andre lover (fastlegeordningen)*, Oslo: Ministry of Health and Care Services.

Propper, C. (2000) 'The demand for private health care in the UK', *Journal of Health Economics* 19: 855–76.

Propper, C. (2018) 'Competition in health care: Lessons from the English experience', *Health Economics, Policy and Law* 13: 492–508.

Ringard, Å., Saunes, I. S. and Sagan, A. (2016) 'The 2015 hospital treatment choice reform in Norway: Continuity or change?', *Health Policy* 120: 350–5.

Rommetvedt, H., Opedal, S., Stigen, I. M. and Vrangbæk, K. (2014) *Hvordan har vi det i dag da? Flernivåstyring og samhandling i norsk og dansk helsepolitikk*, Bergen: Fagbokforlaget.

Saunes, I. S., Karanikolos, M. and Sagan, A. (2020) 'Norway: Health system review', *Health Systems in Transition* 22: i–163.

Schiøtz, A. (2003) *Folkets helse – landets styrke 1850 – 2003*, Oslo: Universitetsforlaget.

Skudal, K. E., Sjetne, I. S., Bjertnæs, Ø. A., Lindahl, A. K. and Nylenna, M. (2016) *Commonwealth Funds undersøkelse av helsetjenestesystemet i elleve land: Norske resultater i 2016 og utvikling over tid*, Oslo: Folkehelseinstituttet.

Statistics Norway (2020) Available at: https://www.ssb.no/statbank/table/05375/

Tollånes, M. C., Knudsen, A. K., Vollset, S. E., Kinge, J. M., Skirbekk, V. and Øverland, S. (2018) *Sykdomsbyrden i Norge i 2016. Tidsskrift for Den norske legeforening.*

Ursin, G., Skjesol, I. and Tritter, J. (2020) 'The COVID-19 pandemic in Norway: The dominance of social implications in framing the policy response', *Health Policy and Technology* 9: 663–72.

Vaglum, P. (2020) 'Hva gjør Legeforeningen for å avskaffe foretaksmodellen?', *Tidsskrift for Den norske legeforening.* Available at: https://doi.org/10.4045/tidsskr.19.0723

Veggeland, N. (2018) 'Fastlegeordningen og reformer. Innspill om offentlig ansettelse', *Tidsskrift for Velferdsforskning* 21: 59–68.

Vrangbæk, K. (2009) 'The political process of restructuring Nordic health systems', in Magnussen, J., Saltman, R. B. and Vrangbæk, K. (eds) *Nordic Health Care Systems: Recent Reforms and Current Policy Challenges*, Berkshire: Open University Press.

The Mediterranean macro-region

6 Italy

Giovanna Vicarelli

Introduction

Italy is characterised by having changed its welfare model four times in its 150 years of existence as a nation-state (since 1861). It has transitioned from a 'residual welfare' model as characterised by Titmuss (1974) in the Liberal era (1861–1921) to an industrial 'authoritarian' achievement-performance model in the Fascist government (1922–43) and from an industrial 'democratic' achievement-performance model in the years of the First Republic (1945–77) to an institutional redistributive model starting from 1978, during the Second Republic. For a long period, therefore, families, ecclesiastical networks, entrepreneurial paternalism and the various modes of self-protection at work assumed responsibility for meeting healthcare needs. It was only with the establishment of the National Health Service (NHS) (Law 833/1978) that the State assumed direct responsibility, albeit with significant changes during the 1990s and the first part of the 2000s, due to the application of New Public Management (NPM) policies. Before and after the Covid-19 pandemic, the major political debate focused on how the NHS should be transformed and whether it should come back to a residual or industrial achievement-performance welfare model or towards a revitalisation of the NHS.

This chapter will focus on the transformation of the Italian healthcare system from a process-oriented perspective that is primarily inspired by the historical institutionalism approach. The latter underscores how institutions emerge from, and are embedded in, temporal processes through path dependence and divergence at critical historical junctures (Pierson, 2004). It also draws on the contributions within neo-institutionalism linked to a neo-Weberian approach that emphasise the institutional logics which are so valuable in depicting social transformations. In particular, it is intended to detail how the growth and expansion of new logics in healthcare led to the valorisation of different actors, behaviours and governance structures. As Scott and colleagues (2000) have shown, since the 1990s, even when the concept of doctors and their patients was replaced by healthcare providers and consumers, professional, bureaucratic and market logics intermingled, with one supplanting but not eliminating the other. As such, institutional logics focus the

DOI: 10.4324/9781003139799-11

attention of key actors on a particular set of central problems and solutions (Powell and Bromley, 2015).

The genesis of the National Health Service

The first health law (Law 5849) in united Italy dates back to December 1888. At the end of the nineteenth century, coinciding with the industrialisation and urbanisation of the country, the very high infant mortality rates, the growing number of persons unfit for military service, the high morbidity of women and men of working age and the spread of cholera throughout the country forced the governments in office to legislate on health matters (Vicarelli, 1997a). A 'residual welfare model' consistent with the dominant liberal principles was codified. The family and main Catholic charity associations (*Opere Pie* initially), as well as the forms of solidarity linked to entrepreneurial paternalism and mutual aid societies, were identified as the natural channels for enabling the survival of citizens. At the same time, healthcare assistance to the poor was extended by making it compulsory for municipalities to provide this. This task was added to that of protecting hygiene, for which a new professional figure – the public health officer – was created. Within this framework, the legislation on malaria was enacted in 1907, the Order of Physicians was established in 1910, rules were introduced regulating the employment of women and children, and the National Maternity Fund was established in 1910 to protect public order and the provision of minimum guarantees to a population increasingly engaged in factory work.

It is not surprising therefore that the Fascist government, from 1922 onwards, could boast of giving the country its first real package of health policies. In fact, it created in 1925 an almost universal institute – the National Maternity and Childhood Organisation – supporting maternity and childhood; it launched compulsory insurance against tuberculosis (1927); it started the mutualistic system (1927); it systematised the hospital sector (1938); and it issued compulsory health insurance (1943). An industrial 'authoritarian achievement-performance model' of welfare was therefore created, which provided for the integration of the middle and working classes into the new Fascist state through corporatist health funds with different occupational categories, as well as the exaltation of domestic and family work (Vicarelli, 1997b).

From 1948 onwards, the Republican state chose the path of continuity rather than discontinuity with the past. It left unchanged the industrial achievement-performance model of welfare created by the Fascist government and gradually extended it to the entire population. At the same time, there was a revaluation of the traditional systems of self-protection (family, kinship and territorial community) which were given the task of responding to new healthcare needs. In short, the Republican state proposed an industrial 'democratic achievement-performance model' based on health coverage to those who had a guaranteed job or to social groups who, in a client-based and particularistic way, managed to obtain protection.

During the 1960s and 1970s, the demand for a 'universalistic model' developed, in opposition to the previous system. This demand was supported by different collective actors and spontaneous movements: confederal trade unions, left-wing parties, associations of public health and occupational doctors, associations of psychologists and social workers, feminist and student movements and the anti-psychiatric movement. The NHS was formed in December 1978, 30 years after the birth of the Republic. Law 833 was passed not only after an intense ideological competition between right and left political parties but also after an economic and financial crisis of the mutual societies. The inequalities in healthcare coverage and services, institutional fragmentation, duplication of treatment and waste of human and financial resources were the results of political choices taken by successive different governments over the years. The latter considered healthcare as a tool for social consensus, a major reservoir of employment opportunities and a means of hidden party financing. With the establishment of the NHS, therefore, Italy created an institutional redistributive welfare model, the fourth mode of health protection since the years of its constitution in 1861 as a nation state (Vicarelli, 1997b; Giorgi and Pavan, 2021).

Main health reform trends

A very difficult implementation (1978–92)

The late approval of Law 833/1978 placed Italy in a very special position in the western panorama of welfare systems. In fact, while the country had finally arrived at a public and universalistic system, a process of transformation of welfare policies was taking place, based on the neo-liberal experiences implemented by British governments (Enthoven, 1988, 1993; Radcliffe and Dent, 2005; Saltman, Bankauskaite and Vrangbæk, 2007). It is from this political model and its financial and organisational tools, centred on NPM, that the reform process of western healthcare systems developed, framing the implementation of law 833/78.

In Italy, since its inception, though, the NHS has experienced a growing discord with its socio-political and cultural environment. The middle and upper-middle classes wanted to reduce public protection or at least make it more flexible. In fact, for the first time, the health market seemed to be able to hold its own without public support, finding in the new technologies and the new health needs adequate tools and demands for its expansion. The pressure expressed by these social groups was met with the demands of the traditional autonomous middle classes such as traders and small artisans. The latter hoped to escape the constraints imposed by public health protection which they had hitherto enjoyed at no particular cost. This alignment of the upper classes and the self-employed middle classes was in contrast to the homogenisation of wage labour. Teachers, public and private employees, social and health workers, technicians and guaranteed workers called for the implementation of the NHS. At the same time, they also called for a greater economic rigour in health spending as well as more involvement of Catholic and voluntary associations (Ascoli and Pasquinelli, 1993).

Given this situation, it is not surprising that, instead of proceeding swiftly with the creation of the NHS, all its stages were made difficult and complex: the necessary financial resources were reduced; the time required to issue the implementing regulations was prolonged; and processes for amending Law 833 were immediately prepared. In addition, three mechanisms have had the greatest influence on the implementation of the new healthcare system: first, a regulatory mechanism due to the contradictions inherent in Law 833 as a result of the compromises that were reached among different actors (at parliamentary and governmental level) over the long period of its genesis; second, an institutional-organisational mechanism due to the difficulties in transforming the structures of the mutualist systems into the new forms provided for by Law 833; third, an implementation mechanism linked to the asymmetries that occurred between what was provided for by the regulations and what was actually implemented, in the absence of a system for monitoring and evaluating the implementation of the law.

A public policy of managed competition (1992–95)

It was in this context that, at the beginning of the 1990s, a health policy approach based on 'managed competition' emerged (Vicarelli, 2005). In a period of great economic difficulty, Legislative decree 502/1992 (the first neo-liberal reform) was issued without any scientific or political debate, as the result of an imposition by the 1992–93 Amato government (made up of the Christian Democrats, the Socialist Party, the Social Democratic Party and the Liberal Party) and the Liberal minister of health, De Lorenzo. However, in the following months, the decree came under political attacks and was rethought – soon leading to its amendment by legislative decree 517/1993 (the second neo-liberal reform). This turnaround should be interpreted in light of the institutional crisis known as *Tangentopoli*, in which the new government lasted only until 1994; while the newspapers revealed the illicit accumulation of funds by Minister De Lorenzo's father and by the General Director of the Italian Medicine Agency, Poggiolini, and while the minister himself was being investigated, the highest representatives of the government parties entered a destructive parabola at an institutional and political level.

As a result, citizens' dissatisfaction grew rapidly and the new technical government, chaired by Azeglio Ciampi, considered it necessary to modify the liberal rules laid down in Legislative decree 502/1992. In other words, the article of the decree introducing the possibility for citizens to leave the NHS by choosing mutualistic or private protection was modified. However, the managed competition drawn from the Thatcher reforms was reaffirmed and the Italian NHS was corporatised and regionalised. The local health authorities (ASLs) and hospitals (AOs), controlled by the regions, replaced the local health units controlled by the municipalities. Experiments on analytical and economic accounting, new forms of planning and control and the accreditation of public and private services were carried out.

Three mechanisms played a role in the definition of these policies. First of all, there was an asymmetry between regulatory frameworks and real actions: scandals producing an institutional change were generated from below, based on the work of local magistrates who identified behaviours completely different from those legitimised and codified. Second, there was a wide institutional permeability: in a climate marked by a strong revaluation of the market, competition became a pivotal element in the reorganisation of the public sector. The slogan 'more market and less state', long supported by the Liberal Party and the Socialist Party at the end of the 1980s, became an accepted concept even by opposition parties in face of the evident moral and institutional decline of public structures. Third, there was a mode of rational imitation whereby managed competition became a means of giving continuity to public control, but with the application of market rules in a healthcare system suffocated by corruption.

Attempts at administrative cooperation (1996–2001)

The period immediately following 1992–93 was characterised by great political and institutional uncertainty. The revision of Legislative decree 502/1992 was disliked by the entrepreneurial high and middle classes and their new political spokespeople. It is no coincidence that, in the political elections of 1994 and 1996, the Radical Party and the Northern League called for the abolition of compulsory registration with the NHS. Moreover, the centre-right group (*Polo delle Libertà*) proposed 'a welfare state with fewer functions, fewer responsibilities and therefore lower costs' (Ferrera, 1984:7). The centre-left coalition (*Ulivo*), on the other hand, aimed at rationalisation of the NHS based on a pre-established package of health services, the stability of expenditure and a federalist organisation.

The prevalence of this latter coalition in the spring of 1996 seemed to show that the dependent middle classes had the upper hand over other social forces. However, the picture was much more complex due to the narrow margin of victory and the consequent political weight of the opposing forces; the corporate interests of the medical class; the desire of regions and municipal authorities to play a leading role; the demands for recognition of voluntary associations, and the latent dissatisfaction of citizens. It was in this context that Legislative decree 229/1999 (the third neo-liberal reform) was issued, at the behest of the D'Alema government in power from 1998 to 1999, made up of a political coalition of the *Ulivo, Partito dei Comunisti Italiani, Unione Democratica per la Repubblica and Indipendenti.*

The package of services and benefits that the NHS intends to provide to all citizens in a universalistic manner was facilitated by Health Minister Rosy Bindi. This reform aimed to make the NHS more efficient, fairer and more human, while remaining within the limits of the corporatisation and region-alisation of the system. More generally, the new decree aimed to overcome managed competition in the name of 'managed cooperation'. All the players in the NHS were called upon to participate in a new health pact. However, physicians had to be involved exclusively in the NHS. This means that they have to choose whether to remain in public service with the associated finan-cial and career penalties or to give commitment to the health service with the possibility of entering private practice within the public system. This rule, which was strongly opposed by the professions and trade unions, led to great conflict and ultimately Bindi's dismissal as minister.

The years of regional neo-centralism (2001–08)

On 18 October 2001, after a long regulatory process, reform of Constitutional Law 3 (the fourth neo-liberal reform) was enacted, emphasising the region-alisation of the NHS. The new wording of Article 117 broadened the powers of the regions in health matters, leaving the determination of the Essential Levels of Care (LEA) to the exclusive competence of the State. Article 119 guaranteed the financial autonomy of the regions (including autonomy of income and expenditure), providing an equalisation fund as a tool to maintain the provision of services at uniform levels throughout the national territory. The reform was a concession by the centre-left government to the Northern League. However, it was implemented very slowly by the right and left gov-ernments that alternated during the first decade of the year 2000. This meant that the implementing regulations were issued a decade late. Consequently, the regions found themselves with limited autonomy, especially from an eco-nomic and financial point of view. All these produced a process of regional centralisation, resulting in a reduction of ASLs and autonomy of the AOs.

   Overall, from 2001 to May 2008, Italy experienced a period of weak and contradictory governance of the healthcare sector, which was led by the Min-istry of Economy. The serious financial situation of the health services in many regions (especially in the South) led the Ministry of Economy to initiate a binding monitoring of regional budgets with the obligation to implement policies to contain costs and reorganise the health services (Mapelli, 2012).

The years of the economic and financial crisis (2008 to 2019)

The beginning of the 2008 economic crisis in Italy coincided with the start of another centre-right government led by Silvio Berlusconi which held office from 2008 to 2012 based on a political coalition consisting of *Partito delle Libertà, Lega Nord and Movimento per le Autonomie*. The Ministry of Health was merged with the Ministry of Labour and Social Policies. Min-ister Sacconi explicitly pursued the idea of revising the relationship between public and private in favour of the latter. In concrete terms, it was only in 2011 that the government decided to intervene in healthcare spending with a planned cut of €7.5 billion. However, during that year, the economic situation seemed to be deteriorating and Berlusconi was forced to resign.

Mario Monti's new technical government from 2011 to 2013 planned to intervene on four fundamental aspects of the health system: further reducing financing, limiting pharmaceutical spending, reducing beds and hospitalisation rates and providing for new primary care facilities. The aim was, at least in the short term, to ensure a generalised reduction in the supply of services with performance directly entrusted to the regions, as well as a reduction of the workforce engaged in the NHS – producing a worsening of working conditions (Dirindin, 2012). All the following five successive governments of the centre-left and centre-right – namely, the Letta, Renzi, Gentiloni, Conte and Conte II governments with different coalitions – followed this trend. Until 2019, therefore they operated with a gradual and systematic reduction of the material and non-material resources of the NHS without any policy of recalibration in relation to the welfare system. This was unlike what happened in the same period in most Central and Northern European countries (Pierson, 2001; Ferrera and Hemerijck, 2003).

The impact on the architecture of the system

As a result of the policy processes highlighted here, in 2019, the NHS contained four fundamental distortions (Vicarelli and Giarelli, 2021). Two of these were of an institutional and structural nature, in so far as they were linked to the NHS regionalisation and health inequalities in the country, while two were of a functional and cultural nature, in so far as they related to the prevalence of hospital services and the low incidence of preventive services. These distortions revealed that there had been a reduced and modified implementation of the NHS since the 1990s, which affected both its institutional and universalistic character and its effectiveness in protecting the health of citizens.

Institutional and structural distortions

The first two distortions were identified within the increasing regionalism of the NHS and its consequences in terms of the universalism of health services and benefits. In the early 1980s, at a time of the genesis and cultural acceptance of the 'strong universalism underpinning the NHS', many believed that health and healthcare inequalities, at a territorial level, were likely to be gradually surmountable (Spina and Vicarelli, 2020). However, the process of regionalisation, which had developed since the 1990s, created conditions that limited the homogenising trends of the previous period. The possibility for regions to reach differentiated levels in the guarantee of the LEAs led to strong territorial differences (see Table 6.1).

In this period, therefore, the concept of 'selective universalism' was the one that seemed to be the most politically useful. This concept resolved the

Table 6.1 Different essential levels of care by regions and services in Italy in 2017

	Hospital Services	Prevention Services	Territorial Services
Piedmont	84,14	92,90	84,05
Aosta Valley	74,38	64,12	34,52
Lombardy	77,13	86,84	77,05
Liguria	79,99	73,94	84,16
Veneto	83,67	80,75	95,10
P.A. Trento	94,75	83,56	82,45
P.A. Bolzano	73,97	53,37	44,82
FVG	80,72	53,18	74,02
Emilia Romagna	88,51	93,03	86,82
Tuscany	94,27	87,07	82,67
Umbria	80,59	92,89	67,91
Brands	69,84	69,00	78,51
Lazio	70,78	86,18	57,99
Abruzzo	67,92	66,36	63,76
Molise	40,66	74,18	31,25
Campania	44,83	72,51	55,16
Apulia	65,90	66,21	64,60
Basilicata	72,56	78,69	49,86
Calabria	50,63	65,49	47,35
Sicily	73,05	50,20	74,87
Sardinia	63,74	76,36	35,16

Colour coding:

Score >80	Score 50–60
Score 70–80	Score 40–50
Score 60–70	Score<40

Source: Corte dei Conti (2020).

contradiction between the universalist principles underlying the 833 law and the different responses given by Italian regions to health preservation. Since 2007, this trend underwent a further phase linked to the request for increased autonomy by some Central and Northern regions – that led to the devaluation of lesser performing territories (generally those of the South), based on the idea that they did not have to be helped to achieve greater levels of territorial equity (Rodriguez-Pose, 2017). From this viewpoint, there emerged a proposal for 'reduced or sufficient universalism' (Fourie and Rid, 2017). This process involved many actors – not least governments and regional bureaucracies that were not always able to guarantee the LEAs, especially in Southern Italy and political parties (mainly those of the centre-right party) that were increasingly opposed in their universalistic conceptions of welfare in healthcare.

These different choices resulted in different health expenditures. The total health expenditure in 2019 was €2,590 per capita. At the regional level, the highest values were recorded in Aosta Valley and Trentino Alto-Adige in the North (€3,091 and €2,995) and at the opposite extreme are Campania (€2,216.40) and Apulia (€2,320) in the South. The difference between the region with the highest and the one with the lowest expenditure was 1.4 times or €875.40 (CREA, 2020). On the other hand, the share of public financing on health expenditure in Italy has been progressively decreasing over the years. In 2019, this value was 74.1%, which was lower than that of Eastern European countries (74.5%) and Western Europe (80.5%). In Italy, the offer of services by low-cost companies and cooperatives (especially in the field of dental care) was increasingly evident. Nor should we overlook the use of supplementary mutuality linked to the health funds, which in recent years have received increasing attention (Giarelli and Giovannetti, 2019). In fact, entrepreneurs see health benefits as a way to avoid much more onerous commitments in terms of salaries or new forms of work organisation. According to some surveys, the recourse to the services of the funds until 2010 did not appear to be a substitute for public protection; on the contrary, in recent years, this aspect became dominant (Pavolini, Ascoli and Mirabile, 2013).

It is not surprising that in the face of such differences in welfare, strong inequalities in health remained. In 2015, the average life expectancy in Italy reached 80.1 years for males and 84.6 years for females – 2.2 and 1.3 years, respectively, higher than the figure for Europe as a whole. Within the peninsula, however, life expectancy changed depending on the place of residence: in 2015, a male born in Trentino-Alto Adige was more likely to survive by 2.7 years than a resident of Campania. Several regions in the South showed limited longevity (in Sicily 79.4 years and in Molise and Calabria 79.6 years). Aosta Valley, with an average male life expectancy of 78.8 years, was the only area in the North to be at the bottom of the league table (ISTAT, 2019). Moreover, in 2014–15, about 20 out of every 100 residents suffered from two or more serious chronic diseases, with significant regional variability.

Functional and cultural distortions

Functional and cultural distortions can be summed up in the concept of hospital-centrism and medicalisation. On one hand, the enhancement in life expectancy and chronic illnesses should have led to increasing forms of territorial and home-based services with the inclusion of family, community and neighbourhood networks. On the contrary, in 2018, hospital expenditure accounted for 44% of the total Italian health expenditure, against 39% in the European Union (EU) (28% in Germany, 38% in France and 39% in Sweden) (OECD, 2020). Long-term care accounted for 6% of spending in Italy, compared to 8% in the EU – a figure that varies widely, with spending at 27% in the Netherlands and only 2% in Greece. During the 1990s and early 2000s, professional groups, especially doctors, played a key role in these figures. They opposed both the reallocation of resources (from the hospital to the community) and new forms of empowerment of other health professions and the direct involvement of patients and families.

On the other hand, the medicalisation of health impacted in different ways. First of all, it did so in the tangential relevance of prevention in the complex of health services. Despite being included in the LEA as the third macro-area (after community and hospital care), expenditure on prevention in Italy represented 4.4% of public health spending (against 8% in the EU in 2018). However, per capita expenditure was €137.1 in Italy, while it was €194.5 in the United Kingdom (UK) and €177.7 in Germany (European House Ambrosetti, 2020). The limited financial resources allocated to prevention also impacted the limited capacity for action of the Prevention Departments of the health authorities, whose staff have been greatly reduced in the last decade (Tagliavento and Vicarelli, 2021). This orientation towards illness was expressed, at the level of health services, in the prevalence of an organisational model based on the so-called 'waiting medicine' after the onset of pathology. Despite experimentation with new models of care such as the Chronic Care Model inspired by a new 'initiative medicine', their diffusion was still rather limited. General practice itself, which in Italy was fairly well represented with 72 general practitioners (GPs) per 100,000 residents (in comparison with 70 GPs in Germany, 75 GPs in the UK and 90 GPs in France 90), (OECD, 2020) was not exempted from this cultural mode. Here strong responsibility must be attributed to the medical culture focused on demographic transition (and therefore the end of the pandemic age) with a consequent devaluing of collective prevention in favour of individual prevention.

The devaluation of human resources

The four distortions mentioned earlier have been accompanied by policies to ration NHS resources. The price of reduced funding was to be paid by the healthcare workforce through a freeze on bargaining and salary increases; an increase in working hours, running against European legislation; and a reduction in senior positions. In consequence, in 2009, there were 9,691 directors of Complex Structures at the pinnacle of their professional careers, in contrast to 2019, when there were 6,629 such directors, a 31.5% reduction. Moreover, the number of Heads of Simple Structures (the level immediately below) decreased from 18,536 in 2009 to 10,368 in 2019, a reduction of 44% (ANAAO-ASSOMED, 2021). The workforce of the NHS more generally saw a sharp decline in permanent positions (reduced by 6,348 doctors and dentists and 10,373 nurses from 2010 to 2017) and an increase in the average age of such senior personnel from 43.5 years from 2001 to 50.7 in 2018 (Vicarelli, 2020). Moreover, in 2019, according to data from the Annual Treasury Account, 2.9% of hospital doctors (3,123 with a prevalence in the Northern and Central regions) decided to leave their jobs in the public sector or move to territorial services in search of an economic improvement and quality of life (ANAAO-ASSOMED, 2021). Capital investments were also limited resulting in the negative impact on technological innovations, in particular computerisation and digital technologies, which were capable of improving the efficiency and effectiveness of the NHS, as well as the quality of professional work (CREA, 2017, 2018).

How far the neo-liberal reforms changed the National Health Service

In Italy, the neo-liberal reforms were applied simultaneously with the implementation of the NHS. Created in 1978, the Italian NHS underwent its first neo-liberal reform in 1992. The following reforms (1993, 1999 and 2001) took place in a very short time. In just ten years, in fact, the different governmental coalitions proposed to pass from a competitive system to a cooperative one and from this to regional centralism within a broad retrenchment logic. Therefore, on the one hand, the slowness in arriving at an institutional redistributive model (passing through various forms of welfare system) and, on the other, the rapidity of the changes have thwarted a balanced construction of health protection. The result is a much more complex picture than that of central and northern European countries. In Italy, regulatory changes have taken place within the same welfare model and over a longer period of time. More specifically, health protection entered an era of permanent austerity (in the 1990s) in conditions of great institutional changes (corporatisation and regionalisation) and with great political instability (at both the national and regional levels). Unfavourable demographic trends (the rapid ageing of the population) aggravated this situation.

Although formally universalistic and institutional, the Italian healthcare model seems, in recent years, to be strongly displaying a family-based matrix and a tendency to return to an industrial achievement-performance model or even residual model. It is not surprising, in this context, that before the pandemic, many people in Italy foresaw a slow but inexorable destructuring and devaluation of the NHS due to economic difficulties, the increased ageing and chronic illness of the population and the greater expenditure requirements linked to new drugs and the use of improved medical technologies (Longo and Ricci, 2020). This ignores the citizen/patient side of the equation in that the formulation of a patient-centred health system was out of the scope of the reform package. Therefore, the universalism of the Italian healthcare system and the role of the state appear even more formal in 2019 than in the past, with a very high level of territorial and social inequalities. In this sense, the thesis that decentralisation leads to better functioning of the NHS, repeatedly upheld by NPM's supporters, has not been verified. The regionalisation of healthcare was not accompanied by a process of thorough implementation of new management models, nor better results in terms of effectiveness and efficiency of the NHS in all Italian regions.

In summary, the change that has taken place as a result of neo-liberal policies does not seem to be an effective 'directive change' wanted and supported by central governments (Powell and Wessen, 1999). Reform proposals hardly ever arise from wide-ranging planning, based on the collection and evaluation of data and knowledge regarding the real functioning of the country's health services. They tend to respond to the financial imbalance of the state (for example, decree 502/92) as well as to different ideological positions taken by political parties (for instance, decree 517/93). This mode of action largely reflects a peculiar feature of the Italian public administration: the absence of a bureaucratic class that is aware of its function and prepared to adequately exercise it. At the same time, the political class continues to make instrumental use of the administrative apparatus, bending it to its own particularistic ends (Vicarelli, 2010a). Another specific feature of the Italian public policy environment is the existence of political forces that are ready to use the NHS in a corrupted way, even after the Tangentopoli period (Galli della Loggia, 2010). Due to the lack of a strong impetus from central government, the transformations can be considered simply as an 'adaptive change' (Powell and Wessen, 1999). The regionalisation and the corporatisation, as well as the retrenchment policies, have been driven by local political coalitions and economic lobbies.

If we take into account the actions of some occupational and professional groups, as well as certain non-governmental actors (including groups such as the Catholic Church and the mafias), it is easy to sustain the notion of 'integrative change' as lying at the heart of the neo-liberal reforms (Powell and Wessen, 1999). In Italy, a prominent role in the construction and transformation of the health system has always been played by the Catholic Church. Since the 1990s, it emphasised horizontal subsidiarity forms and the commitment of volunteers in the health sector, supporting a dense network of private health structures both in hospitals and in territorial rehabilitation services (Della Porta and Vannucci, 2007). Moreover, in such decentralised contexts, the mafias also demonstrate their ability to infiltrate both the public and private health systems. If in the former, they act to offer their members favours and job opportunities, in the latter, they move with direct objectives of money laundering or pure enrichment (Mete, 2011, 2013).

Within this framework, the medical profession played a central but ambivalent role (Vicarelli, 2010b). What is striking is the attempt by doctors to participate in the management of local health systems (Vicarelli, 2016). A survey focused on the main journals of their major trade union associations showed that they have been focusing on managerialism in the first part of the 2000s. Subsequently, however, these associations do not hide their progressive disappointment, and intolerance, towards managerial concepts. All these are especially so when cuts to healthcare are proposed in a top-down, linear manner with wide-ranging repercussions for professional activity (Fassari, 2003). However, recent research has demonstrated that doctors have internalised a hybrid professional model (Kuhlmann et al., 2015; Kurunmaki, 2004; Noordegraaf, 2015; Saks, 2016, 2018) where managerial characteristics merged with the traditional manner of practice (Spina and Vicarelli, 2021).

It was in these same years that the presence of physicians in the political roles of control of regional healthcare (through boards and presidencies), as well as in the top positions of the ASLs and AOs, increased. This appears to be a strategic response by physicians, who are interested in regaining control of healthcare by becoming managers and policymakers themselves. Nurses, on the other hand, do not constitute a professional category in Italy that can sustain such processes of change (Ministero della salute, 2012; Cergas, 2013). They are, in fact, undersized in number compared to other European countries and with a limited economic and social status. As a result, their voice remains very limited even when they bear the brunt of the cuts and reorganisation processes of the health service. In the background are the citizens who, although showing a growing interest in the health service, are still overwhelmed by the economic crisis of 2008, leading to their voice being even less heard than in the past. On the other hand, the Italian family continues to be considered by the centre-left and centre-right coalitions as one of the most solid actors in health protection, despite its transformations and its reduced ability to cope with economic difficulties (Saraceno, Benassi and Morlicchio, 2020).

Conclusion: the future of the Italian NHS

Starting from 31 January 2020, when Italy decreed a state of national emergency, the country faced the Covid-19 pandemic with a healthcare system that has been reduced and weakened by the neo-liberal policies of previous decades. Compared to the aforementioned distortions, the policies of the Covid-19 era were driven by the need to contain contagions in ways that are mainly mitigatory, given the great impact of the pandemic – especially in northern regions (Vicarelli and Giarelli, 2022). However, there was an attempt to reverse the trend of the previous two decades, to contain regional autonomy and strengthen prevention and territorial services. Nonetheless, health and mortality differentials, which made the pandemic even more evident, were not reduced by such policies, but were instead increased by them

(Vicarelli and Neri, 2021). In both cases, these policies were largely affected by path dependency processes (Vicarelli and Neri, 2021). The capacity for the innovative formulation of the associated objectives and tools was seriously affected by the structural rigidities of the ministerial and regional health apparatuses, as well as the contingencies of the controversial political coalitions governing the country. The management of the pandemic has in fact been dealt with by two different governments: the first is a coalition government led by Giuseppe Conte until February 2021 and the second is a government of national unity led by Mario Draghi. The latter issued the National Recovery and Resilience Plan (PNRR) in April 2021 to take advantage of European funds made available by the Next Generation EU programme.

In the PNRR, Mission 6, which is dedicated to health and healthcare, there are two components. The first aims to strengthen healthcare in the territory and in the home as well as to homogenise them through the introduction of a shared organisational model based on structural, organisational and technological standards issued in May 2022 (DM71). In addition, a new institutional set-up for health, environmental and climate prevention is to be established by 2022. The second component addresses the modernisation of the technological-digital infrastructure and the strengthening of bio-medical research. In both components, the aim is to address and solve the low levels of prevention and home care (cultural and functional distortion), affecting regional differences and their effects (institutional and redistributive distortion). In doing so, the PNRR seems to look more to the past, trying to solve old ills of the *Servizio Sanitario Nazionale* without addressing a future that requires greater predictive capacity with respect to post-pandemic health and care needs.

During the Covid-19 pandemic, different public and private actors claimed to want to strengthen the NHS, reversing the trend of recent decades. According to some scholars, two factors suggest that this change could be possible. The first is the presence of an organised policy community (experts, managers, trade unions and professional representatives) able to use the crisis to reinforce the NHS. This can be realised thanks to funds coming from the Recovery and Resilience Plan. The second factor is linked to the nature of the pandemic and its symbolic and emotional dimension (Birkland, 1998; Razetti, 2020). This is supported by the fact that every health reform in Italy has taken place at the same time as a major political and economic crisis in the country. However, to be certain of proceeding with rapid and effective policies, it would be necessary to bring about substantial changes in interest groups, especially professional ones (doctors and other health professions have been waiting for a long time for greater valorisation), in institutional governance (by modifying the difficult relationship between the state and the regions), in the private market of health services (today it is growing and much more competitive than in the past), and in the voice of civil society (whose forms of political and associative representation are currently quite weak).

Finally, it should be emphasised that a reversal of trends of this nature requires more far-reaching changes to be long lasting. The transition to a new configuration of the NHS means the creation of a new 'welfare configuration', a complex way of regulating and protecting health. This calls into question transformations in the dominant political philosophy (new forms of state interventionism after the neo-liberal age), in market dynamics (new chains of productivity and value after the anomic digital globalisation of recent decades) and in community actions and values (new forms of participation and social commitment after the hedonistic individualism of past years). At the moment, no empirical evidence allows us to affirm that the exceptional nature of the crisis created by the Covid-19 pandemic enables the reinforcement of the public healthcare system. It will be the policies and strategic actions of the coming years that will give us a better indication of this.

References

ANAAO-ASSOMED (2021) *Lavorare in ospedale? No, grazie. Oltre 3000 medici in fuga nel 2019. Lostudio Anaao*. Available at: www.anaao.it/content.php?cont=31733

Ascoli, U. and Pasquinelli S. (eds) (1993) *Il Welfare Mix in Italia. Stato sociale e terzo settore*, Milan: Franco Angeli.

Birkland, T. A. (1998) 'Focusing events, mobilization, and agenda setting', *Journal of Public Policy* 18(1): 53–74.

Cergas, N. (ed) (2013) *Essere infermieri oggi. Ricerca della Commissione Europea delle professioni sanitarie della C.E.S.I. I risultati italiani dell'inchiesta*, Milan: Cergas-Nursind.

Corte dei Conti (2020) *Rapporto 2020 sul coordinamento della finanza pubblica*. Available at: www.quotidianosanita.it/allegati/allegato5380690.pdf

CREA (2017) *XIII Rapporto Sanità. Il cambiamento della Sanità in Italia fra transizione e deriva del sistema*, Rome: CREA.

CREA (2018) *XIV Rapporto Sanità. Misunderstanding*, Rome: CREA.

CREA (2020) *XVI Rapporto Sanità. Oltre l'emergenza: verso una "nuova" vision del nostro SSN*, Rome: CREA.

Della Porta, D. and Vannucci, A. (2007) *Mani impunite. Vecchia e nuova corruzione in Italia*, Roma-Bari: Laterza.

Dirindin, N. (2012) 'Salvaguardare il sistema di welfare, riconvertire le risorse', *Politiche Sanitarie* 13(2): 94–108.

Enthoven, A. (1988) *Theory and Practice of Managed Competition in Health Care Finance*, Amsterdam: North-Holland.

Enthoven, A. (1993) 'The history and principles of managed competition', *Health Affairs* 12(1s): 24–48.

European House-Ambrosetti (2020) *XV Meridiano Sanità. Le coordinate della salute. Rapporto 2020*. Available at: www.ambrosetti.eu/wp-content/uploads/RAPPORTOMS15low.pdf

Fassari, C. (2003) 'Manager e medico: più odio che amore', *Management Medico* 5: 2.

Ferrera, M. (1984) *Il welfare state in Italia*, Bologna: Il Mulino.

Ferrera, M. and Hemerijck, A. (2003) 'Recalibrating Europe's welfare regimes', in Zeitlin, J. and Trubek, D. (eds) *Governing Work and Welfare in a New Economy: European and American Experiments*, Oxford: Oxford University Press.

Fourie, C. and Rid, A. (eds) (2017) *What Is Enough: Sufficiency, Justice, and Health*, New York: Oxford University Press.

Galli della Loggia, E. (2010) *Tre giorni nella storia d'Italia*, Bologna: Il Mulino.

Giarelli, G. and Giovannetti, V. (eds) (2019) *Il Servizio sanitario nazionale italiano in prospettiva europea. Una analisi comparata*, Milan: Franco Angeli.

Giorgi, C. and Pavan, I. (2021) *Storia dello Stato sociale in Italia*, Bologna: Il Mulino.

ISTAT (2019) *La salute nelle regioni italiane – Bilancio di un decennio (2005–2015)*, Rome: ISTAT.

Kuhlmann, E., Blank, R. H., Bourgeault, I. L. and Wendt, C. (eds) (2015) *The Palgrave International Handbook of Healthcare Policy and Governance*, London: Palgrave Macmillan.

Kurunmaki, L. (2004) 'A hybrid profession: The acquisition of management accounting expertise by medical professionals', *Accounting, Organizations and Society* 29: 327–47.

Longo, F. and Ricci, A. (2020) 'Le fratture generate dal Covid-19: quali priorità strategiche per la sanità italiana?', in *CERGAS – Bocconi Rapporto OASI 2020*, Milan: Egea.

Mapelli, V. (2012) *Il sistema sanitario italiano*, Bologna: Il Mulino.

Mete, V. (2011) 'Lo spergiuro di Ippocrate. Mafia, politiche e carriere nel campo della sanità in provincia di Reggio Calabria', in Sciarrone, R. (ed) *Alleanze nell'ombra*, Rome: RES-Donzelli.

Mete, V. (2013) 'Mafie ed aree grigie nel campo della sanità', *Rivista delle Politiche Sociali* 2012(4s): 227–41.

Ministero della Salute (2012) *Il personale del sistema sanitario italiano 2010*, Rome: Ministero della Salute.

Noordegraaf, M. (2015) 'Hybrid professionalism and beyond. (New) forms of public professionalism in changing organizational and societal contexts', *Journal of Professions and Organization* 2(2): 187–206.

Organisation for Economic Cooperation and Development/European Union (2020) *Health at a Glance. Europe 2020: State of Health in the EU Cycle*, Paris: OECD Publishing.

Pavolini, E., Ascoli, U. and Mirabile, M. L. (eds) (2013) *Tempi moderni: il welfare nelle aziende in Italia*, Bologna: Il Mulino.

Pierson, P. (ed) (2001) *The New Polities of the Welfare State*, Oxford: Oxford University Press.

Pierson, P. (2004) *Politics in Time: History, Institutions, and Social Analysis*, Princeton, NJ: Princeton University Press.

Powell, F. D. and Wessen, A. F. (eds) (1999) *Health Care Systems in Transition: An International Perspective*, Thousands Oaks, CA: Sage.

Powell, W. W. and Bromley, P. (2015) 'New institutionalism in the analysis of complex organizations', in Wright, J. D. (ed) *International Encyclopedia of the Social and Behavioral Sciences*, 2nd edition, Volume 16, Oxford: Elsevier.

Radcliffe, J. and Dent, M. (2005) 'Introduction: From new public management to the new governance?', *Policy and Politics* 33(4): 617–22.

Razetti, F. (2020) *Il Coronavirus e i nervi scoperti del welfare italiano*. Available at: www.secondowelfare.it

Rodríguez-Pose, A. (2017) 'The revenge of the places that don't matter (and what to do about it)', *Cambridge Journal of Regions, Economy and Society* 11(1): 189–209.

Saks, M. (2016) 'A review of theories of professions, organizations and society: The case for neo-Weberianism, neo-institutionalism and eclecticism', *Journal of Professions and Organization* 3(2): 170–87.

Saks, M. (2018) 'The medical profession, enterprise and the public interest', in Saks, M. and Muzio, D. (eds) *Professions and Professional Service Firms*, Abingdon: Routledge.

Saltman, R., Bankauskaite, V. and Vrangbæk, K. (eds) (2007) *Decentralization in Health Care*, London: European Observatory on Health Systems and Policies.

Saraceno, C., Benassi, D. and Morlicchio, E. (2020) *Poverty in Italy: Features and Drivers in a European Perspective*, Bristol: Policy Press.

Scott, W. R., Ruef, M., Mendel, P. and Caronna, C. (2000) *Institutional Change and Healthcare Organizations: From Professional Dominance to Managed Care*, Chicago: University of Chicago Press.

Spina, E. and Vicarelli, G. (2020) 'Disuguaglianze e SSN: una contraddizione irrisolvibile?', *Politiche Sociali/Social Policies* 1: 77–102.

Spina, E. and Vicarelli, G. (2021) 'Verso un nuovo professionalismo medico', *Salute e Società* 1: 55–71.

Tagliavento, G. and Vicarelli, G. (2021) 'La pandemia da SARS-CoV-2 e il sistema di prevenzione in Italia', in Favretto, A. R., Maturo, A. and Tomelleri, S. (eds) *L'impatto sociale del Covid-19*, Milan: Franco Angeli.

Titmuss, R. (1974) *Social Policy: An Introduction*, London: Allen & Unwin.

Vicarelli, G. (1997a) *Alle radici della politica sanitaria in Italia. Società e salute da Crispi al fascismo*, Bologna: Il Mulino.

Vicarelli, G. (1997b) 'La politica sanitaria tra continuità e innovazione', in Barbagallo, F. (ed) *Storia dell'Italia repubblicana Volume III: L'Italia nella crisi mondiale. L'ultimo ventennio*, Torino: Einaudi.

Vicarelli, G. (2005) 'Control, competition and cooperation in European health systems: Points of contact between health policy and industrial policy', in Di Tommaso, M. and Schweitzer, S. (eds) *Health Policy and High-Tech Industrial Development*, Cheltenham: Edward Elgar.

Vicarelli, G. (2010a) 'Du centralisme napoléonien au fédéralisme administratif. Les processus de décentralisation du système sanitaire en Italie', *Revue Sociologie Santé* 32: 23–57.

Vicarelli, G. (2010b) *Gli eredi di Esculapio. Medici e politiche sanitarie nell'Italia unita*, Rome: Carocci.

Vicarelli, G. (2016) 'Les médecins italiens à l'épreuve du management: régulation, Négociation et négation', in Ferreol, G. (ed) *Médiations et Régulations*, Louvain-la Neuve: EME édition.

Vicarelli, G. (2020) 'La valorizzazione delle risorse umane nel sistema sanitario nazionale: un principio disatteso', *La Rivista delle Politiche Sociali* 3: 75–96.

Vicarelli, G. and Giarelli, G. (eds) (2021) *Libro Bianco. Il Servizio Sanitario Nazionale e la pandemia da Covid-19: Problemi e proposte*, Milan: Franco Angeli.

Vicarelli, G. and Giarelli, G. (2022) 'Tackling the Covid-19 pandemic: The Italian National Health Service in a comparative perspective', *Rassegan Italiana di Sociologia* 3: 555–84.

Vicarelli, G. and Neri, S. (2021) 'Una catastrofe vitale? Le scelte di politica sanitaria per far fronte al Covid-19', *Politiche Sociali/Social Policies* 2: 233–54.

7 Spain

Ana M. Guillén and Sigita Doblytė

Introduction

This chapter deals with the analysis of the evolution of the Spanish National Health Service (NHS) during the last 40 years. The analysis is theoretically underpinned by the neo-Weberian and neo-institutionalist approaches to the study of public policy in general (Heclo, 1974; March and Olsen, 1984; DiMaggio and Powell, 1991) and healthcare policies in particular (Immergut, 1991).

The Spanish case is of much interest for at least two reasons. First, the healthcare system was developed under authoritarian rule for 30 years (1943–75) and under a further period of transition to democracy (1976–82) before the inception of an NHS in 1986. During this 40-year interval, a health insurance system (HIS) was built, based on two major sets of reforms (see Guillén, 2000). A compulsory health insurance scheme *Seguro Obligatorio de Enfermedad* (SOE) was introduced in 1943, covering a small proportion of salaried (industrial) workers. The scheme expanded coverage to many other categories of workers in subsequent decades and was transformed into a proper social security scheme in 1963 (implemented from 1967 onwards) through the Basic Law of Social Security, namely the so-called *Asistencia Sanitaria de la Seguridad Social* (ASSS).

By 1975, the year of the demise of Francisco Franco and the onset of the process of transition to democracy, population coverage was over 80%. Still, what bears more salience in order to understand future developments is that, despite its Bismarckian conservative-corporatist root, the ASSS was organised as one single health fund, in stark difference to other HISs such as the German, French or Italian, where separate health insurance funds were established for different categories of workers, enjoying different conditions for access and packages of services. As argued by Guillén (2010), the existence of a single health fund for all workers was to ease the transition from an HIS to an NHS when such a move was undertaken in the early 1980s.

Furthermore, the ASSS was organised under a gate-keeping structure so that, in Spain, reference to higher levels of care has always been in the hands of primary doctors. As this is a very prevalent characteristic among NHSs, it can be considered a facilitating factor for the transformation into an NHS.

DOI: 10.4324/9781003139799-12

Against this, some of the conservative-corporatist traits have tended to resurface during the last four decades. One salient example is that while universal coverage was attained *de facto* under the NHS (even including residents and undocumented immigrants), it was not until 2011 that it was sanctioned *de jure* on the basis of citizenship, the principle of access remaining tied to the status of worker or dependant on a worker.

The second reason of interest is that the Spanish NHS is also peculiar as to its marked regionally decentralised character. Devolution of healthcare competencies to autonomous regions started in 1982 with the transference of powers to Catalonia and was completed in 2003 with the devolution of responsibilities to the last ten, out of 17, autonomous regions. In comparison with Italy, not only the intensity of decentralisation has been greater but also devolution did not take place immediately, but this was negotiated bilaterally by the corresponding autonomous region and the central state in a period lasting for 20 years. Hence, one can talk of an asymmetric, long-lasting process in the Spanish case, resulting in the final establishment of independent regional healthcare systems, all represented in the Interterritorial Council of Healthcare (*Consejo Interterritorial de Salud*) (Rico Gómez, 1997; Moreno Fuentes, 2012). This second characteristic of the Spanish healthcare system bears much importance to understanding inequalities among regions and the difficulties encountered in the process of decision-making at the national level, difficulties and problems which have come to the fore, especially during the recent Covid-19 pandemic.

The origins of the National Health Service

The Spanish National Health System (*Sistema Nacional de Salud*) is predicated, despite the use of the term 'system' rather than 'service', on the basic principles of an NHS, the terminology responding more to the fact that its inception meant the inclusion of all pre-existent healthcare networks into a single institution. Within it, the funds that assist public employees, the armed forces and the judiciary, and the funds or Mutualities for occupational diseases and labour accidents, count on different organisational and provision arrangements (Bernal-Delgado et al., 2018). The HIS built under the Francoist regime turned into an NHS service in the late 1980s. While the first steps of the health policy reform coincided with the Spanish transition to democracy (1975–82), especially the broadening of population coverage and services, the more pressuring claims in other policy areas (the reform of the political institutions, above all), uncertainty due to the economic oil crises or the power of the anti-reformist groups (in particular, physicians) pushed the formal shift to 1986, when the General Healthcare Law was finally passed (Guillén, 2002; Guillén and Cabiedes, 1997).

The passing and enactment of the 1986 Law – that is, the creation of the NHS – were enabled by a range of political, economic and social transformations such as the formal recognition of universal access to healthcare in the 1978 Constitution, the legitimation needs of the new democratic political regime, the presence of left-wing parties in the government, the democratisation of decision-making processes and the positive economic cycle in the late 1980s (Guillén, 2002; Guillén and Cabiedes, 1997). Likewise, as noted in the introduction, the maturity of the existing system in terms of the breadth, depth and scope of coverage, coupled with its governance through a single unified sickness fund, further facilitated the transition. That is, publicly provided health services and population coverage were wide in 1975 (81.4% of the population covered), when the Francoist Dictatorship ended, and more so in 1985 (95.4% of the population). The basic healthcare structure had also been reformed by then (Royal Decree 137/1984), including a new geographical division into health areas with their corresponding primary healthcare centres that replaced the old *ambulatorios* (Bernal-Delgado et al., 2018; Guillén and Cabiedes, 1997).

In light of this, the General Healthcare Law 'produced little change in the short term and rather tended to preserve and expand what already existed' (Guillén and Cabiedes, 1997:326). It did, however, convey more qualitative paradigmatic transformations that were implemented incrementally. This included healthcare financing progressively from general taxation, which came to fully replace social security contributions by 1999 (García-Armesto et al., 2010; López-Casasnovas, Costa-Font and Planas, 2005). Universalisation of access was completed in 1989 when the beneficiaries of the previous poor relief network were incorporated into the NHS (Petmesidou and Guillén, 2008).

The scope and depth of coverage were explicitly established for the first time in 1995, with its revisions afterwards. The publicly financed common-benefit basket includes a comprehensive package of primary and specialised healthcare services, which are free at the point of use, except outpatient pharmaceutical prescriptions that require co-payments. Yet it excludes optical products, dental care (with the partial exception of children and pregnant women), spa treatments, psychoanalysis or hypnosis, among others (Bernal-Delgado et al., 2018). Service delivery is undertaken by health centres, which provide primary and paediatric care and act as gatekeepers to specialised care, and hospitals, which offer inpatient care and integrate specialist outpatient consultations (except outpatient mental health services provided in mental health centres). They are mostly publicly owned. Yet some regions (for instance, Catalonia) partially contract primary services out to private providers; likewise, many of smaller hospitals within the network of public utilisation are private (López-Casasnovas, Costa-Font and Planas, 2005; García-Armesto et al., 2010).

The 1986 Law also outlined the legal basis for the decentralisation process. The regions' demand for political and administrative autonomy was, in turn, another key factor that contributed to the reform and definition of the NHS as 'the grouping of the services of the autonomous regions suitably coordinated by the state' (Petmesidou and Guillén, 2008:108). The Spanish NHS, therefore, consists of 17 sub-systems or regional systems that enjoy autonomy over provision, governance and funding. The latter is guaranteed from their general budgets, which come from taxes devolved by the central government and based on a weighted per capita criterion, from regionally retained taxes (especially in the Basque Country and Navarre) and other transfers to fully cover regional needs (Bernal-Delgado et al., 2018). The regions must follow the basic national legislation, which, among others, includes the provision of the aforementioned common-benefit package that can be complemented with additional services on their own initiative. The central government, nevertheless, maintains its authority over certain areas such as the aforementioned basic national legislation, general coordination of the NHS, pharmaceutical policy or international health issues.

The main health reform policies

In parallel with the system consolidation, concerns about the growth of healthcare expenditure were increasingly present, which led to several recalibration reforms already in the 1990s (Guillén and Cabiedes, 1997). This further accelerated in the 2000s after the devolution had been completed, and in particular, after the onset of the recent economic and financial crisis. Decentralisation has allowed for healthcare adaptation to the needs of local populations and has greatly enhanced innovation (Petmesidou and Guillén, 2008). At the same time, such processes contributed to regions' 'never-ending race to match the advancements of the nearby autonomous communities' (Ventura and González, 2013:61), and, in turn, resulted in cross-regional inequities and persistent financial deficits generating issues of sustainability (Bernal-Delgado et al., 2018; Petmesidou, Pavolini and Guillén, 2014; Repullo, 2014).

From 2003 onwards, that is after the completion of devolution, reform policies began a search for a balance between devolution and national coordination that would guarantee equity and efficiency of the system in light of increasing, yet uneven, spending across the regions. The Cohesion and Quality Act in 2003 was one of such attempts (García-Armesto et al., 2010). The key role of coordination was assigned to the Interterritorial Council, which consists of 34 representatives of the national and 17 regional health ministries and which is to develop national strategies and to monitor quality standards. However, its consensus-based policymaking process severely limits its role due to the difficulties to reach agreements between members from different political orientations and with different regional needs (Ventura and González, 2013). Besides, decisions take the form of recommendations and are not legally binding.

In the climate of harsh austerity after the onset of the latest economic crisis, nevertheless, pressures towards the re-centralisation became greater (Bernal-Delgado et al., 2018; Del Pino and Pavolini, 2015; Moreno Fuentes, 2019). Re-centralisation of more stringent conditions on regional expenditure was implemented unilaterally by the central government by means of different legal norms at the peak of the crisis in 2012, setting caps on regional budget deficits. Furthermore, in the same year, population coverage was restricted through a backlash to corporatist principles of entitlement and limiting the access of undocumented immigrants to emergency services.

Likewise, rapidly increasing pharmaceutical spending throughout the 1990s and 2000s led to several rationalisation measures undertaken at different points in time and directed towards the control of pricing and pre-scription practices (for example, the regulation of reference prices, prescrip-tion by active ingredient or use of generics) (Petmesidou and Guillén, 2008). Although well-evidenced and designed, such measures did not have a sub-stantial effect on the pharmaceutical expenditure prior to the crisis, which questions their implementation (Repullo, 2014). After the onset of the cri-sis, several laws were, in turn, passed aiming at reducing pharmaceutical expenditure in the whole territory, including stronger control of pharmaceu-tical prices and purchases by the central government.

Another area that the reform policies have focused on is public health (Bernal-Delgado et al., 2018). Devolved to all of the regions in the late 1970s to early 1980s, the system was governed regionally long before healthcare services were decentralised (García-Armesto et al., 2010), except certain cen-tralised policies such as health alerts and epidemiological surveillance. In the absence of common legislation that defines public health service governance and provision, territorial inequalities remain significant and particularly rel-evant in the case of non-communicable disease prevention (Bernal-Delgado et al., 2018; Spanish Economic and Social Council, 2020). The General Law on Public Health in 2011, therefore, attempted to fill the gap and to find an equilibrium between such devolution and equity, albeit with limited success.

The Law upgraded the coordination mechanism for epidemic surveil-lance and enforced a common package of public health benefits enacted in the entire country and aimed at both individuals (services mostly integrated to the primary care level) and the entire population (Bernal-Delgado et al., 2018). Such benefits included the (failed) establishment of a single vaccina-tion calendar and strategies for cancer screenings, among others. Despite this pursuit for efficiency and quality, and due to its timing, the implementation of the 2011 Law has been hindered by the need to reduce public expendi-ture (Petmesidou, Pavolini and Guillén, 2014). Thus, the defined instruments were not developed and public health remained a low priority, receiving approximately 1% of total health expenditure (Spanish Economic and Social Council, 2020). The first wave of the Covid-19 pandemic, in turn, uncovered such unpreparedness and underinvestment. Since then, however, Spain has improved its capacity for testing, detection and surveillance at the regional level, and coordination at the national level (Sierra Moros et al., 2021).

To sum up, health reform policies over the past decades have been mainly implemented incrementally and intended to rationalise medical practice rather than to ration services. In particular, the reforms in the 1990s aimed at management innovation, whereas coordination and cohesion after devolu-tion dominated thereafter in the 2000s (García-Armesto et al., 2010). After the onset of the crisis, nevertheless, the necessity for cost containment was more present and urgent (Petmesidou, Pavolini and Guillén, 2014; Moreno Fuentes, 2019), which led to the increasing role of central government in the allocation of financing resources. In the following section, we in turn con-sider the impact of these reforms on equity of access, quality and efficiency by discussing available statistical data on a range of indicators addressing the infrastructure of the system and population's health.

The impact of reforms

To begin with, total health expenditure – as a share of both Gross Domestic Product (GDP) and per capita (see Table 7.1) – had been growing until 2009, when it reached 9% of GDP for the first time. Rationalising reforms undertaken under economic prosperity, therefore, seem to have had a limited effect on the spending, although they might have slowed it down. After the onset of the crisis, total health expenditure remained stable and close to the European Union (EU) average of 9.9% in 2018. Yet the latest reforms did decrease health spending per capita from 2009 to 2014, when it returned to grow and recovered the 2009 level in 2018. Worrying is the evolution of the composition of public expenditure by the level of care. Figure 7.1 shows how increases were mainly directed to specialised care, while they were kept much lower and stable in the case of primary care, this latter remaining the 'poor sister' of the NHS, an issue which is always problematic but much more so in the face of a pandemic.

Public health expenditure per capita also dropped in the period between 2009 and 2014. Although returning to grow since then, it has not reached its highest level registered in 2009 – per capita either as a share of total health expenditure (decreased from 75% to 70% in 2018) or as a share of GDP (6.3% in 2018). It is also lower than the EU average, which reached 79% of total health expenditure and 7.8% of GDP in 2018 (OECD, 2021). This, therefore, signals that the reforms, success in decreasing public health expenditure might have been achieved by shifting the cost to the user, through the gradual privatisation of risk. The proportion of health expenditure falling on users' shoulders was lowest in 2009, but increased to more than 22% since then, which is substantially higher than the EU average of less than 16% (OECD, 2021). Such privatisation of risk is particularly evident in health spending per capita, which has been steadily increasing since 1995, notwithstanding the crisis.

As discussed in the previous section, the pharmaceutical policy was one of the areas frequently approached in order to decrease public health expenditure. The laws aimed at both the supply and demand sides by seeking to reduce prescribed pharmaceutical prices and quantities, on the one hand, and by increasing co-payments, on the other hand. Following earlier patterns, public pharmaceutical expenditure dropped in the crisis period but has returned to slowly grow since 2014, which signals a positive but fast fading effect of the measures in terms of both volume and price (López-Valcárcel and Barber, 2017; Spanish Economic and Social Council, 2020). Figure 7.2 demonstrates that the average annual growth of public expenditure on prescribed medicines was indeed negative in the period 2009–13, yet out-of-pocket spending has dramatically increased in the same period, or, to be precise, in 2012 and 2013. In other words, the effect of the shift of costs to the user – through increased co-payments for working-age people and their

Table 7.1 Healthcare expenditure and resources in Spain

	1995	2000	2003	2006	2009	2012	2015	2018
Total health expenditure as a share of GDP	7%	6.8%	7.6%	7.8%	9.1%	9.2%	9.1%	9%
Total health expenditure (THE)[1]	1821	2123	2561	2848	3176	2917	3021	3195
Public health expenditure[1] (share of THE)	1312 (72%)	1515 (71.4%)	1821 (71.1%)	2054 (72.1%)	2385 (75.1%)	2103 (72.1%)	2154 (71.3%)	2249 (70.4%)
Out-of-pocket expenditure[1] (share of THE)	441 (24.2%)	516 (24.3%)	575 (22.5%)	599 (21%)	604 (19%)	636 (21.8%)	673 (22.3%)	708 (22.2%)
Practising doctors per 1,000 population	2.75[2]	3.14	3.22	3.62	3.6	3.82	3.85	4.02
Practising nurses per 1,000 population	3.26[2]	3.54	4.29	4.46	4.95	5.24	5.29	5.87
Curative care hospital beds per 100,000 population	299.73	289.33	269.91	260.90	252.70	244.32	248.05	249.67

Source: OECD (2021); Eurostat (2021a).

1 Constant PPPs (2015) per capita, in US dollars.
2 1996 data.

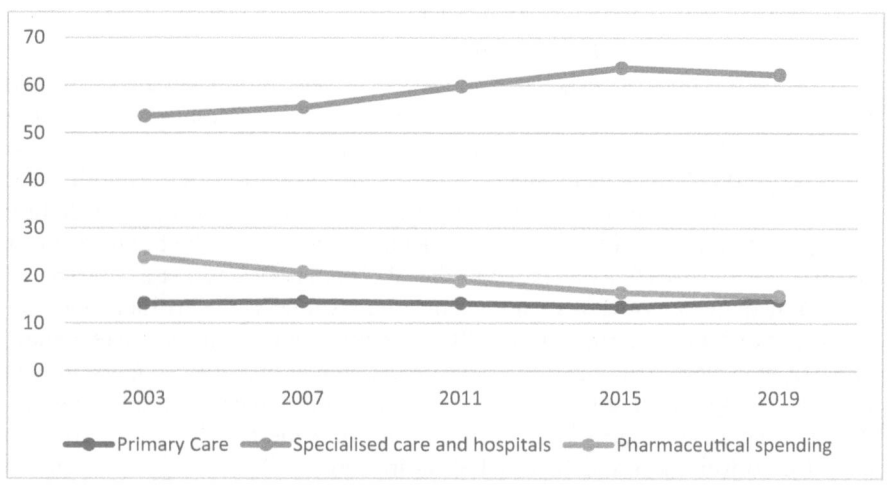

Figure 7.1 Percentage distribution of public health expenditure in Spain

Source: Ministerio de Sanidad, Consumo y Bienestar Social (2021); own elaboration.

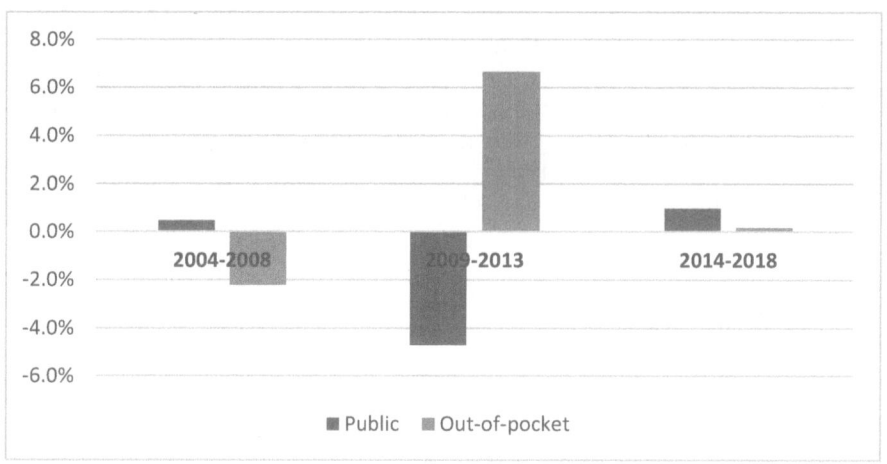

Figure 7.2 Average annual growth of expenditure on prescribed medicines in Spain (constant PPPs per capita in 2015, US dollars)

Source: OECD (2021); own elaboration.

introduction for pensioners – seems to have been stronger than pharmaceutical price control or rationalisation of prescription practices.

The measures on the supply side, in particular after the onset of the crisis, also targeted human and physical resources. There has been a trend towards less curative care beds (Table 7.1), which may owe more to the epidemiological shift towards chronic diseases rather than to the policies *per se*, and is very likely to

increase in the future due to the Covid-19 pandemic and the sequels of the infection on patients having suffered from it. While there was a small drop from 2012
to 2014, the number of beds has stabilised since then (approximately 250 beds
per 100,000 population). It is, however, substantially lower than the EU average
of nearly 400 beds. In the meantime, the number of practising doctors or nurses
has been gradually increasing since 1995. Yet the growth rates during the years
of harshest austerity were close to zero, or, in some cases, negative. In light of
said epidemiological shift, which is particularly relevant in the Spanish society
that has the highest life expectancy in the EU (Bernal-Delgado et al., 2018), the
most immediate outcome of spending cuts on personnel is the prolonged waiting
times (López-Valcárcel and Barber, 2017), for the demand for services remains
stable or may even grow due to greater distress under austerity. The mean waiting times for specialist consultation or elective surgery have indeed been gradually increasing (see Figure 7.3): from 54 days in 2006 to 81 days in 2019 for
specialist consultation and from 81 days in 2003 to 115 in 2019 for elective
surgery, and it is likely to substantially deteriorate due to the coronavirus pandemic. In addition, interregional variation of waiting times is large (Bacigalupe
et al., 2016; Spanish Economic and Social Council, 2020).

The increased privatisation of risk, long waiting times or insufficient number of hospital beds and doctors may have adverse effects on the population's
health due to inequities of access or declines in healthcare quality, although
their contribution is difficult to quantify, as well as taking time to affect. To
tentatively do so, we consider a number of objective and subjective indicators addressing healthcare quality and equity of access. First, treatable and
preventable mortality rates – that is, mortality that can be avoided/delayed
with timely and effective healthcare or illness prevention – have been rapidly
decreasing (Table 7.2) and are much below the EU average (Bernal-Delgado

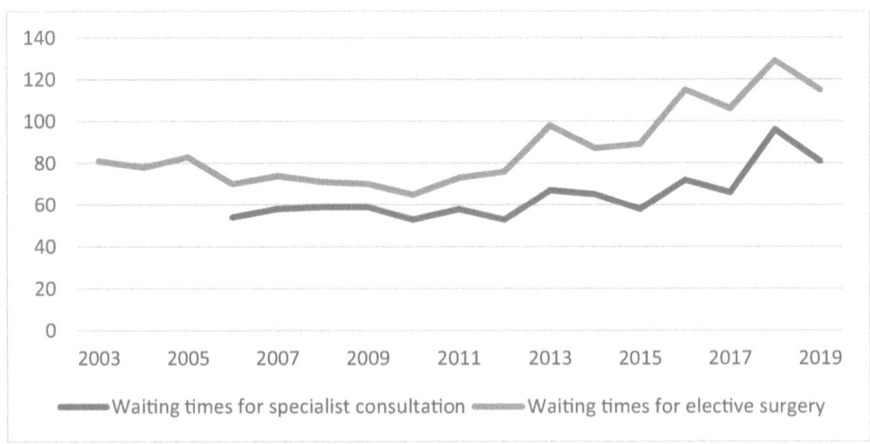

Figure 7.3 Mean waiting times in days in Spain

Source: Ministerio de Sanidad, Consumo y Bienestar Social (2021); own elaboration.

Table 7.2 Selected indicators on population health in Spain

	1995	2000	2003	2006	2009	2012	2015	2018
Life expectancy at birth	78.1	79.3	79.7	81.1	81.9	82.5	83.0	84.0[2]
Healthy life years at birth	na	na	Na	63.8	62.7	65.3	64.0	69.9[2]
Treatable mortality rate	na	80	76	68	62	56	53	51[3]
Preventable mortality rate	na	142	133	118	107	98	93	90[3]
Infant mortality rate[1]	5.5	4.4	3.9	3.5	3.3	3.1	2.7	2.7
Maternal mortality rate[1]	3	3.5	4.5	2.9	3.4	2.2	3.6	1.9
Self-perceived health as very good or good	na	na	Na	67.7%	70.6%	74.3%	72.4%	75.2%[2]
Unmet medical needs for health-system reasons	na	na	Na	0.6%	0.5%	0.7%	0.6%	0.2%
Unmet needs for dental care for financial reasons	na	na	Na	3.6%	4.6%	6.5%	4.9%	4.6%

Source: Eurostat (2021a, 2022); OECD (2021); Ministerio de Sanidad, Consumo y Bienestar Social (2021).

1 Per 100,000 live births.
2 2019 data.
3 2017 data.

et al., 2018). Infant and maternal mortality rates, which may likewise depend on healthcare quality to a certain degree, pursue a similar favourable trend. This good population's health is further supported by self-perceived health. Although the proportion of population perceiving their health as good or very good slightly decreased in 2013–2016, the trend is upward and above the EU average.

Self-reported unmet medical needs for health-system-related reasons might also signal inequities of access due to low affordability and availability of services through time (waiting times) or geographical barriers (Petmesidou, Guillén and Pavolini, 2020). While slightly increasing during the crisis, unmet medical needs have remained very low in Spain: 0.2% compared to the EU average of 2% in 2019 (Eurostat, 2021a). However, unmet needs for dental examination due to financial barriers, in particular, follow a different pattern. Not only did they increase during the crisis, but they also continue to double the EU average to date and are tightly related to individuals' income (Doblytė and Guillén, 2020). Since dental care is excluded from the common-benefit package, such unmet needs are related to income reductions rather than to the decreased scope of the health system. It does, nevertheless, point to gaps in it, and that cost containment might have hindered the further expansion of services.

To sum up, good perceived health, decreasing amenable and preventable mortality rates or very low unmet medical needs allow for a conclusion that equity of access and quality of healthcare remain high. The cost containment measures have not substantially affected these underlying principles of the Spanish NHS, nor have they negatively impacted the population's health (Bernal-Delgado et al., 2018; Petmesidou, Guillén and Pavolini, 2020). Yet territorial inequalities in access to health services continue to exist (Moreno Fuentes, 2012; Petmesidou, Pavolini and Guillén, 2014; Spanish Economic and Social Council, 2020). Some of such inequalities among regions were already present prior to the process of decentralisation; some surged and were exacerbated henceforth. This was due especially to asymmetric regional financing rules, thanks to which, for example, the Basque Country and Navarre enjoy a special and advantageous status. However, inequalities in access and the incidence of unmet medical need are intense; in fact, territorial equity of the NHS is significant both among and within regions. The trend towards increasing waiting times and the shift of cost to users of services also raise concerns, for this suggests that cost reduction has been achieved not necessarily by means of increased efficiency but by diminishing the public sector *per se* (Petmesidou, Guillén and Pavolini, 2020).

The institutional impact of neo-liberal health reforms

Neo-liberal health reforms have been pretty absent in Spain thus far and, when introduced, they have tended to affect the supply side rather than the demand one, thus bearing a lesser impact on equity. Over the past decades, the reforms *on the supply side* have aimed at controlling cost (decreasing expenditure or slowing down its increase rates) or at boosting performance, and as such, efficiency, albeit by means of different measures.

From the 1990s onwards, programme agreements, which settle certain quantity and quality of activity for agreed resources between the purchaser of services (centralised or regionalised) and the provider/manager of each health area, or prospective hospital budgeting both were introduced and can be viewed as performance-based instruments to achieve higher efficiency (Cabiedes and Guillén, 2001; Petmesidou and Guillén, 2008). In the meantime, the introduction of free choice of general practitioners during the same decade was to encourage primary healthcare physicians' performance by linking the number of patients they attract to financial incentives (Petmesidou and Guillén, 2008). In practice, however, the part of remuneration that depends on the number of patients is negligible and thus questions its effectiveness. In the 1990s, therefore, the main health reforms followed 'a trend towards prospective budgeting, implying stronger accountability and performance-based financing by a monopsony' (Cabiedes and Guillén, 2001:1211). Since 1997 too, some new hospitals have adopted the form of public foundations or public enterprises in order to endorse them with greater managerial flexibility and autonomy.

The few measures introduced *on the demand side*, which directly affect users of services by transforming the breadth, scope and depth of coverage, have been mainly implemented after the onset of the last crisis. Due to the unpopularity of such reforms among the electorate and opposition by the unions or users' associations, earlier proposals to institute, for instance, additional user charges were few and mainly unsuccessful (that is, the 1991 *Abril Report*, derived from the works of a parliamentary commission, that, among other measures, proposed the introduction of pharmaceutical co-payments for the retired population) (Cabiedes and Guillén, 2001). The closeness in time between the creation of the NHS and the initiation of the austerity period caused by the run-up to the Euro might have contributed to this strong opposition towards such reforms (Petmesidou and Guillén, 2008). While the establishment of a benefit package that included a positive and negative list of services in 1995 or the approval of a negative list of pharmaceuticals in 1993 may be viewed as cost-control measures on the demand side, such lists were hardly restrictive and did not diminish the scope or depth of coverage (Guillén and Cabiedes, 1997).

While the initial decades of the 2000s were rather devoted to enhancing cohesion and improving coordination among regional health services, as already pointed out, things were to change soon after the outbreak of the 2008 crisis. Already in 2011, under socialist rule, salary cuts for public employees were introduced (representing a large part of personnel in the health system), increased working hours, the freeze of new contracts (the reposition rate was established at 8%) or restructured and downsized some hospitals, among others (Doblytė and Guillén, 2020; López-Valcárcel and

Barber, 2017; Petmesidou, Pavolini and Guillén, 2014). The Ministry of Finance took over financial control to monitor uneven and disproportionate growth of health expenditure, to enforce certain targets and sanctions, and in turn, to improve health system sustainability (Bernal-Delgado et al., 2018; Del Pino and Pavolini, 2015).

The magnitude of the crisis and a new conservative government taking office in 2012 meant further move in the demand side. In particular, Royal Decree 16/2012 re-established the social insurance principle as the basis of entitlement to healthcare, and in turn, restricted access for undocumented adult immigrants limiting it to pregnancy and emergency care (Petmesidou, Pavolini and Guillén, 2014). Previously all irregular immigrants could access the public system under the only condition of being signed in a municipal census. The reform meant that around 870,000 people were to be deprived of their personal health cards. Besides the violation of the universality principle, its cost-effectiveness was criticised, for early detection of infectious diseases, or severe mental disorders, among others, can be more efficient (Repullo, 2014). Furthermore, the Decree introduced a co-payment on prosthesis, diet therapies and non-urgent sanitary transportation.

Reactions against these measures were intense and numerous among associations pro public healthcare provision and health personnel unions. The new co-payments were never enforced. The minister of health announced in 2014 that the intention of the government was to leave them unapplied (El Mundo, 13 January 2014). This means that the Spanish NHS remains free at the point of use, the only existent co-payments concerning outpatient prescription drugs. Since the passing of the Royal Decree, and especially after the regional elections of May 2015, almost all regional governments reacted against the reform on criteria for access to healthcare, either by passing legislation to lessen its consequences or by refusing implementation (López-Valcárcel and Barber, 2017; Petmesidou, Guillén and Pavolini, 2020). As of July 2018, the new socialist government fully reversed the 2012 legislation, and access was *de jure* re-universalised.

Royal Decree 16/2012 also re-centralised decision-making process regarding the benefit package. The common package to be implemented by all the regions and decided by the Interterritorial Council now consists of the basic (core services that are fully publicly funded), supplementary (outpatient pharmaceutical prescription, orthoprosthesis provision or non-emergency medical transport, among others) and accessory packages (non-essential services, not specified yet). The latter two imply cost-sharing that is centrally regulated. In the meantime, the regions may decide upon the complementary package, if they can justify the need for new services to the Interterritorial Council and guarantee their sufficient financing, once the common-benefit package is covered (Bernal-Delgado et al., 2018).

As a result of such re-definition of the benefit package, and in order to reduce pharmaceutical expenditure, the cost-sharing mechanism for outpatient pharmaceutical prescription that forms part of the supplementary package was also modified through the same Royal Decree. Co-payments were increased, but, at the same time, linked to users' household income levels (Doblytė and Guillén, 2020). The retired population, previously exempted from cost-sharing, was now obliged to pay a certain level of co-payment (namely 10%), albeit with a monthly cap. While the linking of co-payment to household income appears to be a more equitable approach, an absence of exemptions or monthly caps for the non-retired population may nevertheless result in financial barriers to healthcare for lower-income groups (Petmesidou, Guillén and Pavolini, 2020). Population contestation was also intense, as data collected by the Centre for Sociological Research (2021/22) show. This is why legislation on co-payments on outpatient prescription medicines was relaxed in December 2020 through the State Budget Law: several groups, including people receiving the minimum living wage or pensioners with an annual income below EUR11,200, were exempted from pharmaceutical co-payments.

To sum up, neo-liberal measures have affected mostly the supply side at the management level up to the onset of the last economic crisis. Reform during the economic crisis was addressed by reducing spending on both human and physical resources and placing caps on regional expenditure, together with the introduction of several measures affecting the demand side. These latter, nonetheless, either failed to be implemented (new co-payments), were legally reverted (population coverage) or lessened (co-payments on outpatient pharmaceuticals). Hence, the balance allows to conclude that the Spanish NHS remains as such. However, as we show in the next section, some creeping developments, together with the stress-test posed by the pandemic, may well endanger future sustainability.

Future sustainability

In order to assess future sustainability of the Spanish NHS, this section first deals with demographic and epidemiological trends and then focuses on the cultural and socio-political contexts.

Demographic and epidemiological trends

Spain is an ageing society, the proportion of population aged 65 years and more standing at nearly one-fifth of the whole population and only slightly below the EU-27 average in 2018, which can also be said of the proportion of population aged 80 and over (Table 7.3). However, due to longer average life expectancy and to lower fertility rates, population ageing is expected to be more intense in Spain in the coming years (see projections in Table 7.3). This generates a higher incidence of both chronic and degenerative diseases. Unsurprisingly, official data on mortality show that 45% of deaths were caused by cancer and heart diseases, while other degenerative and chronic illnesses account for the remaining bulk of causes of death (Table 7.4). Increasing

Table 7.3 Selected indicators on demographic transformations in Spain

		1995	2008	2018	2030[2]	2040[2]	2050[2]
Population aged 65 and more (%)	Spain	15.0	16.4	19.2	23.8	29.1	32.7
	EU-27[1]	14.8[3]	17.3	20.0	24.2	27.6	29.5
Population aged 80 and more (%)	Spain	3.3	4.5	6.2	7.3	9.3	12.3
	EU-27[1]	na	4.4	5.7	7.2	9.2	11.3
Median age of population	Spain	35.2	39.2	43.6	48.0	49.7	50.1
	EU-27[1]	na	40.6	43.4	46.1	47.7	48.2
Fertility rate	Spain	1.2	1.4	1.3	1.3	1.4	1.4
	EU-27[1]	na	1.6	1.5	na	na	na

Source: Eurostat (2021b, 2022).

1 From 2020.
2 Baseline projections.
3 EU-28.

Table 7.4 Mortality by causes in Spain in 2018

	Number of deaths	*Share of deaths*
Cancer/malignant neoplasms	108,526	25.4%
Heart diseases	83,744	19.6%
Cerebrovascular diseases	26,420	6.2%
Alzheimer disease	14,929	3.5%
Chronic lower respiratory diseases	14,607	3.4%
Pneumonia and influenza	12,267	2.9%
Accidents	11,530	2.7%
Diabetes mellitus	9,921	2.3%
Kidney diseases	7,629	1.7%
Hypertensive heart disease	4,998	1.2%
Parkinson disease	4,583	1.1%
Chronic liver disease	4,001	0.9%
Intentional self-harm	3,541	0.8%
Sepsis	3,040	0.7%
Intestinal ischemia	2,846	0.7%
Other causes	115,499	27%

Source: Ministerio de Sanidad (2021).

survival periods for patients affected by malignant neoplasms and cardio and cerebrovascular diseases will but intensify the demand for healthcare in upcoming years.

The cultural and socio-political context

Spaniards show a medium to high level of satisfaction and trust in their NHS. A general reluctance to pay more taxes for social protection improvements was detected by Calzada and del Pino (2019) and related to lower availability of resources in households during the past crisis together with a deterioration of the image of the fiscal system. In fact, prior to the crisis in 2005, 69.2% of citizens were in favour of exchanging fiscal support for better services (Calzada, 2007). Longitudinal changes in public opinion may be ascertained through the *Centro de Investigaciones Sociológicas* (CIS) time series of the Health Barometer. A detailed analysis can be found in Guillén and Luque (2020), covering the barometers issued from 2005 to 2018, while the corresponding ones for 2019 demonstrate continuity. The analysis comprises three axes, namely, the opinion of citizens on the functioning of the NHS, preferences for public or private provision, and public perceptions on the equity of healthcare provision.

According to the CIS Healthcare Barometer, in 2018, citizens considered that the main aspects of the NHS in need of change and the most pressing problems to be solved include, prominently, waiting lists (86.8%), followed by congestion of emergency services (67.7%), shortages of time devoted to patients in consultations (38.8%) and co-payments on outpatient prescription drugs (36.4%). Despite this, the degree of satisfaction with the NHS has remained pretty stable during the last 15 years. On a 1–10 scale, the average score has kept close to 6.5 since 2008, although slightly under such figure in the years 2014 (6.31) and 2015 (6.38), namely the years most affected by severe budgetary cuts due to the austerity-driven policies enacted during the crisis.

As to the level of care, the evolution of satisfaction is also pretty stable, with a slight decrease for the hospital and emergency care levels in the central years of the crisis (2013–2015). Again, on a scale ranging from 1 to 10, the greatest level of satisfaction goes to primary care (an average of 7.3 since 2011). At the opposite extreme are emergency services (6.0), while specialised care and hospital care score in between with an average of 6.8. However, while satisfaction remained stable, citizens' perceptions of the functioning of the system worsened significantly during the peak crisis years and consequent pressure on public expenditure. In fact, as compared to the previous five years, the percentage of citizens perceiving defective functioning grew from very low figures (around 10%) to 43.1% in emergency care, 37.3% in specialised care, 35.6% in hospital care and 29.7% in primary care (data for 2014). Such percentages tended to decrease during the crisis recovery period.

The opposite may be ascertained, though, as to perceptions of the quality of services received, that remained stable, around 75% evaluating it as good or very good, especially at the primary and hospital care levels. Health professionals are also valued very positively (7.7 over 10 in primary care and 7.37 in specialised and hospital care). Where citizens perceived a clear worsening trend was in the domain of waiting lists: those considering they had deteriorated went from 10% in 2010 up to almost 40% in 2014, to then fall to 24% in 2018. This does not match the real evolution of waiting lists, which, as noted earlier, have grown steadily since 2008.

The majority of interviewees consider that gender is not a differentiating factor, also applying to age intervals, socio-economic status or nationality of origin. Conversely, only 40% of respondents perceive that access to services is the same in rural areas as compared to urban ones. Last but not least, the highest inequalities perceived are those among the autonomous regions, even prior to the Great Recession (García Burgos et al., 2009). However, it has to be noted that satisfaction with services at the regional level is very weakly linked with the level of financial and human resources devoted to healthcare in each region, which, subject to further research, rather points to issues of organisation and management of regional services (Campos et al., 2016).

Nonetheless, closely related to the real growth of waiting lists and despite expressed perceptions is another indicator demonstrating that citizens are aware of such problems, namely the proportion of users now contracted to a private insurance premium. Again, in accordance with the data gathered by CIS Healthcare Barometers, this percentage grew from 7.9% in 2004 to 13.7% in 2018. To this, a further 3.5% of citizens enjoying double coverage in the same year through private premiums paid by companies have to be added. Data provided by the insurers' association even provide a higher figure, around 20% (UNESPA, 2019). The two main reasons put forward by individual contractors were those of reaching care quicker (77.9%) and getting specialised attention without referrals from primary doctors (37.3%).

Independent of the enjoyment of a private premium on top of public access, if citizens could choose between public and private provision, a large majority (over two-thirds) would prefer the former, with the exception of specialised care (only 55%). Nonetheless, it is to be underscored that, despite the high level of stress that the latest crisis imposed on the NHS, the percentage of citizens who would opt for public care grew significantly during the crisis. The reasons consist of higher technological assets and resources in general, better skills among public health professionals and better and clearer information on specific health problems. Against this, private services are preferred on the basis of higher comfort and a swifter reach of specialised services.

While it is still too early to ascertain the impact of the pandemic on citizens' attitudes to and perceptions of the Spanish NHS, one could claim that, in a nutshell, the majority of Spanish citizens remain attached to public provision in both good and bad times, especially in the case of serious illness and this despite growing waiting lists. A hypothetical explanation is that, when in dire straits, the presence of public services may be better valued, for shrinking disposable income entails lower opportunities to access private services. However, the increase in the number of individual private premiums is a matter of concern: it implies mounting inequalities between those able to pay for them and thus enjoy double coverage and those unable to do so.

Conclusion

Over the last four decades, the Spanish healthcare system has managed to weather many storms successfully. A complex transformation from an HIS built under a dictatorship into an NHS was first achieved, in parallel with the process of transition to a democracy. Soon after, when the new NHS was still less than a decade old, the run-up to the Euro-imposed austerity policies. Second, severe economic crises had to be faced, starting with the oil crises up to the recent Great Recession. Third, the system has shown a low degree of permeability to neo-liberal measures that were introduced mainly to the supply side for purposes of rationalisation, management, cohesion and coordination gains. Last but not least, while harsh austerity brought about by the need to appease the markets and comply with EU conditionality by means of budgetary cuts and the adoption of retrenchment measures, unmet medical needs and inequities grew as they were very much avoided.

However, the strains of the last 30 years have taken their toll. Especially during the most recent period, increasing waiting lists have led to a growing proportion of the population contracting private insurance premiums and overuse of emergency services. The share of public health expenditure has also shown a downward trend. Both of these developments speak of an increased effort by citizens and of a loss of equity between those who can resort to private provision and those whose income does not allow them to do so. On top of this, both perceived and objective increasing differences and dissimilarities can be ascertained among regional healthcare services.

To close, the Spanish NHS can still be termed as both equitable and efficient. Furthermore, satisfaction with, and trust in, it remains high. Still, the challenges for the future are immense. These are derived from projected even more intense ageing of the population than the current trend, and the corresponding consequences in terms of morbi-mortality patterns. The pandemic, even when fully over, will also mean increased pressure on the system, given the many long-term conditions that Covid-19 patients are suffering. Spain will need to further experience a tough period of recovery due to imbalances in public accounts and the coronavirus-induced economic crisis, which is most likely going to lead to even more intense consequences than the Great Recession. Given that poverty and shortage of economic resources in households are associated with worsening health conditions, a vicious circle may well occur.

While it is yet far too soon to know if the Spanish NHS will be able to weather yet another major storm, what is apparent is that the near future is plagued with severe challenges. The pandemic has revealed, as everywhere else, where the weakest points lie. As in any other healthcare system, in varying degrees, Covid-19-induced pressures have meant that too little attention and resources have been devoted to public health and far too much to the specialised and hospital levels, to the detriment of primary services. The coronavirus crisis has also brought to the fore the need for improved socio-sanitary care (as different from acute care) aimed at those suffering from chronic ailments.

References

Bacigalupe, A., Martín, U., Font, R., González-Rábago, Y. and Bergantiños, N. (2016) 'Austeridad y privatización sanitaria en época de crisis: Existen diferencias entre las comunidades autónomas?', *Gaceta Sanitaria* 30(1): 47–51.

Bernal-Delgado, E., García-Armesto, S., Oliva, J., Sánchez-Martínez, F. I., Repullo, J. R., Peña-Longobardo, L. M., Ridao-López, M. and Hernández-Quevedo, C. (2018) 'Spain: Health system review', *Health Systems in Transition* 20(2): 1–179.

Cabiedes, L. and Guillén, A. M. (2001) 'Adopting and adapting managed competition: Healthcare reform in Southern Europe', *Social Science and Medicine* 52: 1205–17.

Calzada, I. (2007) '¿Qué Estado de Bienestar queremos? Las opiniones de los ciudadanos sobre cómo son y cómo deberían ser nuestras políticas sociales', *Zerbitzuan, Revista de Servicios Sociales del Gobierno Vasco* 42: 103–14.

Calzada, I. and Del Pino, E. (2019) 'En lo bueno y en lo malo. Las opiniones de los españoles hacia las políticas sociales durante la crisis y más allá', *Documento de Trabajo 4.5 del VIII Informe FOESSA*. Available at: www.foessa.es/viii-informe/

Campos, M. S., Fernández-Montes, A., Gavilán, J. M. and Velasco, F. (2016) 'Public resource usage in health systems: A data envelopment analysis of the efficiency of health systems of autonomous communities in Spain', *Public Health* 138: 33–40.

Centro de Investigaciones Sociológicas *Barómetros Sanitarios*. Available at: www.cis.es/cis/opencm/ES/11_barometros/index.js

Del Pino, E. and Pavolini, E. (2015) 'Decentralisation at a time of harsh austerity: Multilevel governance and the welfare state in Spain and Italy facing the crisis', *European Journal of Social Security* 17(2): 246–69.

DiMaggio, P. J. and Powell, W. W. (eds) (1991) 'Introduction', in Powell, W. W. and Dimaggio, P. J. (eds) *The New Institutionalism in Organizational Analysis*, Chicago: University of Chicago Press.

Doblytė, S. and Guillén, A. M. (2020) 'Access compromised? The impact of healthcare reforms under austerity in Lithuania and Spain', *Social Policy and Society* 19(4): 521–37.

Eurostat (2021a) *Public-use Database of the Statistical Office of the European Union: Health*. Available at: https://ec.europa.eu/eurostat/web/main/data/database

Eurostat (2021b) *Public-use Database of the Statistical Office of the European Union: Population Projections*. Available at: https://ec.europa.eu/eurostat/web/main/data/database

Eurostat (2022) *Public-Use Database of the Statistical Office of the European Union: Demography, Population Stock and Balance*. Available at: https://ec.europa.eu/eurostat/web/main/data/database

García-Armesto, S., Abadía-Taira, M. B., Durán, A., Hernández-Quevedo, C. and Bernal-Delgado, E. (2010) 'Spain: Health system review', *Health Systems in Transition* 12(4): 1–295.

García Burgos, J., Stoyanova Matrakova, M., Fuente, I. A. and de la Oteo García, I. (2009) 'La percepción de los enfermos crónicos y de los usuarios asociados sobre el Sistema Nacional de Salud', *Biblioteca Lascasas* 5(1). Available at: www.index-f.com/lascasas/documentos/lc0390.pdf

Guillén, A. M. (2000) *La construcción política del sistema sanitario español: de la postguerra a la democracia*, Madrid: Ex Libris.

Guillén, A. M. (2002) 'The politics of universalisation: Establishing national health service in Southern Europe', *West European Politics* 25(4): 49–68.

Guillén, A. M. (2010) 'Defrosting the Spanish welfare state: The weight of conservative components', in Palier, B. (ed) *A Long Good-Bye to Bismarck: The Politics of Welfare Reforms in Continental Welfare States*, Amsterdam: Amsterdam University Press.

Guillén, A. M. and Cabiedes, L. (1997) 'Towards a National health service in Spain: The search for equity and efficiency', *Journal of European Social Policy* 7(4): 319–36.

Guillén, A. M. and Luque, D. (2020) 'La opinión pública sobre el sistema sanitario español', *Panorama Social* 30: 125–43.

Heclo, H. (1974) *Modern Politics in Britain and Sweden: From Relief to Income Maintenance*, New Haven, CT: Yale University Press.

Immergut, E. (1991) *Health Politics: Interests and Institutions in Western Europe*, Cambridge: Cambridge University Press.

López-Casasnovas, G., Costa-Font, J. and Planas, I. (2005) 'Diversity and regional inequalities in the Spanish "system of healthcare services"', *Health Economics* 14: S221–35.

López-Valcárcel, B. G. and Barber, P. (2017) 'Economic crisis, austerity policies, health and fairness: Lessons learned in Spain', *Applied Health Economics and Health Policy* 15: 13–21.

March, J. and Olsen, J. (1984) *Rediscovering Institutions*, New York: The Free Press.

Ministerio de Sanidad (2021) *Patrones de Mortalidad en España, 2018*. Available at: www.sanidad.gob.es/estadEstudios/estadisticas/estadisticas/estMinisterio/mortalidad/docs/Patrones_Mortalidad_2018.pdf

Ministerio de Sanidad, Consumo y Bienestar Social (2021) *Indicadores Clave Sistema Nacional de Salud*. Available at: http://inclasns.msssi.es/main.html

Moreno Fuentes, L. (2012) 'Políticas sanitarias en perspectiva comparada. Descentralización, mercados y nuevas formas de gestión en el ámbito sanitario', in Del Pino, E. and Rubio Lara, M. J. (eds) *Los Estados de Bienestar en la encrucijada. Políticas Sociales en perspectiva comparada*, Madrid: Tecnos.

Moreno Fuentes, L. (2019) 'Crisis económica y crisis de modelo en el Sistema Nacional de Salud', *VIII Informe FOESSA Documento de trabajo 4.7*. Available at: www.foessa.es/

Organisation for Economic Cooperation and Development (2021) *Public-Use Database of Organisation for Economic Cooperation and Development: Health Dataset*, Paris: OECD. Available at: https://stats.oecd.org

Petmesidou, M. and Guillén, A. M. (2008) '"Southern-style" national health services? Recent reforms and trends in Spain and Greece', *Social Policy and Administration* 42(2): 106–24.

Petmesidou, M., Guillén, A. M. and Pavolini, E. (2020) 'Healthcare in post-crisis South Europe: Inequalities in access and reform trajectories', *Social Policy and Administration* 54(5): 666–83.

Petmesidou, M., Pavolini, E. and Guillén, A. M. (2014) 'South European healthcare systems under harsh austerity: A progress-regression mix?', *South European Society and Politics* 19(3): 331–52.

Repullo, J. R. (2014) 'Cambios de regulación y de gobierno de la sanidad', *Informe SESPAS, Gaceta Sanitaria* 28(S1): 62–8.

Rico Gómez, A. (1997) *Descentralización y reforma sanitaria en España (1976–1996): Intensidad de preferencias y autonomía política como condiciones para el buen gobierno*, Doctoral dissertation, Autonomous University of Madrid. Available at: https://repositorio.uam.es/handle/10486/131121

Sierra Moros, M. J., Monge, S., Suarez Rodríguez, B., García San Miguel, L. and Simón Soria, F. (2021) 'COVID-19 in Spain: View from the eye of the storm', *The Lancet Public Health* 6(1): E10.

Spanish Economic and Social Council (2020) 'Memoria sobre la situación socioeconómica y laboral de España 2019', *Colección Memorias* 27. Available at: www.ces.es

UNESPA (2019) *Informe Estamos Seguros 2018*. Available at: www.estamos-seguros.es/informe-estamos-seguros/

Ventura, J. and González, E. (2013) 'Spain: Quo vadis? From cost containment to structural reforms', in Pavolini, E. and Guillén, A. M. (eds) *Health Care Systems in Europe Under Austerity: Institutional Reforms and Performance*, Basingstoke: Palgrave Macmillan.

8 Portugal

Joana Almeida

Introduction

In line with other Western European countries, and after several decades of dictatorship and a transition to democracy, Portugal successfully established a (quasi-)universal healthcare system, which was heavily shaken by the 2008 financial crisis. Just as it was recovering, it has seen the lasting impact of the coronavirus pandemic, which prompted 'the worst global economic recession since World War II' (Schiller and Hellmann, 2021:1). Since its inception, the country's public healthcare system has seen the implementation of reforms and public health strategies over the last four decades – the gradual adoption of neo-liberal policies since the 1990s being the most significant. The World Health Organization (WHO) (2018:13), however, has stated, 'Portugal has a strong record in development of health plans and strategies, and weaknesses in local approaches to implementation'.

The aim of this chapter is to assess the main changes and challenges in the Portuguese national healthcare service over the last four decades, and their impact on the public and other actors, such as the state, the medical profession and other healthcare workforce. To achieve this, a brief overview of the current socio-demographic context of the country will be presented, followed by an introduction to the Portuguese National Health Service (NHS), its structure and organisation. The main health policy reform strategies in primary, secondary and continuing care services will be addressed. Health policymaking in the context of the 2008 financial crisis and the Coronavirus pandemic will also be discussed. The chapter finishes by looking at the extent to which the Portuguese healthcare system is sustainable and will continue to be in a post-pandemic society. The analysis will be undertaken by using a neo-Weberian approach, which emphasises market conditions and power relations within and between professions and the state in the provision of services. This is complemented by a neo-institutionalist framework, in which the role and logics played by transnational governance structures become prominent.

DOI: 10.4324/9781003139799-13

The inception and development of the Portuguese National Health Service

Portugal has a population of 10.29 million (including Madeira and the Azores) (Instituto Nacional de Estatística, 2019) and has seen an increased life expectancy at birth since the turn of the century, lying slightly above the European Union (EU) average (81.9 compared to 80.9 years in 2017). Nonetheless, the gender and social class gap in life expectancy has been prevalent – with women living 6.2 years longer than men and those from lower socio-economic backgrounds living less than those from higher socio-economic ones. This is highlighted by the Organisation for Economic Cooperation and Development and European Commission (OECD, 2019).

The country has been a member state of the European Union (EU) since January 1986, and like many other EU countries, it has witnessed an ageing demographic – 21% of the population were aged 65 and over in 2017 – together with a fall in the fertility rate (now 1.38 births per woman) and an increased prevalence of chronic illness and co-morbidities (53% of the population aged 65 and over reported living with at least one chronic condition in 2017) (OECD and European Commission, 2019; WHO, 2020a). This has been accentuated by increasing emigration particularly among the younger educated generation since the 2008 financial crisis, and persistent gender, socio-economic and health inequalities (Sakellarides et al., 2014; OECD and European Commission, 2019). The current Covid-19 crisis will have further important consequences for Portuguese society. Even before this, the WHO (2018) stated that Portugal's population was expected to fall to 7.5 million by 2080.

The Portuguese NHS (*Serviço Nacional de Saúde* – SNS) was established in 1979 by Act 56/79, after the Carnation Revolution and in the context of the international crisis of the 1970s (Hespanha, 2019). It is a (quasi-)universal, almost free, and tax-financed welfare system, also subsidised by a social security system. The SNS complements social and private voluntary insurance schemes. Social insurance schemes can be traced back to pre-SNS healthcare provision, are occupation-based and cover about one-fifth to a quarter of the population (Barros, Machado and Simões, 2011); rather like those found elsewhere in continental Europe and parts of Latin America, they are principally enhanced social entitlements (health subsystems) for state-employed professionals such as teachers, the police, military, and some financial workers, who have greater choice of healthcare provision. Officially a universal public healthcare system, private voluntary healthcare insurance and out-of-pocket payments play a significant role in public healthcare expenditure in the country, providing access to private hospital care and ambulatory consultations (OECD and European Commission, 2019) for 10–20% of the population (Barros, Machado and Simões, 2011). This tripartite overlapping public, social and private mechanism comprises the healthcare security system. This system offers, or attempts to offer, integrated care, including health promotion, disease prevention, the diagnosis and treatment of the population, and medical and social rehabilitation (Assembleia da República Portuguesa – ARP, 1979:2357).

The SNS is managed centrally by the Ministry of Health and, at the regional level, by different local, public and private healthcare providers which operate under the supervision of five autonomous Regional Health Administrations (*Administrações Regionais de Saúde* – ARS) created in 1993 (Simões et al., 2017). A total of 308 municipalities and 3,091 sub-municipal localities represent the local level of government (Jalali, Bruneau and Colino, 2020; OECD and European Commission, 2019). The Directorate-General of Health (Direção Geral da Saúde – DGS) is a public body of the Ministry of Health which guides, monitors and regulates the healthcare field. Although the Ministry of Health controls, regulates and supervises the SNS, the decentralisation of tasks and of SNS management is a key principle included in the 1976 Constitution, the SNS Act and the Health System Act 95/2019. Article 6 of the 1976 Constitution states:

> [T]he state is unitary and the way in which it is organised and functions shall respect the autonomous island system of self-government and the principles of subsidiarity, the autonomy of local authorities and the democratic decentralisation of the Public Administration.
>
> (ARP, 2005)

Article 19 of the SNS Act also states that the SNS should promote the decentralisation of decision-making and the involvement of the service user in the planning and management of services (ARP, 1979). The Health System Act 95/2019 (which replaced the Health System Act 48/90 and Decree-Law 185/2002 which set the rules for private–public partnerships within the SNS) also states that the SNS has a regional organisation and participatory and decentralised management (ARP, 2019a).

Pereira (2011) highlights three phases of primary healthcare services in Portugal: the first phase was started prior to the SNS foundation, with the creation of the Health Centres (*Centros de Saúde* – CS) in 1971, which should be the first point of contact of the service user and should provide the best care to a family unit by the same professional and in each geographic area. This phase was particularly focused on strengthening public health in the country, by implementing sanitary measures and vaccination plans to tackle infectious diseases. Public health and hospital physicians and nurses were the main providers of care in the CS, since it was only in 1983 that the specialty of general practitioner was created and granted jurisdictional closure through Legislative Order 97/83, thus marking the second phase of the SNS. The second phase was also highly centralised by the General Directory of Primary Healthcare Services. It was as a reaction to too much centralisation that the third phase emerged, in 1999, through Decree-Law 157/99, which set the rules for the restructuring of the CS, and the establishment of Functional Units (*Unidades Funcionais* – UFs) such as the Family Health

Units (*Unidades de Saúde Familiar* – USFs), the Community Care Units and the Public Care Units, all with some functional, organisational and technical autonomy and composed of multidisciplinary teams. This restructuring, however, only happened in 2005, through Decree-Law 88/2005 which restored Decree-Law 157/99 after failed attempts at reform of primary healthcare services. In 2005, the Health Centres Clusters were then created, which include one or more CS and the USFs, and were decentralised from the ARS. The 2005 primary healthcare reform which restructured the CS and created the USFs was one of the most successful public health service reforms in Portugal since democratisation (Biscaia and Heleno, 2017).

In August 1990, the publication of the Health System Act 48/90 strengthened the regulatory role of the state and the relationship between the public, social and private sectors in healthcare provision, by setting up conventions and partnerships. A good example is hospital care which operates in the public and private sectors in the country. At the turn of the century, with the introduction of Law 27/2002 and Decree-Law 188/2003 and following EU New Public Management policy strategies, some SNS-run hospitals were given autonomous management, including decision-making power over financial, technical, and human resources and financial incentives to productivity and quality of care provision (ARP, 2003), thus allegedly increasing market competition. This resulted in 34 hospitals being corporatised and 31 named Entrepreneurial Public Entities (*Entidades Públicas Empresariais* – EPEs), expecting in return higher efficiency and cost-containment (Jardim, 2006). Public–private partnerships in the managing of hospital facilities and provision of healthcare services for long contractual periods (up to 30 years) were also established by Decree Law 185/2002.

Another good example of state partnership is continuing care. The delivery of efficient continuing healthcare services in Portugal has traditionally been a delicate area, which goes back to the 1980s, with the creation of private social solidarity institutions (WHO, 2020a). Further initiatives were developed throughout the 1990s, but it was only at the turn of the century that long-term care measures became more prominent. The 2004–10 National Health Plan identified palliative care as a priority area, focusing on intervention, organisation, and training in palliative care. In 2006, through Decree-Law 101/2006 and in recognition of demographic changes of the Portuguese population, the Ministry of Health created the National Network for Long-Term Integrated Care (Rede Nacional de Cuidados Continuados Integrados – RNCCI), in partnership with the Ministry of Labour, Solidarity and Social Security, directed to patients who needed post-hospital care (follow-ups, short-, medium- and long-term hospital recovery, rehabilitation and/or palliative care), through referral from primary or secondary healthcare services. Among the principles of the RNCCI were the 'proximity of care provision, through the empowerment of integrated services in the community' and the 'multidisciplinary and interdisciplinarity in the provision of care' (ARP, 2006:3858). The involvement of the service user and their carers in the care plan, provision of care and treatment process was also highlighted.

Expanding and coordinating long-term care were then a measure taken by the Ministry of Health through the implementation of the National Palliative Care Program 2011–13 (*Programa Nacional de Cuidados Paliativos –* PNCPs) in 2010, regulated by the RNCCI. The Development Strategy for the PNCPs 2011–13 called for a multi- and interdisciplinary approach to palliative care, implying the inclusion of the informal carers in the care plan to educate not only the service users but also themselves, in relation to their vulnerability throughout the palliative care process, and to provide physical, psychological and emotional support to the service user (Unidade Missão para os Cuidados Continuados Integrados, 2011). With care needs increasing, the palliative care response was improved with the creation of the National Commission for Palliative Care (CNCP) which coordinates the Palliative Care National Network (ARP, 2012). The RNCCI programme introduced important reforms in the provision of long-term care services in the country, resulting from strong cooperation between the SNS, the social service sector (mostly by the Holy House of Mercy) and private institutions (Baptista and Perista, 2018). The WHO (2020a), however, includes Portugal among those countries with a general provision of palliative care, still lacking a comprehensive palliative care provision, when compared with countries like the United Kingdom, Canada, Switzerland or France, that are at the forefront of palliative care, at a stage of its advanced integration into mainstream service provision. Figure 8.1 shows how, despite recent partnerships, long-term care is under-resourced and the average spending in the sector in 2019 was well below the OECD average.

Austerity policies enacted after the 2008 financial crisis reduced public financial resources for Portuguese health services and investment shrank (WHO, 2018), thus affecting their efficiency, delivery and quality. In May 2011, due to the country's elevated level of public debt, the Portuguese government signed a Memorandum of Understanding (MoU) with the Troika (the European Commission, European Central Bank and the International Monetary Fund), in exchange for a loan of €78 billion. The MoU included a

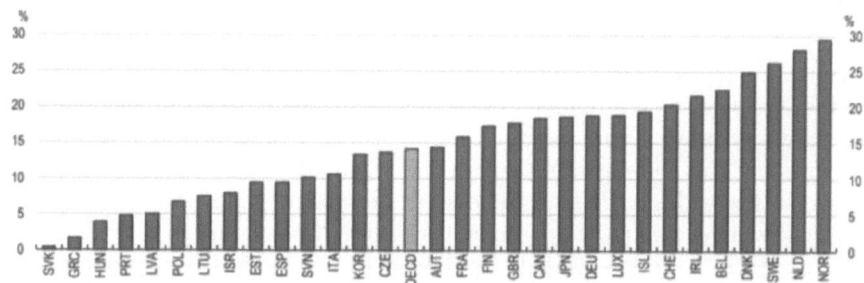

Figure 8.1 Spending in the long-term care sector in 2019 or latest year available
Source: OECD (2021b).

readjustment programme with punitive austerity measures to increase cost-containment, efficiency and regulation, directed to different sectors including health, which lasted until mid-2015. Consequently, expenditure on health was reduced, with some healthcare services in hospitals even forced to shut down (Jalali, Bruneau and Colino, 2020); there were salary cuts in the public sector and state pensions, the unemployment rate increased to a peak of 17.9% in January 2013, and the exodus of critical healthcare workforce such as nurses and medical doctors to other countries was and remains a national problem, causing a decline of this healthcare workforce in the country.

The main financial and post-financial crisis reforms of the SNS have been controversial, as some of these reforms, imposed by European and international bureaucratic institutions, were rejected by the state itself from 2015, while some of the proposed SNS state reforms are yet to be achieved. It is to these post-2011 reforms and their effect on the Portuguese healthcare system that we now turn.

The financial and post-financial crisis reforms of the *Serviço Nacional de Saúde*

Among the strategies that the Portuguese right-wing coalition government at the time used to try to recover its financial and political autonomy after the 2011 MoU was the implementation of reforms to rationalise service use and control public expenditure. Across sectors, including healthcare, many of those reforms were ostensibly based on improving regulation, governance, accountability and inclusivity. However, the main drivers were cost-cutting, with a coterminous extension of managerialism as a rebalancing mechanism in the pharmaceutical market set out in the MoU. According to the agreement, Portuguese physicians, the only health professionals in the country with the authority to prescribe, were to be instructed by the government to prescribe the least costly, generic medicines available following international prescription guidelines. This was to be combined with an enhanced monitoring system for drug prescriptions and a new complementary diagnostic exams prescription measured 'in terms of volume and value' (European Commission and Directorate-General for Economic and Financial Affairs, 2011:18). This increasing external control of the medical profession by the Portuguese state and the Troika represented a loss of professional autonomy and discretion and a marked shift towards greater economic and political influence for the state and supra-state organisations (Saks, 2016).

The MoU also contended that the Portuguese government had to strengthen primary and hospital care by rationalising services (European Commission and Directorate-General for Economic and Financial Affairs, 2011). This was done through the overall increase of SNS user charges, cuts in tax allowances and in health-benefit schemes, the increase in the number of USFs, to reach the more-needed population and tackle health inequality, and the diversion of service users from unnecessary visits to specialist and emergency services to primary care. The reinforcement of measures to guarantee increasing competition among private healthcare providers and to 'reduce by at least 10 per cent the overall spending (including fees) of the NHS with private providers delivering diagnostic and therapeutical services to the NHS by end 2011 and by an additional 10% by end 2012' (European Commission and Directorate-General for Economic and Financial Affairs, 2011:19) is also mentioned in the MoU. The power of the ARS in setting the rules for the provision of private healthcare providers shifted to the Troika, in compliance with the European competition rules of this provision. Finally, the move of some hospital care services to community care was also highlighted. Once again, these reforms suggest the existence of different and wider structures of power beyond the professions and the state, changes in power dynamics, and increasing institutional competition, in theory at least, between multiple ecologies, such as healthcare professions, the Portuguese state, the SNS, private healthcare providers, the EU and international decision-making groups. Because of the MoU implementation, not only professional autonomy but also state, financial and political autonomy decreased until 2015.

During the implementation of the Troika's austerity measures, the demand for healthcare services decreased due to a considerable disinvestment in access to healthcare in the country, resulting in a decline of the volume of healthcare services in the SNS, public health sector and mental health services. Health sector expenditure fell from 9.8% of General Domestic Product (GDP) at the end of 2010 to 9% in 2015 (Nunes and Ferreira, 2018). Contributing to this were the policies enacted to control pharmaceutical expenditure, such as the reduction in prices of generics and compulsory e-prescription, allowing for better monitoring and auditing of doctors and pharmacies and the increasing availability of the cheapest medicines in pharmacies (European Commission, 2014).

According to the European Commission's report on Portugal's performance, the austerity reforms led to an increase in the number of USFs from 326 in 2010 to 397 in 2013, and the number of people without a family doctor decreased from 17% to 14%; the development of telemedicine and of an electronic platform of medical records accessed by primary care providers and hospitals also contributed to a more cost-effective use of the country's healthcare services (European Commission, 2014). The reorganisation and streamlining of the hospital network, with the reclassification of hospitals, also led to budgetary savings; the reforms of the public-sector health insurance sub-system, with an increase of the beneficiaries' contributions and a decrease of state contributions, and a revision of services covered and reimbursed resulted too in cost-efficiency improvements. The report concludes that austerity reforms produced significant savings, but there were still challenges ahead to create financial gains to pay the overdue debt. It was during austerity that seven complementary and alternative medicines (CAM) gained statutory regulation in the country through Act 71/2013, although they are not widely available through the SNS, and some are still in a transitional state as they have not achieved full regulation since then (Almeida and Barros, 2020).

In November 2015, however, António Costa's Socialist Party formed an alliance with three anti-EU, and more radical left-wing parties, the Portuguese Communist Party, the Left Bloc Party and the Ecologist Party known as 'The Greens'. Taking office as a majority government, they aimed to ease austerity and reverse some of the most negative aspects of the Troika-mandated fiscal retrenchment. Costa's government no longer needed external assistance but had to deal with the consequences of the punitive measures imposed by the Troika's package. An agreement between Costa's Socialist Party and each of its government allies was signed, proposing a reversal of all Troika's austerity measures. For example, this joint position included policies to fight social and economic inequality and impoverishment. The government agreed to increase the national minimum wage by 20%; it also raised the state pension and decreased income taxes for employees. In addition, it proposed to safeguard public services by banning new privatisations; increasing taxes on large firms; strengthening the SNS by boosting its financial, technical and human resources; and registering every single citizen with a family doctor and nurse, a project which had never been successfully completed despite previous attempts to do so.

The abolition of SNS user charges, seen as an obstacle to accessing public healthcare services, was also considered, and each agreement called for political decentralisation (De Sousa and Da Costa, 2015; Partido Socialista and Partido Ecologista Os Verdes, 2015; Partido Socialista and Bloco de Esquerda, 2015). Through these agreements, the *geringonça* (a pejorative term used by other parties to refer to the coalition) aimed to reverse the economic and social degradation caused by the punitive measures enacted by the previous right-wing government and the Troika and to restore governmental financial and political power and autonomy. The Health System Act 95/2019 (which replaced Act 48/1990 and Decree-Law 185/2002), for example, initiated the introduction of new rules for the establishment of new public–private partnerships in the healthcare sector, which became temporary or supplementary, and for cases of justified need.

The impact of the anti-austerity measures of the *geringonça* was reflected in a sharp fall in the unemployment rate from 16.3% in 2013 to a single-digit rate in 2017 (8.9%) and to 6.1% in 2021 (Instituto Nacional de Estatística, 2020), reflecting a decrease in the public deficit, and increasing economic activity and health expenditure growth (OECD and European Commission, 2019). By 2017, state expenditure on health had decreased to 66.4%, while healthcare expenditure per capita increased (although still below the EU average), mainly due to an increase in out-of-pocket spending (one of the highest among OECD and EU countries), which counted for 27.5% of total healthcare gains (OECD, 2016; OECD and European Commission, 2019). The *geringonça* proved to be an effective machine, enacting large-scale reform without clashing with the Troika's fiscal rules, proving it is possible to be 'in and against' the EU and to remain and reform (Wainwright, n.d.). By 2018, the Euro Health Consumer Index ranked the country 13th out of 35 countries, just behind Germany and France. It scored well in overall outcomes (although suicide rates and MRSA infections received red scores), accessibility to services, and patient rights and information areas. However, it still scored lower in pharmaceuticals, prevention (red scores were still flagged for alcohol misuse and traffic deaths), and the range and reach of services provided (with red scores for caesarean sections, percentage of dialysis effected outside clinics, and equity of the healthcare system) (Health Consumer Powerhouse, 2018).

In October 2019, a new centre-left Socialist government was elected with 36% of the votes. This time, there was no formal agreement with the other left-wing parties but instead the Socialist Party took up office alone as a minority government, until January 2022. This new government maintained the programme of the coalition which preceded it in dealing with the impact of austerity policies, as well as with the impact of Brexit on the country's economy, the rise of populist parties and the significant effect of the new and unexpected infectious disease caused by the coronavirus on the healthcare system. The expectation of another international crisis due to the Covid-19 pandemic, which may surpass the 2008 monetary crisis, is not a bright scenario for the SNS, which has become vulnerable again to pressure for rationalisation and cost containment as austerity measures. As Shaaban, Peleteiro and Martins (2020) have stated, during previous economic crises, the Portuguese healthcare sector became politically and financially vulnerable and a target for budget cuts, due to its size and the high potential for improved performance. In January 2022, an early general election triggered by a rejection of the proposed state budget for 2022 took place, and Costa's Socialist Party won a parliamentary majority for the first time. The main reason for this electoral success was the way the previous Costa's minority government handled the pandemic – not least through its positively regarded vaccination programme. On 7 July 2022, the new SNS Statute (Decree-Law 1171/ XXII/2021) was approved by the Council of Ministers (replacing the one in place since 1993), with the main aim of implementing all aspects of the Health System Act 95/2019, by reinforcing the role of the SNS and setting up a new SNS Executive Directorate (Lusa, 2022). We turn now to the way the SNS has been affected by and responded to the Coronavirus pandemic.

Covid-19: its effects on the *Serviço Nacional de Saúde* and population health

Covid-19, declared as a pandemic by the WHO (2020c) on 11 March 2020, has had an enormous impact on healthcare systems globally. The SNS has long been focused on non-communicable diseases (Varanda, Gonçalves and Craveiro, 2020). Therefore, it was not prepared to mitigate the effects of new unexpected infectious diseases efficiently and rapidly such as SARS-CoV-2. Varanda, Gonçalves and Craveiro (2020) argue that the powerful sense of local community was a main asset in the country in handling the Covid-19 pandemic; the mobilisation of the population in implementing lockdown measures started before the President of the Republic Marcelo Rebelo de Sousa's first declaration of the state of emergency on 18 March 2020, which lasted until 2 May 2020 under pressure from civil society. Following many other European countries, the Portuguese government published population measures in its National Plan for preparing and responding to coronavirus (*Plano Nacional de Preparação e Resposta à Doença por Novo Coronavírus* [Covid-19]) on 11 March 2020. This consisted of the lockdown of the population at home except for some key workers, the use of antiseptic products and face masks, social distancing, and quarantine (Direção Geral da Saúde, 2020) – and, more recently, a national vaccination programme. The DGS also created Taskforce COVID-19, which included health specialists and experts to advise and work on the pandemic and coordinate the vaccination plan, which started in December 2020.

A 2020 population-wide survey conducted by the Portuguese Medical Council (PMC) and the Portuguese Association of Hospital Administrators (PAHA) on the impact of Covid-19 revealed that 81% of the participants felt very positive about the work of medical doctors and nurses during the pandemic. Here, a significant majority expressed high levels of trust in the provision of care by medical doctors, healthcare centres and public hospitals, although 73% felt that healthcare investment had not been sufficient. These relatively high levels of trust can be illustrated by the high vaccination rate against coronavirus – one of the highest among OECD countries (OECD, 2021b). Furthermore, in November 2020, the user charges were abolished for medical consultations and complementary diagnostic exams in primary healthcare by Decree-Law 96/2020. However, WHO (2022b) data also show disruption in emergency and outpatient primary care services for non-Covid-19 conditions, cancer screening and treatment, elective surgery, rehabilitative care, routine immunisation coverage and misuse of antibiotics to treat Covid-19, all leading to a backlog of care.

In European countries heavily hit by the 2008 financial crisis and the Troika's radical measures in countries such as Portugal, the Covid-19 impact has been particularly evident where the government has traditionally struggled to provide adequate services. In the Portuguese case, latent problems have existed with the accessibility and quality of mental health services, the number of inpatient hospital beds, community care and long-term, chronic care services, and medical human, technical and digital resources. OECD (2021a, 2021b) data show how the percentage of the population with above-basic overall digital skills was very low and below the OECD average in 2019. According to such data, unmet need for mental healthcare lies at 63.5%, although there is no comprehensive dataset available capturing the extent of demand for mental health services in Portugal. The recent Global Burden of Disease Study in 2019 (Castelpietra et al., 2022) also corroborates these data on the mental health status of young people aged 10–24 years in the period between 1990 and 2019 in the country, by concluding that, out of 31 European countries, Portugal has the highest burden of common (depression and anxiety) and severe (schizophrenia and bipolar disorder) mental health conditions.

Unmet need is driven by financial pressures, waiting times, inefficient SNS transport, lack of telemedicine services and an extremely limited mental health workforce capacity and community-based support. Another survey showed an increasing vulnerability to mental health problems due to financial and job disruption, work–family balance issues and unsettled routine – and highlighted how informal networks of aid, entrenched familism and third sector institutions have prevented the Covid-19 pandemic from being more damaging to people's lives (Magalhães et al, 2020). Figure 8.2 shows that over 20% of the population reported symptoms of psychological distress before the pandemic, one of the highest rates across Europe. Burnout syndrome among Portuguese medical doctors and nurses was already a frequently reported issue before the pandemic, often associated with poor working conditions (Marôco et al., 2016) – and, with coronavirus, incidences of burnout syndrome have persisted (Serrão et al., 2021). The scientific brief of the WHO (2022a) based on early evidence of the pandemic's impact on the mental health and well-being of the world's population shows how Covid-19 has indeed led to an increase of mental health problems among service users and healthcare workers and how this increased risk for suicidal behaviours, particularly among the most vulnerable.

One of the consequences of the post-crisis cost-containment measures in the Portuguese healthcare sector was the lowering of the number of curative care beds. In 2020, Portugal had one of the lowest numbers of curative care beds (3.5) per 1,000 inhabitants when compared to other OECD countries (OECD, 2022). Furthermore, the number of people without a family doctor has also increased during the pandemic to a total of 1,050,000 (Lusa, 2021). In addition, only 9% of the population had a telemedicine consultation during the

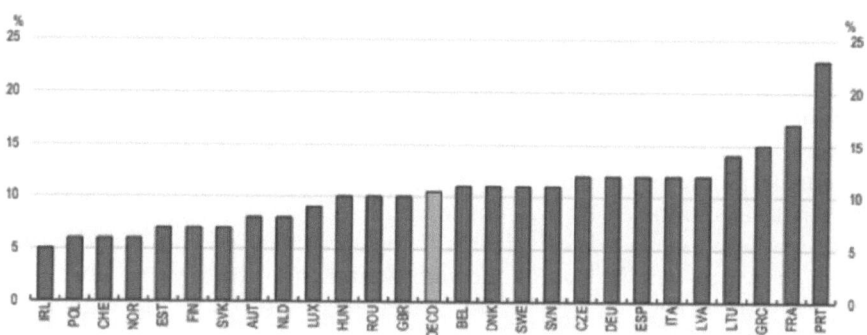

Figure 8.2 Prevalence of psychological distress among the population aged 16 and over in 2018

Source: OECD (2021b).

crisis, mostly by phone (95%) (PMC and PAHA, 2020). Finally, although the Portuguese government has shown a preoccupation with extending care to service users with permanent functional impairments, such as mental health conditions, the fragile elderly and the terminally ill, the WHO (2020a) highlights that there are still persistently high rates of institutionalisation of the chronically ill, geographical inequalities, limited accessibility, long waiting lists, a high proportion of hospital readmissions without ambulatory contact and very limited digital platforms allowing for effective data management and cooperation between the SNS and the social service sector. In addition, the strong association between chronic and informal care (provided mainly by female family members) has helped to reinforce the absence of comprehensive state services (Baptista and Perista, 2018), a dynamic which has been exacerbated by the pandemic crisis.

Portugal will receive around €61 billion over 2021–29, in particular from the EU's Recovery and Resilience Facility and the Cohesion Policy funds (OECD, 2021b), to recover from the pandemic. Portugal's Recovery and Resilience Plan provides for a resilient SNS, including the expansion of the healthcare network in rural areas, the reform of mental health policies and the digitalisation of the healthcare system. The analysis now turns to the future sustainability of the SNS.

The future sustainability of the *Serviço Nacional de Saúde*

The WHO (2018) and the Observatório Português dos Sistemas de Saúde (2014) note that, despite significant changes in interprofessional work over the last four decades, Portuguese health service provision remains very doctor-centred and hospital-centred. The WHO (2018) calls for a greater variety of healthcare workers within the system, with more diverse skills, and a better configuration of health professionals to meet the needs of a growing elderly population with complex and chronic co-morbidities. For example, there is a need to sustain long-term care services with an effective number of long-term care workers, with proper training, empowerment and better remuneration of less qualified support work providers such as healthcare assistants. According to the OECD (2021b), Portugal has one of the lowest numbers of long-term care workers, as shown in Figure 8.3, and about 60% of these workers have minimum education levels, as Figure 8.4 illustrates.

Furthermore, as shown by the Covid-19 pandemic, the Portuguese welfare state is supported by a strong welfare society. Political commitment to address the unmet needs of informal carers will be the key to tackling high rates of institutionalisation of the elderly and the mentally and chronically ill. The Bill in February 2019, with measures to support and regulate the duties and rights of long-term informal carers and patients approved by the Council of Ministers, has been a step further (Comunicados do Conselho de Ministros, 2019), but this should be further developed in a post-pandemic, more sustainable SNS, with a broader awareness of long-term, chronic and palliative care.

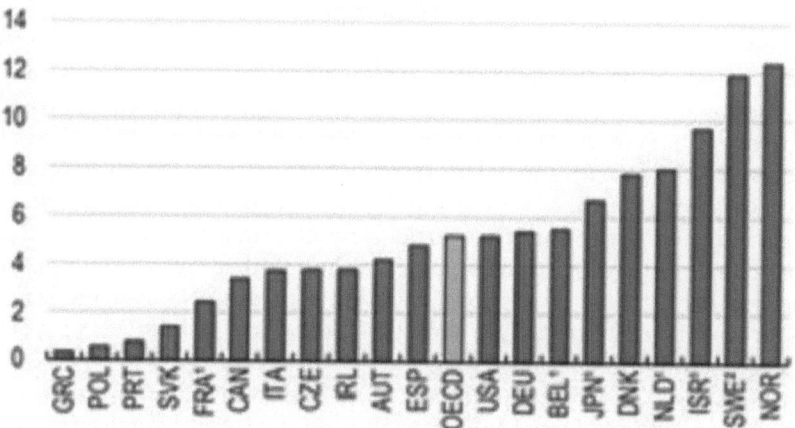

Figure 8.3 Number of long-term care workers per 100 individuals aged 65 or more in 2019 or latest year available

Source: OECD (2021b).

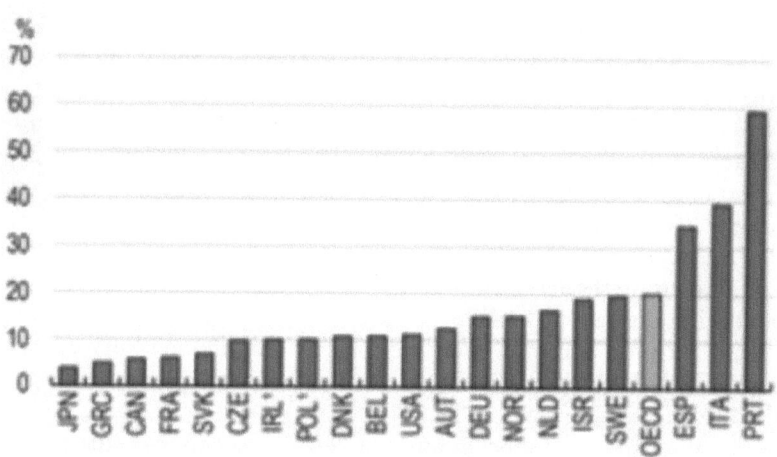

Figure 8.4 Percentage of long-term care workers with lower secondary school education in 2019 or latest year available

Source: OECD (2021b).

Boosting community-based care and interventions should also be a priority. For example, Perelman and colleagues (2018) suggest greater involvement of primary care centres in the prevention and treatment of mild mental health conditions such as depression by using psychosocial interventions (moving away from pharmaceuticals), as well as general practitioners (GPs) and nurses and psychologists and mental health workers. Community-based care and multi-disciplinary teams that go beyond the GP, psychiatrist and nurse are also recommended for severe mental illness, since they allow for lower stigma, better reinsertion and fewer readmissions. The Portuguese Psychology Council Review of the SNS Statute (Ordem dos Psicologos Portugueses, 2021) provides an alert for the need to increase the number of psychologists within the SNS and highlights that mental healthcare remains a neglected area in the country, particularly at primary care level and after the pandemic; according to the Council, although there was a slight increase in the number of these professionals working for the SNS over the last four years (from 917 in 2018 to 1,063 in 2021), there are still only 2.5 psychologists per 100,000 population.

To boost community care services, it is important to commit to decentralisation of services. Despite decentralisation measures being mentioned in the Portuguese Constitution and in some of the most important healthcare Acts in the country, according to the 2000 Sustainable Governance Indicators (Jalali, Bruneau and Colino, 2020), Portugal is one of the most centralised Western European countries. Few responsibilities are decentralised, thus explaining the extremely low levels of subnational public expenditure. For example, OECD and European Commission (2019) data show that the subnational government expenditure in Portugal only accounts for 13.3% of total public expenditure (compared to an EU average of 33.6%) or 5.9% of GDP (compared to an EU average of 15.3%). Although the country has taken some measures towards decentralising some competences to local authorities through Law 50/2018 and Decree-Law 23/2019 (ARP, 2018, 2019), authors like Abrantes (2019) have argued that this has been an illusory decentralisation, meaning an administrative transference of power without the corresponding transference of financial resources, which remain under the control of central government. Furthermore, for decentralisation to be successful, it is essential to equip the service providers with digital technologies and upskill the population digitally. The Digital Transition Action Plan was launched in April 2020 with the aim of digitalising the state services and private companies and upskilling the population through digital inclusion and literacy and digital education.

The WHO (2020b), in its coordinated global research roadmap for coronavirus, supports research priorities which can pre-prepare healthcare systems for the next epidemic. Shaaban, Peleteiro and Martins (2020) state that the Covid-19 crisis poses an important challenge to the Portuguese government in regard to retaining the current healthcare workforce and avoiding future shortages. The exodus of healthcare workers has traditionally been a problem in the country, mainly due to precarious working conditions and remuneration – more so in a post-pandemic society where countries with more developed economies might be attracting healthcare providers due to their shortages in medical human resources. Shaaban, Peleteiro and Martins (2020) also recommend that healthcare spending should focus on the development of specialities such as anaesthesiology, radiology and emergency room medicine, where valuable skills to treat infectious diseases like Covid-19 lie. They think too that there should be more public health medical doctors, which represent only 1.5% of all physicians, as well as medical disaster specialists. Furthermore, the new SNS statute (República Portuguesa, 2021) includes plans to increase professional motivation and attract healthcare professionals to rural areas, with a potential impact on tackling geographical inequalities in health.

Health promotion to prevent and control disease is another area for improvement. The National Health Plan 2012–20 did focus on health promotion, education and well-being and presents as goals the reduction of premature mortality (70 years and under) to below 20%, the increase of life expectancy at 65 years of age by 30%, the reduction of smoking rates among those aged 15 and over, and the control of excess weight and obesity among children. The 2012–20 National Health Plan and the new SNS statute also introduce the concept of co-production in health, where citizens, professionals, the different administrative sectors of the SNS and other interested parties contribute to governing health (Direção Geral da Saúde, 2015; República Portuguesa, 2021).

Finally, rethinking the use of language in the country's health policymaking is also important, more so if the future direction is towards multi-professionalism, integrative healthcare, collaboration and workforce equity. One of the recommendations of the OPP (2021) to the new SNS Statute Proposal is to reconsider the use of the word 'medic'; for example, expressions like 'medical personnel', 'medical action' and 'medical activity' should be replaced by 'health personnel', 'medical and health action' and 'medical and health activity'.

Conclusion

This chapter has presented a case study of the Portuguese NHS to illustrate the effect of increasing neo-liberal and austerity measures within the healthcare sector in a Western European context over the last 40 years. As previously stated, the Portuguese public healthcare system was set up in the 1970s as a (quasi-)universal, almost free and tax-financed welfare system, subsidised by a social security system. Nowadays, the SNS is still tax-financed and subsidised by a social security scheme, but still not fully grounded on the principles of universal accessibility and health coverage, free at the point of delivery. The tripartite public, social and private health insurance system has coexisted and created significant inequalities in terms of healthcare coverage. The pre-SNS health subsystems continue to cover several employees who have access to a wider choice of providers and higher reimbursement levels. Neo-liberal and austerity policies imposed by the Troika during the 2008 financial crisis included the increase of SNS user charges, and although one of the goals of the *geringonça* was to abolish these fees, this was only achieved in Costa's minority government and during the peak of the pandemic. Furthermore, there are healthcare services that are still not fully covered by the SNS, due to geographical inequalities, or where out of pocket spending and the role of the private sector is very high (as in dental or mental healthcare, for example).

The 2008 financial crisis and the intervention of the Troika in the country are a clear example of an attempt to move to more transnational modes of governance and regulation that go beyond the classic neo-Weberian state–profession relationship where professions are protected by the state usually through professional regulation. Such health professions were able to regulate market conditions through forms of exclusionary closure, thus limiting the opportunities of outsiders and leading to an increase in their income, status and power (Brock and Saks, 2016). However, the multiple logics at play during the crisis shifted some of the traditional power of the state and professions to transnational organisations, even though during the *geringonça* government and during the peak of the Covid-19 pandemic, the state claimed some of its powers back to demonstrate that it was fit to govern the country.

The complex intersecting levels that the state and its different administrative sectors, the professions, the patients and public, private organisations and transnational institutions such as the EU and the WHO have had to engage in during the coronavirus pandemic is another good example of the hybrid regulatory and managerial control present in neo-liberal policies in the West. On one hand, the Portuguese government needs to regulate and empower more professionals to diversify the SNS workforce, promote interprofessionalism, and turn SNS careers more attractive and improve workforce equity; on the other hand, the Portuguese state needs to delegate power to its sub-national levels of governance and decentralise. However, it also needs to align itself with transnational and multinational organisations and follow pandemic and post-pandemic guidelines.

The Covid-19 crisis has also exposed areas where the government has traditionally struggled and created new opportunities for new investments and reforms of the SNS. For example, Costa's newly elected government has the task of meeting the goals of the country's Recovery and Resilience Plan and the new SNS Statute. How the interaction between this complex network of actors will unfold in a post-pandemic society with the long-term effects of coronavirus should be the focus of future analysis.

References

Abrantes, R. D. (2019) 'Decentralization and (de)politization in Portugal: Descentralização e (des)politização em Portugal', *Perspectivas – Journal of Political Science* 20: 33–44.

Almeida, J. and Barros, N. (2020) 'Complementary and alternative medicine as an invisible health support workforce', in Saks, M. (ed) *Support Workers and the Health Professions in International Perspective: The Invisible Providers of Health Care*, Bristol: Policy Press.

Assembleia da República Portuguesa (1979) *Lei no. 56/79 – Sistema Nacional de Saúde*, 15 Setembro. Diário da República, 1, Série, 214, 2357–63. Available at: 369864 (dre.pt)

Assembleia da República Portuguesa (2003) *Decreto-Lei no.* 188/2003, 20 agosto. Diário da República, I Série-A, 191, 5219–30. Available at: 654581 (dre.pt)

Assembleia da República Portuguesa (2005) *Constituição da República Portuguesa. VII Revisão Constitucional.* Available at: Constituição da República Potuguesa (parlamento.pt)

Assembleia da República Portuguesa (2006) *Decreto-Lei no. 101/2006*, 6 junho. Diário da República, Série I-A, 109, 3856–65. Available at: 353934 (dre.pt).

Assembleia da República Portuguesa (2012) *Lei de Bases dos Cuidados Paliativos.* Lei no. 52/2012, 5 Setembro. Diário da República no. 172, 1, série, 5119–24. Available at: 0511905124.pdf (dre.pt).

Assembleia da República Portuguesa (2018) *Lei no. 50/2018.* 16 agosto. Diário da República no. 157/2018, Série I, 4102–8. Available at: Lei 50/2018, 2018–08–16 – DRE.

Assembleia da República Portuguesa (2019a) *Lei no. 95/2019 Lei de Bases da Saúde*, 4 setembro. Diário da República, 1 Série 214, 2357–63. Available at: Lei 95/2019, 2019–09–04 – DRE.

Baptista, I. and Perista, P. (2018) *ESPN Thematic Report on Challenges in Long-Term Care. Portugal*, Brussels: European Commission. Available at: PT_ESPN_thematic report on LTC.pdf

Barros, P. P., Machado, S. R. and Simões, J. de A. (2011) 'Portugal: Health system review', *Health Systems in Transition* 13(4). Available at: HiT_Portugal web version.indd (who.int)

Biscaia, A. R. and Heleno, L. C. (2017) 'Primary health care reform in Portugal: Portuguese, modern and innovative', *Ciência e Saúde Coletiva* 22(3): 701–12.

Brock, D. and Saks, M. (2016) 'Professions and organizations: A European perspective', *European Management Journal* 34: 1–6.

Castelpietra, et al. (2022) 'The burden of mental disorders, substance use disorders and self-harm among young people in Europe, 1990–2019: Findings from the Global Burden of Disease study 2019', *The Lancet Regional Health – Europe* 16(100341).

Comunicados do Conselho de Ministros (2019) *Comunicado do Conselho de Ministros de 7 de fevereiro de 2019.* Available at: Comunicado do Conselho de Ministros de 7 de fevereiro de 2019 – XXI Governo – República Portuguesa (portugal.gov.pt).

De Sousa, J. and Da Costa, A. G. (2015) *Posição Conjunta do PS e do PCP sobre a Solução Política*, 10 Novembro. Available at: posicao_conjunta_pcp_ps_sobre_situacao_politica.pdf

Direção Geral da Saúde (2015) *Plano Nacional de Saúde. Revisão e Extensão a 2020.* Lisbon: DGS. Available at: Plano-Nacional-de-Saude-Revisao-e-Extensao-a-2020.pdf (netdna-ssl.com).

Direção Geral da Saúde (2020) *Plano Nacional de Preparação e Resposta à Doença por Novo Coronavírus (COVID-19)*, Lisbon: DGS. Available at: Plano-de-Contingência-Novo-Coronavirus_Covid-19.pdf (min-saude.pt)

European Commission (2014) *The Economic Adjustment Programme for Portugal 2011–2014*, Occasional Paper 202, Brussels: European Union. Available at: The Economic Adjustment Programme for Portugal. 2011–2014 (europa.eu).

European Commission and Directorate-General for Economic and Financial Affairs (2011) *Portugal: Memorandum of Understanding on Specific Economic Policy Conditionality*, 17 May.

European Observatory on Health Systems and Policies, and European Commission. (2019) *State of Health in the EU: Portugal. Country Health Profile 2019*. Available at: 85ed94fc-en.pdf (oecd-ilibrary.org).

Health Consumer Powerhouse (2018) *Euro Health Consumer Index 2018*. Available at: EHCI-2018-index-matrix-A3-sheet.pdf (healthpowerhouse.com).

Hespanha, P. (2019) 'The impact of austerity on the Portuguese national health service, citizens' well-being, and health inequalities: Crisis, austerity and health inequalities in Southern European countries', *E-Cadernos CES* 31: 43–67. Available at: The Impact of Austerity on the Portuguese National Health Service, Citizens' Well-Being, and Health Inequalities (openedition.org).

Instituto Nacional de Estatística (2019) *Resident Population 2019*. Available at: Statistics Portugal – Web Portal (ine.pt).

Instituto Nacional de Estatística (2020) *Employment Statistics*. Available at: Statistics Portugal – Web Portal (ine.pt).

Jalali, C., Bruneau, T. C. and Colino, C. (2020) *Portugal Report: Sustainable Governance Indicators*. Available at: 2020 Portugal Country Report | SGI Sustainable Governance Indicators (sgi-network.org).

Jardim, A. L. (2006) 'An overview of the healthcare system in Portugal', *ICU Management and Practice* 6(3). Available at: An-overview-of-the-healthcare-system-in-portugal.pdf

Lusa (2021) 'Estudo revela quebra de 40% nas urgências e de 25% nas cirurgias num ano de pandemia', *Lusa*, 7 July. Available at: Estudo revela quebra de 40% nas urgências e de 25% nas cirurgias num ano de pandemia – SIC Notícias (sicnoticias.pt).

Lusa (2022) 'New statute provides "strategic solutions" for under pressure health service', *Lusa*, 6 July.

Magalhães, P., Gouveia, R., Lopes, R. C., Silva, P. A., et al. (2020) *O Impacto Social da Pandemia*. Estudo ICS/ISCTE Covid-19, Abril. Available at: Microsoft Word – Relatório geral final.docx (ulisboa.pt).

Marôco, J., Marôco, A. L., Leite, E., Bastos, C., Vazão, M. J. and Campos, J. (2016) 'Burnout em profissionais da saúde portugueses: Uma análise a nível nacional', *Acta Médica Portuguesa* 29: 24–30.

Nunes, A. M. and Ferreira, D. C. (2018) 'Reforms in the Portuguese health care sector: Challenges and proposals', *International Journal of Health Planning and Management* 34: e21–e33.

Observatório Português dos Sistemas de Saúde (2014) 'Saúde – Síndroma de negação', *Relatório de Primavera*, OPSS. Available at: Relatorio Primavera 2014–28junho1.pdf (justnews.pt).

Ordem dos Psicólogos Portugueses (2021) PARECER OPP – Projecto de Decreto-Lei que aprova o Estatuto do Serviço Nacional de Saúde (SNS) | DL 1171/XXII/2021, *Ordem dos Psicólogos Portugueses*, 16 November. Available at: parecer_opp_projecto_de_decreto_lei_que_aprova_o_estatuto_do_servi__o_nacional_de_sa__de.pdf (ordemdospsicologos.pt).

Organisation for Economic Cooperation and Development (2016) 'Health policy in Portugal', *OECD Health Policy Overview*, July.

Organisation for Economic Cooperation and Development (2021a) *A New Benchmark for Mental Health Systems: Tackling the Social and Economic Costs of Mental Ill-Health*, Paris: OECD Publishing.

Organisation for Economic Cooperation and Development (2021b) *OECD Economic Surveys: Portugal.* Available at: Portugal-2021-OECD-economic-survey-overview.pdf

Organisation for Economic Cooperation and Development (2022) *Hospital Beds (Indicator).* Available at: https://data.oecd.org/healtheqt/hospital-beds.htm

Organisation for Economic Cooperation and Development and European Commission (2019) *Key Data on Local and Regional Governments in the European Union,* Pris: OECD.

Partido Socialista and Bloco de Esquerda (2015) *Posição Conjunta do PS e do Bloco de Esquerda sobre Solução Política,* 10 Novembro. Available at: 8ff33d1130d43cc d3f9ae27d27d70561_4a5ed0a4f3450cb56e076d8070ed3d96.pdf (rtp.pt).

Partido Socialista and Partido Ecologista Os Verdes (2015) *Posição Conjunta do PS e do PEV sobre Solução Política,* 10 Novembro. Available at: PosicaoConjuntaPS_PEV.pdf (osverdes.pt)

Pereira, T. L. de S. (2011) 'Unidades de saúde familiar – A evolução na gestão dos cuidados de saúde primários em Portugal', *Mestrado Integrado em Medicina,* Faculdade de Medicina, Universidade do Porto. Available at: Microsoft Word – Tese Março 2011 (up.pt).

Perelman, J., Chaves, P., de Almeida, J. M. C. and Matias, M. A. (2018) 'Reforming the Portuguese mental health system: An incentive-based approach', *International Journal of Mental Health Systems* 12(25).

Portuguese Medical Council and Portuguese Association of Hospital Administrators (2020) *Estudo à População: Acesso a Cuidados de Saúde em Tempos de Pandemia,* Ordem dos Médicos Portuguesa, Associação Portuguesa dos Administradores Hospitalares. Available at: saudeemdia.pt

República Portuguesa (2021) *Projeto de Decreto-Lei que aprova o estatuto do serviço nacional de saúde (SNS).* Available at: Consulta – ESTATUTO DO SERVIÇO NACIONAL DE SAÚDE (consultalex.gov.pt).

Sakellarides, C., Castelo-Branco, L., Barbosa, P. and Azevedo, H. (2014) 'The impact of the financial crisis on the health system and health in Portugal', in *European Observatory on Health Systems and Policies,* Geneva: WHO. Available at: The impact of the financial crisis on the health system and health in Portugal (eapn.pt).

Saks, M. (2016) 'A review of theories of professions, organizations and society: The case for neo-Weberianism, neo-institutionalism and eclecticism', *Journal of Professions and Organization* 3(2): 1–18.

Schiller, C. and Hellmann, T. (2021) 'Major differences in the conditions for successful COVID-19 crisis management', *Governance in International Perspective,* Policy Brief 2021/01. Available at: SGI Policy Brief (sgi-network.org).

Serrão, C., Duarte, I., Castro, L. and Teixeira, A. (2021) 'Burnout and depression in Portuguese healthcare workers during the COVID-19 pandemic: The mediating role of psychological resilience', *International Journal of Environmental Research and Public Health* 18: 636–48.

Shaaban, A. N., Peleteiro, B. and Martins, M. R. O. (2020) 'Covid-19: What is next for Portugal?', *Frontiers of Public Health,* 21 August. Available at: https://doi.org/10.3389/fpubh.2020.00392

Simões, J. de A., Augusto, G. F., Fronteira, I. and Hernández-Quevedo, C. (2017) 'Portugal: Health system review', *Health Systems in Transition* 19(2). Available at: Health Systems in Transition – Portugal (who.int).

Unidade Missão para os Cuidados Continuados Integrados (2011) *Development Strategy for the National Palliative Care Program National Network for Continuous*

Care 2011–2013, Lisbon: National Health Service Portugal. Available at: V.Válida-Palliative Care-Estratégia Versão INGLÊS.docx (min-saude.pt).

Varanda, J., Gonçalves, L. and Craveiro, I. (2020) 'The unlikely saviour: Portugal's national health system and the initial impact of the COVID-19 pandemic?', *Development* 63: 291–7.

Wainwright, H. (n.d.) *Remain and Reform: The Portuguese Experience of Being 'in and Against' the European Union*, Transnational Institute, London School of Economics. Available at: portugal-report.pdf (europeforthemany.com).

World Health Organization (2018) *Health System Review: Portugal*, Geneva: WHO.

World Health Organization (2020a) *A Coordinated Global Research Roadmap: 2019 Novel Coronavirus*, Geneva: WHO.

World Health Organization (2020b) *Portugal – Country Case Study on the Integrated Delivery of Long-Term Care*, Geneva: WHO.

World Health Organization (2020c) *Director-General's Opening Remarks at the Media Briefing on COVID-19–11 March 2020*, Geneva: WHO.

World Health Organization (2022a) *Mental Health and Covid-19: Early Evidence of the Pandemic's Impact*, Geneva: WHO.

World Health Organization (2022b) *The European Health Report 2021*, Geneva: WHO.

9 Greece

Charalambos Economou

Introduction

In terms of the historical origins of the Greek National Health Service (NHS), at the end of the nineteenth and the beginning of the twentieth century, municipalities and communities controlled the few existing municipal and communal hospitals built and funded by donations from wealthy Greeks and charity organisations, while some large hospital institutions were controlled by the state at national level. The foundation of mutual societies, the establishment of social insurance funds for seamen, miners, civil servants and military personnel, measures for health and safety at work and the obligatory insurance of employees were introduced, but these enjoyed limited success. In 1929, the health department of the League of Nations, after a request from the Greek government, submitted a plan for the sanitary reorganisation of the country, which was never implemented. The first serious governmental action intended to increase coverage of the population involved the establishment of the Social Insurance Organisation (IKA) in 1934, with the aim to provide health and pension coverage to blue- and white-collar workers (Petmesidou, 2020). In 1937, the preconditions for a common framework regarding the organisation and operation of public hospitals and the creation of public primary healthcare services were set (Kyriopoulos and Mossialos, 2021).

The 1950s and 1960s were characterised by the continual growth and expansion of the social insurance sector and social security benefits. A first attempt to establish a Beveridge-type NHS with legislation passed in 1953 failed, and the law was never implemented in practice. Instead, a number of financial institutions, such as banks, established their own insurance funds. Social health insurance (SHI) schemes were also established for public-sector employees, self-employed professionals and farmers (Petmesidou, 2020). In addition, a network of rural medical stations was established. With the exception of the IKA, which developed its own healthcare infrastructure for its insured population mainly in urban areas, all insurance funds contracted healthcare services from private specialist physicians in the case of primary healthcare services and from public or private hospitals in the case of secondary care.

DOI: 10.4324/9781003139799-14

The dictatorship period 1967–74 has been characterised as the 'black box' of Greek political history. Nonetheless, in 1968, the minister of health presented a reform plan to the junta government. Its aim was to develop, organise and decentralise public health services, to unify the funds' regulations and to introduce a primary care system – including general practitioners (GPs) – in rural areas. However, the proposals had no serious implementation into health policy actions (Polyzos, Economou and Zilidis, 2008; Petmesidou, 2020; Kyriopoulos and Mossialos, 2021).

Following the restoration of democracy in 1974, political and social pressures, as well as the growing number of problems in the healthcare system, intensified the need for healthcare reform, making this an issue of high priority (Economou, 2010; Polyzos, Economou and Zilidis, 2008; Petmesidou, 2020; Tountas Stenannson and Fryssiras, 1995). In 1980, a plan presented in the Parliament by the right-wing government of New Democracy minister of health, Spyros Doxiades, faced strong opposition from both the Pan-Hellenic Physicians Association and members of Parliament of the governing party and was rejected, since it was considered as very 'advanced' for its time, promoting socialised medicine and therefore was counter to the liberal principles and philosophy of their party. With the rise of the socialist party (PASOK), which came to power in 1981, the political and social conditions for a radical change were very favourable. The then active Association of Hospital Doctors of Athens and Piraeus demanded a comprehensive national healthcare system, expressing the wishes of the majority of the public. Law 1397/83, which founded the Greek national health system (ESY), marked the beginning of an attempt to organise a public healthcare system in Greece. Primary healthcare (PHC) was to be developed based on rural and urban centres staffed by GPs and governed by a referral system. Secondary healthcare services were to be provided mainly through public facilities, and establishment of new private hospitals was to be prohibited. ESY doctors and other staff would be fully and exclusively employed by the national health system and would be paid by salary.

However, significant portions of the law were never or only partially implemented (Economou, 2010; Petmesidou, 2020; Tountas, Stenannson and Fryssiras, 1995). Urban health centres were never established, resulting in a fragmented primary care delivery system. The unification of health insurance funds never took place. The private health sector remained a crucial agent through the establishment and expansion of private diagnostic centres. A referral system was never implemented. The emphasis was placed exclusively on the supply side trying to expand and strengthen the public sector in the provision of healthcare. The financing side of the health sector, funding sources, resource allocation mechanisms and remuneration methods were totally ignored.

Principal healthcare reforms

Healthcare reforms introduced during the period 1983–2010

Following the introduction of Law 1397/1983, there was an increase in and upgrading of infrastructure and staffing, as well as improvements in quality and access to healthcare, especially in rural areas. However, in significant areas such as the financing of the system, its management and administration, the control of expenditure and the development of PHC services in urban centres, the situation remained generally unchanged. As a consequence, in the early 1990s, the healthcare sector faced a number of serious weaknesses (Economou and Giorno, 2009; Economou, 2010). The absence of cost-containment measures and defined criteria for funding resulted in the sickness funds experiencing economic constraints and budget deficits. The high percentage of private expenditures went against the principle of fair financing and equity in access to healthcare services. Efficiency was in question due to the lack of incentives to improve performance in the public sector. Mechanisms for need assessment and priority-setting were underdeveloped and, consequently, the regional distribution of health resources was unequal. Centralisation of the system was coupled with lack of planning and coordination and limited managerial and administrative capacity. The oversupply of physicians, the absence of a referral system and irrational pricing and reimbursement policies were factors encouraging under-the-table payments and the black economy (Sissouras, Karokis and Mossialos, 1994; Liaropoulos, 1998).

During the same period, the notion of statism, which was predominant in the 1980s, was gradually receding, and the focus of government healthcare policy was on fiscal issues due to macroeconomic constraints and the adoption of cost-sharing arrangements. The aim was to replace state responsibility with social security and the private sector in the delivery and financing of health services. According to the reform introduced in 1992 by the conservative government (Law 2071/1992), social insurance funds were free to contract with any public or private provider. Restrictions on the entry of new private, profit-making hospitals were abolished, and private institutions were given the right to provide emergency pre-hospital care. Incentives to contract with private insurance were given. Co-payment rates for drugs, per diem hospital reimbursement and insurance contributions were increased. Fees were introduced for visits to outpatient hospital departments as well as for inpatient admissions. Law 2194/1994 passed by the socialist government did not abolish rights granted to private clinics, hospitals and diagnostic centres and retained all the aforementioned financial arrangements introduced by the previous conservative government (Economou, 2010; Polyzos, Economou and Zilidis, 2008).

In 1994, the government established various committees composed of international and national experts to examine the shortcomings of the Greek healthcare system and to make proposals for reform, with an emphasis on organisational structure, management and regionalisation of the system, unification of sickness funds, changes in management and financing of hospitals and the establishment of a GPs' network. The outcome was the submission of two reform plans and finally the enactment of Law 2519/1997. However, once again, the political will to implement the reform measures was absent. Political particularism, fiscal constraints and administrative weaknesses posed significant barriers, resulting in the partial implementation or the total abolition of the attempted reforms (Tragakes and Polyzos, 1998).

With the beginning of the new century, the healthcare system was put at the centre of political debate, and a number of reform initiatives were inaugurated. The changes introduced can be categorised into two rounds of reform processes, also corresponding to two different ideological and political perceptions: the first includes legislation passed during 2000–04 by the socialist government and the second covers measures passed during the period 2005–08 by the conservative government.

In 2000, the minister of health put forward a plan of 200 measures and initiated a public discussion on reforms, most of which reflected long-awaited proposals to organise and develop the ESY (Tountas, Karnaki and Pavi, 2002). Law 2889/2001 on the improvement and modernisation of the ESY, provided for the establishment of 17 regional health authorities (PeSYs), new management structures and prospective reimbursement for public hospitals, private afternoon hospital services in public facilities and new employment relations for public hospital doctors. The modernisation of public health services was to be promoted by Law 3172/2003, with the establishment of new agencies and the development of the country's 'Health and Welfare Map' as a tool for rational resource allocation. Law 3029/2002 foresaw for the first time, the creation of a legal framework for the establishment and operation of professional insurance funds as private legal entities. Last but not least, Law 3235/2004 on PHC provided for the optional establishment by social insurance organisations of primary healthcare networks and family doctors, the transformation of social insurance polyclinics into urban health centres and the establishment of new services for home care, post-hospital care and rehabilitation.

However, Laws 3172/2003 and 3235/2004 were abolished due to the change of government that occurred after the elections of 2004. Law 3329/2005 abolished the professional hospital management framework established in 2001 and replaced it with the previous pattern of political administration. The same law simply renamed the PeSYs as 'health region administrations' (DYPEs), and their number was reduced from 17 to 7 in mid-2006. The main characteristic of the 2005–08 period was that the whole political management of health reform was based on a 'muddling through' model, characterised by micro-regulations, without a concrete health policy.

Healthcare reforms in the era of economic and pandemic crisis

The majority of reforms that have occurred in the Greek health system since 2010 have been a direct result of the three Economic Adjustment Programmes

(EAPs) implemented during the period 2010–18 and creditors' pressure for rapid changes. The Greek economy entered a deep, structural and multifaceted crisis in 2010, the main features of which were a large fiscal deficit and public debt, as well as continuous erosion of the country's competitive position. In order to address the problem, the Greek Government accepted a bailout from the European Union, the European Central Bank and the International Monetary Fund (all three known as the 'Troika'), signing up for an initial EAP starting from May 2010. Greece was until August 2018 under its third EAP, with financial assistance for all programmes amounting to €290 billion. EAPs, based on neo-liberal economic assumptions, aimed at reducing the public deficit and debt, and they were implemented under stringent conditions to deliver a set of reforms to fiscal policy, state ownership and market liberalisation. This has required implementation of severe austerity measures, including funding cuts to healthcare, social welfare and education, achieving savings through reductions in the salaries and the number of public-sector staff, reductions in pensions, increases in direct and indirect taxation, privatisation of state-owned enterprises and introducing deregulation of the labour market and flexibility in industrial relations. These reforms can be summarised under three headings: reforms in health insurance coverage; reforms in financing and payment mechanisms; and reforms in the provision of health services (Economou et al., 2015; Economou et al., 2017; Economou, 2018).

Reforms in health insurance coverage

One of the major reforms of the health system was introduced in March 2011 with the unification of the large number of health branches of the social insurance funds and the formation of the National Organisation for the Provision of Health Services (EOPYY), supposed to function as unique purchaser of health services. The benefit packages of the merged in EOPYY funds were standardised and unified to provide the same reimbursable services based on EOPYY's Integrated Health Care Regulation. A reduction in covered benefits took place and since 2014 ceilings were imposed on the activities of doctors contracted with EOPYY (on visits, the value of pharmaceutical prescriptions as well as prescribing diagnostic and laboratory tests). This means that those insured with EOPYY who need a doctor's visit or a prescription must either find a physician who has not reached his or her ceiling, or they will have to pay out-of-pocket payments (OOPs).

The economic crisis – and total deregulation of the labour market via flexible industrial relations policies and redundancies dictated by the Memoranda of Understanding (MoUs) – increased unemployment in Greece and resulted, according to the National Social Insurance Registry, in more than 2.5m people losing their social health insurance rights. Action to address this development was delayed, and the measures implemented during 2013–15 were uncoordinated, insufficient, bureaucratic and stigmatising for the beneficiaries. Therefore, new legislation came into effect in August 2016 by the left-wing government of Syriza (Coalition of the Radical Left) that provided access to care for the uninsured and vulnerable, including those without health coverage, migrants who are legal residents in Greece, children, pregnant women and people with chronic conditions, irrespective of their insurance status.

Reforms in financing and payment mechanisms

According to the MoUs, Greece was obliged to keep public health expenditures below 6%. The imposition of public health spending restrictions and the simultaneous decline in Gross Domestic Product (GDP) observed since 2009 (from €237.5 billion in 2009 to €165.8 billion in 2020) (ELSTAT, 2021a), means that the public health sector is called upon to meet the increasing needs of the population with decreasing financial resources. Between 2010 and 2018, public health expenditure fell from 6.6% to 4.7% of GDP. On the other hand, private health expenditure as a percentage of total health expenditure increased from 31.1% in 2010 to 41.4% in 2018 (see Table 9.1).

Existing user charges and co-payments increased, and new ones introduced with the aim to increase revenues and limit the demand for health services. In 2011 an increase in user charges from €3 to €5 was imposed on outpatient services provided in public hospitals and health centres (abolished in 2015), and in 2012 a €25 patient fee for admission to a public hospital (revoked in 2014), together with an extra €1 for each prescription issued under the ESY were introduced (in 2016 exemptions were introduced regarding the €1 prescription charge to relieve vulnerable groups). In 2011 increases in medication co-payments were also introduced. For many medicines, the co-payment increased from 0% to 10% and for others from 0% to 25%. Furthermore, the patient has been charged the difference between the retail price and the reference price reimbursed by health insurance. In April 2014, calls to make an appointment with any doctor under the National Primary Health Care Network (PEDY) scheme were outsourced to private telephone companies, with charges ranging from €0.95 to €1.65 per minute, thus increasing the financial burden of the patients. From this point of view, a positive evolution was the development by the Social Insurance E-Governance Centre of the e-RDV application launched in January 2017, enabling patients to make an appointment free of charge. Another issue to be considered is co-payments introduced for EOPYY insurees in 2012. While treatment in public hospitals is free of charge, treatment in private clinics contracted with EOPYY presupposes user charges ranging from 30% to 50% of the new system called DRG-KEN implemented in January 2013, and 100% of the doctor's payment. Similarly, for clinical tests provided free of charge in public facilities, the patient is obliged to pay a 15% co-payment in the case of visiting a private laboratory contracted with EOPYY. This undermines equity of access, particularly in regions where due to the inability of public facilities to provide the necessary services, patients are forced to use contracted with EOPYY providers.

Table 9.1 Health expenditure in Greece 2009–19 in millions of euros

GEO/TIME	2009	2010	2011	2012	2013	2014	2015	2016	2017	2018	2019
Total health expenditure (THE)	22,344.6	21,508.3	18,690.7	16,811.4	15,028.2	14,024.4	14,210.2	14,498.4	14,354.8	14,304.1	14,375.7
THE % of GDP	**9.4**	**9.6**	**9.2**	**8.9**	**8.4**	**7.9**	**8.1**	**8.3**	**8.1**	**8**	**7.8**
Public health expenditure (PHE)	*15,265.8*	*14,820.5*	*12,280.4*	*11,113.2*	*9,272.6*	*8,088.3*	*8,182.8*	*8,805.8*	*8,678.4*	*8,357.6*	*8,590.6*
PHE % of GDP	*6.4*	*6.6*	*6*	*5.9*	*5.1*	*4.6*	*4.7*	*5.1*	*4.9*	*4.7*	*4.7*
PHE % of THE	*68.3*	*68.9*	*65.7*	*66.1*	*61.7*	*57.7*	*57.6*	*60.7*	*60.5*	*58.4*	*59.8*
General government	6,115.4	6,475.4	4,202.3	5,082.1	4,638.6	4,210.5	4,087.6	4,519.0	3,985.0	3,916.0	4,108.6
Social Security Funds	9,150.4	8,345.1	8,078.1	6,031.1	4,634.0	3,877.8	4,095.1	4,286.9	4,693.4	4,441.6	4,482.1
Private health expenditure	*7,076.6*	*6,683.7*	*6,375.6*	*5,673.7*	*5,630.9*	*5,753.6*	*5,793.8*	*5,654.9*	*5,650.7*	*5,927.1*	*5,765.3*
Private insurance	484.3	605.6	551.8	554.8	509.7	550.7	569.7	597.0	614.4	666.4	708.4
Household out-of-pocket payment	6,592.3	6,078.0	5,823.8	5,118.9	5,121.2	5,202.9	5,224.1	5,057.9	5,036.3	5,260.7	5,057.0
Rest of the world financing schemes (non-resident)	*2.1*	*4.2*	*34.8*	*24.5*	*124.7*	*182.6*	*233.7*	*37.7*	*25.7*	*19.4*	*19.8*

Source: ELSTAT (2021b).

The pharmaceutical sector also saw a number of measures aimed at containing costs and enhancing efficiency. Overall, reductions in pharmaceutical expenditure were pursued though price reductions, increased rebates and claw backs imposed on private pharmacies and pharmaceutical companies for both inpatient and outpatient drugs, promotion of the wider use of generics and, to some extent, control of the volume of consumption via methods such as prescription control mechanisms and e-prescribing.

Concerning healthcare providers' payment mechanisms, the EAPs impelled Greece to replace the *per diem* financing method of hospitals with a diagnostic related group (DRG)-based one in a very short time period (one year) in order to increase efficiency and rationalise allocation of resources. As a consequence, the new system DRG-KEN has encountered a number of problems. The pricing is based not on actual costs and clinical protocols but on a combination of activity-based costing with data from selected public hospitals, and so-called imported cost weights. Furthermore, the salary cost of those employed in hospitals is not included as they are paid directly through the state budget. So far, four revisions of the system have been made and at the time of writing a total reformulation of it is in process.

In relation to healthcare personnel, in the drive to reduce health system input costs, salary cuts were applied after 2010 to all public healthcare staff, including administrative personnel, doctors, nurses, pharmacists and paramedical staff. Additionally, almost all subsidies to healthcare staff were abolished. Other workforce measures aimed at reducing costs included the non-renewal of contracts for temporary staff employed under fixed-term contracts and a reduction in the replacement levels of retiring staff (for every five people retiring only one will be appointed).

Reforms in the provision of health services

Legislation was passed in 2014, aiming to develop a nationwide PHC service, consisting of health centres, social health insurance outpatient clinics and contracted health professionals. According to Law 4238/2014 all public PHC facilities passed under the jurisdiction of the Regional Health Authorities (YPEs). In addition, the law introduced a referral system based on GPs. However, the staffing of PEDY units remained oriented towards specialised doctors and a gatekeeping system did not come into effect. In general, the implementation of the reform was quite slow due to human and economic restrains and a rather fiscal-driven managerial approach. A new PHC reform was introduced in August 2017. Under the new legislation (Law 4486/2017), PHC services are provided at the first level by local health units (TOMYs) operating as family medicine units staffed by interdisciplinary health teams, and by health professionals who have private practices and contract with EOPYY. At the second level, PHC services are provided by health centres, with the purpose to provide specialised ambulatory care for all patients who are referred by the TOMYs. In addition, central diagnostic laboratories providing laboratory tests and imaging diagnostic services and specialised care centres providing specialised care, special education, physiotherapy and rehabilitation services should also be established in each YPE. Patient registration with a TOMY, gatekeeping mechanisms and a referral system form part of the new delivery framework. An e-health record was also expected to be developed.

The public hospital sector has been targeted as part of major restructuring efforts under the country's EAPs. In July 2011, the government announced a plan to cut the current number of public hospital beds and reduce the number of clinics and specialist units. Public hospital management boards were replaced by a total of 83 councils responsible for the administration of all hospitals. The total number of beds in ESY hospitals decreased from 38,115 in 2009 to 29,550 in 2016. The number of medical departments and units declined by 600 and 15,000 hospital personnel were cut. Furthermore, 500 public hospital beds were set aside for priority use by private insurance companies for their clients. Additionally, changes were to be made to the use of eight small hospitals, which were supposed to be turned into urban health centres, support and palliative care units and hospitals for short-term hospitalisation and rehabilitation. However, progress in implementing the restructuring of these eight hospitals has been limited (Liaropoulos et al., 2012).

In relation to pharmaceuticals, there is a positive list of reimbursed medicines plus a negative list of non-reimbursed medicines, introduced in 2011 and 2012, respectively. An over-the-counter drug list was also introduced in 2012, which contained many medicines that until then had been reimbursed but now required purchasing OOP. Finally, very expensive drugs are provided only through EOPYY and public hospital pharmacies. An e-prescription system for doctors became compulsory in 2012, enabling monitoring of their prescribing behaviour as well as the dispensing patterns of pharmacists. At the same time, prescription guidelines following international standards were issued in 2012, prescribing budgets for individual physicians have been set since 2014 and the use of generic drugs has been promoted.

Concerning dental care, theoretically, the EOPYY scheme for publicly provided dental services should have begun in January 2014. Insured people were to be eligible to receive treatment and compensation for both preventive and clinical treatment, plus prosthetics, with the freedom to choose a dentist from the network of contracted providers. However, because of budgetary constraints and cuts in public health expenditure, this scheme has yet to start.

Reforms in the era of Covid-19

Most of the measures related to health sector introduced during the pandemic in Greece concern preventing transmission, ensuring sufficient physical infrastructure and health workforce capacity, and maintaining essential services (Economou et al., 2021). Following European Disease Centre guidelines, the Greek Ministry of Health implemented a strategy for SARS-CoV-2 based on diagnostic, screening and surveillance testing performed free of charge, as well as on the vaccination programme started in January 2021.

Concerning physical infrastructure, intensive care units (ICU) public beds increased from 565 in the beginning of 2020 to 1,006 at the end of 2020, as a result of converting ICU beds from other wards into Covid-19 treatment wards and building flexible ICUs wards. Furthermore, public–private partnerships to purchase ICU services from the private sector have been established to be utilised whenever deemed necessary to cater for possible future Covid-19 hospitalisation needs. In addition, a contingency plan is in place should the Covid-19 cases increase dramatically, which entails the requisition of private clinics (Waitzberg et al., 2021). In the beginning of October 2020, the Ministry of Health announced the operational expansion of 185 Health Centres and 42 Regional Clinics, to include case management of citizens with coronavirus symptoms as well as the operation of designated Covid-19 health centres on a 24-hour basis exclusively for the screening and management of Covid-19 patients that do not require hospital referral.

In order to boost quickly surge capacity for health workers, professionals already working within the public sector were reallocated from regular hospital wards to specially designated Covid-19 wards, and from primary care settings to hospitals. Another strategy was temporarily enrolling professionals from the armed forces (Waitzberg et al., 2021). Between March and November 2020, more than 6,800 new recruitments of medical (745), nursing (3,867), paramedical and other staff were made. Furthermore, the Ministry of Health announced position openings for 1,421 doctors and 1,209 nursing (and other) staff. Legislation enacted on April 2020 also provides for the employment of private physicians in public hospitals to deal with emergencies for up to two months with the possibility of extending the cooperation for another two months. However, due to emergency needs and the fact that the doctors did not respond in great numbers to the announcement of related new posts, the government on March 2021 forced 200 private physicians to work for the NHS.

On March 2020, in light of the Covid-19 epidemic and the expected increase in demand for hospital services, hospitals were instructed by a Ministerial Decree to revise their surgical case scheduling to accommodate emergency cases only and all elective surgeries in both public and private hospitals were deferred. Only oncology and emergency services remained operational. As of March 2020, patients have the ability to receive regular prescriptions on their mobile device, via text message or e-mail, as the registration for e-prescription was introduced. In addition, a helpline reachable on the number 10306 with experts providing psychological support to people struggling to deal with the impact of the coronavirus pandemic commenced operation on April 2020.

The impact of health reform policies on the architecture of the national health system

Legislative initiatives undertaken in the 1990s and early 2000s did not change the basic architecture of ESY established in 1983. Until 1985, the strong political will along with people's and scientists' expectations were constituted to materialise a huge project of constructions (hospitals and health centres) and other organisational or financial changes. This was not exactly the case of the second socialist period (1985–89), where emphasis was given mainly to doctors' labour relations and payments. There was little effort in securing the effectiveness, the efficiency, the responsiveness and the quality of the system. The beginning of the 1990s had put a strong emphasis on the so-called new-liberal health policy approaches, but there was a weak willingness at least to evaluate health policies or the system itself. The new socialist period (1994–2004) came along with reform and planning policies in health. They were cases of a top-down process by scientists and individuals from several political or union groups in the Ministry of Health, rather than professional or institutional bodies. Unions and members of political parties were coming to and leaving from the planning or policy process, without continuation, consistency, serious dialogue and formulation of contingency plans. However, a remarkable increase of infrastructures, technology and human resources was obvious in the decade of 1994–2004, assisted by European convergence policies through programmes and funds from the European Commission Cohesion Fund. Regulations in the 1990s were impeded in an incremental way, plans to decentralise the system failed to result in a concrete change, and unification of the funds and transferring the international experience of the provider-purchaser split were both not implemented. The core of the reform initiated in the beginning of the 2000s concerning the segregation of financing and health services provision, the establishment of a single financial institution, and the unified provision of PHC services under the authority of ESY, made no progress. The conservative government elected in 2004 started again with the regulations in a muddling through approach; they had never been integrated, especially with the financing and the gatekeeping of the system.

Consequently, until 2010, the Greek health system featured a mixture of public and private services and funding. In the public sector, elements of the Bismarck and the Beveridge model coexisted. In the private sector, supplemental private insurance was playing only a minor role, accounting for only 8% of private medical spending and covering 10% of the population in 2005, while the substantial proportion of private household health spending, which accounted for roughly 40% of total outlays, stemmed from OOP payments rather than from high formal patient contributions to medical costs. The vast majority of hospital care was public, and the supply of outpatient services was fragmented (Economou, 2010).

In 2011, a major restructuring of the health system resulted in the health branches of all SHI funds being combined to form the EOPYY, which would act as the purchaser of medicines and healthcare services for the insured, thus increasing bargaining power with suppliers. Between 2011 and 2014, EOPYY was gradually transformed into a unitary health insurance fund and its role as the sole purchaser of health services was consolidated. A second major restructuring of the health system was introduced in 2017, concerning PHC. In the first phase of implementation, it was planned that 239 TOMYs would be established throughout the country. However, so far, this target has not been achieved, since, once again, elections and the change of the governing party slowed down the whole process (Economou et al., 2017; Economou and Panteli, 2019).

The burst of the Covid-19 crisis in 2020 could be said so far to be another lost window of opportunity for the Greek healthcare system to address long-standing deficiencies. For example, tele-counselling and e-prescription could become enduring tools for developing telemedicine, e-therapies and e-healthcare services (Giannopoulou and Tsobanoglou, 2020). The increase of ICUs and new recruitment of medical, nursing and paramedical staff are also positive evolutions to fill major gaps in the health system. However, there are still gaps. A strategy to enhance community care has not yet been developed. Public health services and primary care are still in the back seat as hospital services are favoured. So far, a strategic reform plan based on new approaches that address all the root causes of communicable as well as non-communicable diseases, including the social determinants of health, environmental factors and behavioural risk is still an exercise on paper.

The impact of health reform policies on the population's health status

It is difficult to assess the effects on the health status of the population arising from the reforms introduced in the health system. This is largely because it is difficult to estimate whether (and to what extent) an observed health effect is attributable to structural and procedural changes in the health system *per se* or to changes in the social determinants of health brought about by the political and economic context.

However, some conclusions can be drawn from various studies conducted. These studies reveal that in the 1980s at least 70% of the total improvements in life expectancy in Greece were due to falling amenable mortality in both sexes, with about half of this improvement due to declining infant mortality. Turning to the 1990s, compared to other countries, amenable mortality made a somewhat smaller contribution than it had in the 1980s, although its impact was still substantial, accounting for about two-thirds of the total increase in life expectancy in both sexes. Much of this change was again driven by falling death rates in infancy, accounting for 36% in women and 47% in men of the observed improvements (Nolte and McKee, 2004). Furthermore, during the period 1998–2003 mortality from amenable causes had fallen by 11% for males and by 17% for females (Nolte and McKee, 2008). Although these studies suggest a positive impact by the Greek healthcare system on the population's health, another study based on data envelopment analysis concludes that the effectiveness of the healthcare system has been eroded. The analysis shows that the performance of the Greek healthcare system, which had ranked between third and fifth among Organisation for Economic Co-operation and Development (OECD) countries in 1990, had fallen to between 12th and 18th place in 2006, depending on whether the resources available for healthcare are measured by the level of spending per capita or proxied by the number of active medical personnel. While in 1990 it was estimated that using healthcare resources as efficiently as the best-performing countries would have increased life expectancy at birth by between 0.8 and 0.9 years, the gap widened to between 1.7 and 3 years in 2006 (Economou and Giorno, 2009).

Eurostat data indicate that from 2010 to 2015, healthy life expectancy in Greece decreased by 2.9 years (from 66.9 to 64 years), while an increase has been observed afterwards, reaching 66 years in 2019. Data also show changes in the self-perceived health of the Greek population. The percentage of those declaring very bad, bad or fair health status increased from 24.4% in 2010 to 26.5% in 2014 (see Table 9.2). The trend was reversed in the next years and those declaring very bad, bad or fair health status decreased to 20.8% in 2019. On the other hand, the percentage of people declaring very good health status was 50.1% in 2010, decreased to 44.3% in 2014 and increased to 46.7% in 2019. The infant mortality rate in Greece was on the decline for decades and was constantly below the EU-28 average. However,

Table 9.2 Self-perceived health of the Greek population

	2010	2011	2012	2013	2014	2015	2016	2017	2018	2019	2020
Very good	49.9	50.6	46.8	45.8	44.8	44.5	44.9	45.0	46.1	46.4	46.3
Good	25.6	25.8	28.0	28.1	28.7	29.9	29.0	28.9	30.2	32.8	32.0
Fair	14.8	14.6	15.8	15.6	15.8	15.6	15.7	15.6	14.5	14.2	14.9
Bad	6.7	6.3	6.6	7.6	7.8	7.3	7.5	8.1	7.2	5.0	5.0
Very bad	2.9	2.7	2.7	2.9	2.9	2.7	2.9	2.3	2.0	1.6	1.8

Source: EUROSTAT (n.d.).

Table 9.3 Cause of mortality in Greece 2010–18 (standardised rates per 100,000 population)

	2010	2011	2012	2013	2014	2015	2016	2017	2018
All causes of death	819.7	801.6	804.3	754.8	747.1	777.4	746.2	761.5	724.4
Diseases of the circulatory system	360.1	343.6	337.4	305.7	288.6	288.4	268.3	277.8	258.4
Neoplasms	196.6	193.5	198.3	200.5	201.7	203	202.9	199.8	196.3
Diseases of the respiratory system	78.3	74.3	76.1	71.1	79.9	89.6	81.1	78.6	70.1
Infectious and parasitic diseases	8.1	7	7.7	7.7	22.3	24	23.9	24.3	22.7
Mental and behavioural disorders	0.7	0.9	0.9	0.9	4.2	7.2	8.5	10.8	11.5
Intentional self-harm	3.1	3.9	4.2	4.5	4.7	4.4	4	4.4	4.7
Motor vehicle accidents	12.3	11.5	10.3	9.5	9.1	11.7	10.4	8.4	8.1

Source: OECD Health Database (n.d.).

this trend was reversed after 2014 and in 2016 infant mortality reached 4.2 per 1,000 live births, 0.6% above the EU28 average, while in 2019 decreased to 3.7 per 1,000 live births.

According to the OECD Health Database, all-cause mortality (standardised rate) decreased in the period 2010–16, from 819.7 to 746.2 deaths per 100,000 population (see Table 9.3). Diseases of the circulatory system, which remain the leading cause of death in Greece, decreased from 360.1 deaths per 100,000 population in 2010 to 268.3 deaths per 100,000 population in 2016. In contrast, the other two main causes of death in the Greek population – neoplasms and diseases of the respiratory system – showed an upward trend in the same period. It is also worth mentioning two other substantial increases in cause-specific mortality: deaths from infectious and parasitic diseases, as well as from mental and behavioural disorders. In addition, although the suicide mortality rate in Greece is among the lowest in the EU, an increasing trend was observed for the period 2010–14, with a slight decrease in 2016. The opposite trend was recorded for motor vehicle accidents, for which a decrease during the period 2010–14 was followed by an increase in 2016.

Concerns have been raised regarding deteriorating standards of medical care because of the severe cuts, and the impact this could have on population health. A recent study has shown that amenable mortality in Greece experienced a small but significant increase in the years after the economic crisis (Karanikolos et al., 2018). Another major study found a significant increase in mortality from adverse events during medical treatment and estimated that there was an increase of more than 200 deaths per month after the onset of the crisis (Laliotis, Ioannidis and Stavropoulou, 2016).

Furthermore, insights on Greece from the Global Burden of Disease Study exploring the period 2000–16 show that, many of the causes of death that increased in the period following the onset of the crisis are potentially responsive to care (for example, HIV, neoplasms, cirrhosis, neurological disorders, chronic kidney disease, and most types of cardiovascular disease). Substantial changes in health loss indicators since 2010 support the interpretation that austerity measures compounded the country's pre-existing health burden. The study highlights that

> steep quantitative changes in mortality trends and qualitative changes in mortality causes with a rise in communicable, maternal, neonatal, and nutritional diseases since 2010 suggest that an effect of the abruptly reduced government health expenditure on population health is likely.
> (Global Burden of Disease Greece, 2018)

The future sustainability of the national health system

The existing structure of SHI does not deliver effective and universal coverage of the needs of the population. Occupational status and social insurance contributions as we knew them until now do not correspond to the new social, economic and productive conditions generated by the crisis and cannot be the sole basis for entitlement. The nature of employment is changing and the typical dependent eight hours full employment is gradually being replaced by different kinds of flexible, part-time, and in many cases unpaid informal work where the employees are involved in a portfolio of activities, challenging the basic core of the insurance relationship and resulting in inadequate contributions. Furthermore, the ability of households to pay taxes is exhausted. Horizontal measures of user charges and co-payments lead to inequities and postponement or non-use of necessary and needed services.

Under the circumstances of a high unemployment rate and decreasing wages and household income, retaining an SHI system in Greece is a choice that deteriorates the health system's ability to achieve the overriding goal of delivering healthcare to those who need it. Instead, the transition to a tax-financed system has the merits of not leaving a large portion of the population with inferior health coverage, of avoiding many of the labour market distortions associated with payroll financing, and of raising revenues in an equitable fashion. The basic characteristics of such a system should be entitlement to the same health services package on the basis of citizenship or legal residency, and the abolition and replacement of employees' and employers' contributions by new sources such as a special health tax on personal income and on enterprises' turnover or added value. As the share of labour in Greece decreases, wage income is insufficient to cover the cost of healthcare. At the same time, the necessity to increase contributions in order to cover the rising needs of the population may imperil the competitiveness of the economy. The spreading of healthcare cost to all factors of production through comprehensive national health insurance financed by progressive taxation of income from all sources, instead of employer-employee contributions, may be considered as a potential solution for protecting the health system objectives and ensuring health system sustainability, especially during an economic recession (Economou, Kaitelidou and Siskou, 2018). However, it is critical to consider that the prerequisite in order for the proposed plan to be sustainable is the effective combating and the elimination of tax evasion.

Aside from the economic context, demographic and epidemiological trends also undermine the sustainability of ESY. Many individuals present with complex symptoms and multiple illnesses because of ageing, a matter that challenges service delivery to develop more integrated and comprehensive case management. In addition, the recent pandemic crisis raised a structural problem of ESY that undermines its ability to cover the health needs of the population – that is, the absence of an adequate PHC network and the underdevelopment of public health services, resulting in disintegrated outpatient healthcare. The doctor-centric, hospital oriented ESY is not suitable for dealing with the threat posed by infectious diseases, especially in the case of a pandemic. The need is for a paradigm shift in the healthcare delivery system, based on the reorganisation of health services around people's needs and expectations and public policy reforms that secure healthier communities, by integrating public health actions with primary care and by pursuing healthy public policies across sectors. This requires new approaches that address all the root causes of communicable and non-communicable diseases, including the social determinants of health and environmental and behavioural risk factors. It also requires a comprehensive aligned health system response as recommended by the World Health Organization, including effective inter-sectoral policies and governance arrangements; a preventive-oriented and integrated approach to service provision; an interdisciplinary working culture of health professionals; and suitable financial and non-monetary incentives (Economou and Panteli, 2019). We now turn to discuss how far the neo-liberal reforms have changed the Greek NHS.

The national health system in the arena of neo-liberalism

The impact of neo-liberalism on the Greek ESY is particularly evident during the first half of the 2010s, when Greece accepted a bailout from the EU, the European Central Bank and the International Monetary Fund, signing up for three EAPs. The reforms that have been taking place in the Greek healthcare system since 2010 and especially in the period 2010–14, by the government of PASOK (2009–12) and the coalition government led by New Democracy (2012–14), have focused mainly on operational, financial and organisational dimensions. This perspective ignored the citizen/patient side of the equation in that the formulation of a patient-centred health system was out of the scope of the reform package. Furthermore, carrying out major changes coupled with extensive financial cuts has proved to be very challenging in terms of both the ability to conduct meaningful reforms and the consequences for service delivery. Overall, the content and the process of reforms have been mainly technocratic/managerial in nature, with insufficient consideration for the broader functioning of the health system and the health needs of the population (Economou et al., 2015; Economou et al., 2017; Economou, 2018).

The general approach of cost-containment measures has taken the form of horizontal cuts rather than a more sophisticated and strategic approach targeting resource allocation, partly because of the pressure exerted by the EAPs to achieve immediate results in health expenditure cuts. Another point to consider is that the side effects of certain measures have not been adequately taken into account. Reform processes may trigger unintended consequences. Examples in Greece include worsening access to care and pharmaceuticals, especially for vulnerable groups of the population; increasing demands for informal payments due to cuts to the already low salaries of health professionals working in the public system, particularly doctors; migration of many young and well-qualified physicians and other healthcare professionals to other countries as a result of the worsening of reimbursement rates, as well as working conditions (Economou et al., 2014; Economou, 2015).

It can be argued that the majority of the reform measures introduced during the first wave of reforms (2010–14) undermined the health system goals. These included the reduction of the scope of essential services covered; the reduction of population coverage and increases in user charges for essential services; increases in waiting times for needed services; horizontal cuts in public health expenditure and attrition of health workers caused by cuts in salaries; reductions in the replacement levels of retiring staff; and migration to foreign labour markets. On the other hand, introduced measures likely to promote health system goals were limited and, in many cases, not well planned and implemented. This category encompasses the establishment of the EOPYY as a single payer to strengthen risk pooling, the introduction of the DRG-KEN system for hospital payment, and price reductions for pharmaceuticals combined with e-prescribing. Finally, a range of essential policy options were neglected, such as strategic purchasing combining contracts with accountability mechanisms, monitoring and transparency measures, public health measures to reduce the burden of disease, shifting from inpatient to day-case or ambulatory care, integration and coordination of primary care and secondary care, and health and social care, the reduction of administrative costs while maintaining capacity to manage the health system, and fiscal policies to expand the public revenue. In addition, the citizen-patient dimension as the basis for shaping a patient-centred health system appeared beyond the scope of the first wave reform package. Furthermore, the effects, intended or unintended, of the measures introduced were not monitored or adequately considered to further shape policy (Economou and Panteli, 2019).

After 2015, and the election of a left-wing government, these neglected issues came to the forefront of the health policy agenda, building on increasing concerns about achieving universal health coverage, reducing barriers in access to health services, and establishing an integrated PHC system (Economou and Panteli, 2019). However, issues for further consideration remain, such as the structure of co-payments for pharmaceuticals and other health services, a ceiling on doctors' treatment activities, the absence of real dental coverage, and the excessive reliance on indirect taxes and high formal and informal OOP payments – making the overall funding of the health sector regressive and inequitable. The substantial pressures on both components of public financing in the Greek system (SHI and state budget) create justified concerns over the mid- and long-term adequacy of funding in the health system. There is a need to rethink and to promote a public debate on the health budget, which must be viewed not as a financial burden but as a developmental tool, with a focus on addressing not only the economic dimensions but also the welfare of citizens. In relation to the health status of the population, it is necessary not only to develop and implement health in all policies, surveillance and monitoring systems and disease registries but also to reach beyond the health system and strengthen research to better clarify the causal mechanisms connecting socio-economic factors with mortality and morbidity from specific diseases. So far, the aforementioned issues have not been addressed by the right-wing government elected in 2019.

In conclusion, the EAPs directly affected the Greek health system (Kentikelenis, 2017). First, austerity measures stipulated the reduction of public health expenditure with negative impacts on the volume and quality of services provided. Second, health insurance coverage and access to services were reduced through increases in user fees and co-payments, reductions in covered benefits, and the imposition of ceilings in the use of services. Third, human resources for health have been affected via hiring freezes, salary cuts and the brain drain. Fourth, the aforementioned impacts of EAPs on the country's health system had negative knock-on effects on population health and unmet medical needs.

The influence of the neo-liberal wave in the political cycle is also obvious in two recent developments. First, even though Covid-19 showed the importance of the public sector in the management of a pandemic crisis and the necessity of a well-developed and integrated system of primary healthcare and public health services, the right-wing government elected in 2019 passed Law 4931/2022 replacing the primary healthcare system introduced in 2017 with a model of public–private partnerships (PPPs) based on doctors privately practising and contracted with EOPYY. Second, a new law passed on December 2022 provides for full-time doctors in the national health system, who serve in public hospitals, under certain conditions, to operate in private practice or to provide medical services in any kind of private businesses that deliver or cover health services, up to twice a week. Furthermore, it gives doctors the possibility of holding part-time positions in the national health system, who will retain the right to alternate employment in the private health sector and to maintain a private practice. The new law also provides for the transfer of private patients after completion of their hospitalisation to national health system hospitals. In providing transport for this service, the hospitals of the national health system may additionally enter into contracts with the owners of licensed private sector ambulances. All the above measures indicate that the intention of the government is to privatise the NHS, based on its neo-liberal ideology. The government has therefore avoided its responsibility to strengthen the national health system by employing permanent healthcare personnel and increasing public health expenditure. The effects of the new provisions will be to increase supply-induced demand, shifting the cost of healthcare provision to patients and minimising the number of services provided in public settings to push patients to make appointments and undergo scheduled visits and surgery in private practices and clinics.

Conclusion

In the case of Greece, the 'why' question posed by Toth (2021) considering the pattern of development of health systems can be answered by the 'path dependence' theory, a version of neo-institutionalism linked to the neo-Weberian approach. According to this theory, choices, events, strategies adopted in the past and institutions, push policy along particular paths, constraining subsequent developments and attempts to change the system face resistance. Policy change is possible under exceptional conditions of discontinuity caused by a major event called 'critical conjuncture' (Oliver and Mossialos, 2005; Toth, 2021).

The Greek case shows that a successful change process must first disrupt the self-referentiality typical of state-political organisations, and such disruption happens mainly through externally generated behaviour-shaping information (Tsoukas and Papoulias, 2005). System-specific deficits do not suffice in explaining health reforms. The economic and the pandemic shock could be seen as 'critical conjunctions' promoting changes, since political actors, decision makers and stakeholders appear to disagree fundamentally over the values and the directions of health reforms. 'Party thinking' blocked the promotion of changes and this is reflected in the numerous health reform initiatives during 1990s and 2000s that were partially or never implemented. The path-dependent character of health policy in Greece, influenced by clientelism, political particularism, the absence of consensus, low administrative capacities, weak civil society and the dominance of the medical profession caused several aspects of the reforms to stray from the original plans (Mossialos, Allin and Davaki, 2005; Davaki and Mossialos, 2005; Nikolentzos and Mays, 2016). In this context, the metaphor of the 'pendulum' is the most appropriate to describe the planning and implementation of health policy. The retrogressive continuous movement from the one side to the other implies that the impulse towards a favourable direction of achieving a higher degree of effectiveness and efficiency has been followed by an impulse towards the diametrically opposite direction and the application of contradictory policy measures (Polyzos, Economou and Zilidis, 2008).

Since the weakness of promoting important health reforming plans in Greece has been riven with intrinsic difficulties, the economic and the Covid-19 pandemic crisis may be seen as external triggers that have helped in creating a momentum for change in the health system. However, this is only one side of the coin. The other side concerns the question about the direction of the changes and their impact on the effective and efficient functioning of the health system, as well as on the equitable access to services. As this chapter pointed out, neo-liberalism has determined the path chosen by most of the Greek governments after 2010.

References

Davaki, K. and Mossialos, E. (2005) 'Plus ça change: Health sector reforms in Greece', *Journal of Health Politics, Policy and Law* 30(1–2): 143–67.

Economou, C. (2010) 'Greece: Health system review', *Health Systems in Transition* 12(7): 1–180. Available at: https://eurohealthobservatory.who.int/publications/i/greece-health-system-review-2010

Economou, C. (2015) *Barriers and Facilitating Factors in Access to Health Services in Greece*, Copenhagen: WHO Regional Office for Europe. Available at: www.

euro.who.int/__data/assets/pdf_file/0006/287997/Barriers-and-facilitating-factors-in-access-to-health-services-in-Greece-rev1.pdf

Economou, C. (2018) 'Greece's healthcare system and the crisis: A case study in the struggle for a capable welfare state', *Anais do Instituto de Higiene e Medicina Tropical* 17(Supplement 1): 7–26. Available at: https://anaisihmt.com/index.php/ihmt/article/view/246/206

Economou, C. and Giorno, C. (2009) *Improving the Performance of the Public Health Care System in Greece*, Paris: OECD Economics Department Working Papers, No 722. Available at: www.oecd-ilibrary.org/docserver/221250170007.pdf?expires=1620032768&id=id&accname=guest&checksum=401C69E4101990426BE14BDBDAB596C5

Economou, C., Kaitelidou, D., Karanikolos, M. and Maresso, A. (2017) 'Greece: Health system review', *Health Systems in Transition* 19(5): 1–192. Available at: www.euro.who.int/__data/assets/pdf_file/0006/373695/hit-greece-eng.pdf

Economou, C., Kaitelidou, D., Katsikas, D., Siskou, O. and Zafiropoulou, M. (2014) 'Impacts of the economic crisis on access to healthcare services in Greece with a focus on the vulnerable groups of the population', *Social Cohesion and Development* 9(2): 99–115. Available at: https://ejournals.epublishing.ekt.gr/index.php/SCAD/article/view/8880

Economou, C., Kaitelidou, D., Kentikelenis, A., Maresso, A. and Sissouras, A. (2015) 'The impact of the crisis on the health system and health in Greece', in Maresso, A., Mladovsky, P., Thomson, S., et al. (eds) *Economic Crisis, Health Systems and Health in Europe: Country Experience*, Copenhagen: European Observatory on Health Systems and Policies. Available at: https://eurohealthobservatory.who.int/publications/i/economic-crisis-health-systems-and-health-in-europe-country-experience-study

Economou, C., Kaitelidou, D., Konstantakopoulou, O. and Vildiridi, V. (2021) 'COVID-19 policy responses for Greece', *COVID-19 Health System Response Monitor*, Copenhagen: European Observatory on Health Systems and Policies. Available at: www.covid19healthsystem.org/countries/greece/countrypage.aspx

Economou, C., Kaitelidou, D. and Siskou, O. (2018) 'A health system in the era of economic crisis and memoranda: Bearing patiently the consequences or grabbing the chance for introducing reforms?', in Saridi, M. and Souliotis, K. (eds) *The Impact and Implications of Crisis. A Comprehensive Approach Combining Elements of Health and Society*, New York: Nova Science Publishers.

Economou, C. and Panteli, D. (2019) *Monitoring and Documenting Systemic and Health Effects of Health Reforms in Greece*, Copenhagen: WHO Regional Office for Europe. Available at: www.euro.who.int/__data/assets/pdf_file/0011/394526/Monitoring-Documenting_Greece_eng.pdf

ELSTAT (2021a). *The Greek Economy*, Athens: Hellenic Statistical Authority. Available at: www.statistics.gr/documents/20181/17120175/greek_economy_21_05_2021.pdf/c931ca4d-3a2a-86ad-745a-c467618115ea

ELSTAT (2021b) *System of Health Accounts 2019*, Athens: Hellenic Statistical Authority. Available at: www.statistics.gr/en/statistics/-/publication/SHE35/-

Eurostat (n.d.) Available at: https://ec.europa.eu/eurostat/data/database

Giannopoulou, I. and Tsobanoglou, G. (2020) 'COVID-19 pandemic: Challenges and opportunities for the Greek health care system', *Irish Journal of Psychological Medicine* 37(3): 1–5. Available at: www.cambridge.org/core/journals/irish-journal-of-psychological-medicine/article/covid19-pandemic-challenges-and-opportunities-for-the-greek-health-care-system/2630DF16917841D7FBB-FAC3453F97BD9

Global Burden of Disease Greece (2018) 'The burden of disease in Greece, health loss, risk factors, and health financing, 2000–16: An analysis of the Global Burden of Disease Study 2016', *Lancet Public Health* 3: e395–e405.

Karanikolos, M., Machenbach, J., Nolte, E., Stuckler, D. and McKee, M. (2018) 'Amenable mortality in the EU – has crisis changed its course?', *European Journal of Public Health* 28(5): 864–9. Available at: https://doi.org/10.1093/eurpub/cky116

Kentikelenis, A. (2017) 'Structural adjustment and health: A conceptual framework and evidence on pathways', *Social Science and Medicine* 187: 296–305.

Kyriopoulos, I. and Mossialos, E. (2021) 'Greece', in Immergut, E., Anderson, K., Devitt, C. and Popic, T. (eds) *Health Politics in Europe: A Handbook*, Oxford: Oxford University Press.

Laliotis, I., Ioannidis, J. P. A. and Stavropoulou, C. (2016) 'Total and cause-specific mortality before and after the onset of the Greek economic crisis: An interrupted time-series analysis', *Lancet* 1(2): 56–65.

Liaropoulos, L. (1998) 'Ethics and the management of health care in Greece: A health economist's perspective', in Dracopoulou, S. (ed) *Ethics and Values in Health Care Management*, Abingdon: Routledge.

Liaropoulos, L., Siskou, O., Kontodimopoulos, N., et al. (2012) 'Restructuring the hospital sector in Greece in order to improve effectiveness and efficiency', *Social Cohesion and Development* 7(1): 53–68. Available at: https://ejournals.epublish-ing.ekt.gr/index.php/SCAD/article/view/8989/9183

Mossialos, E., Allin, S. and Davaki, K. (2005) 'Analysing the Greek health system: A tale of fragmentation and inertia', *Health Economics* 14: 151–68.

Nikolentzos, A. and Mays, N. (2016) 'Explaining the persistent dominance of the Greek medical profession across successive health care system reforms from 1983 to the present', *Health Systems and Reform* 2(2): 135–46.

Nolte, E. and McKee, M. (2004) *Does Health Care Save Lives? Avoidable Mortality Revisited*, London: Nuffield Trust.

Nolte, E. and McKee, M. (2008) 'Measuring the health of nations: Updating an earlier analysis', *Health Affairs* 27(1): 58–71.

Oliver, A. and Mossialos, E. (2005) 'European health systems reforms: Looking backward to see forward?', *Journal of Health Politics, Policy and Law* 30(1–2): 7–28.

Organisation for Economic Co-operation and Development Health Database (n.d.) Paris: OECD. Available at: https://stats.oecd.org/Index.aspx?QueryId=96018

Petmesidou, M. (2020) 'Health policy and politics', in Featherstone, K. and Sotiro-poulos, D. (eds) *The Oxford Handbook of Modern Greek Politics*, Oxford: Oxford University Press.

Polyzos, N., Economou, C. and Zilidis, C. (2008) 'National health policy in Greece: Regulations or reforms? The Sisyphus myth', *European Research Studies* 11(3): 91–118. Available at: www.ersj.eu/repec/ers/papers/08_3_p7.pdf

Sissouras, A., Karokis, A. and Mossialos, E. (1994) 'Greece', in Organisation for Economic Co-operation and Development (ed) *The Reform of Health Care Systems. A Review of Seventeen OECD Countries*, Paris: OECD.

Toth, F. (2021) *Comparative Health Systems. A New Framework*, Cambridge: Cambridge University Press.

Tountas, Y., Karnaki, P. and Pavi, E. (2002) 'Reforming the reform: The Greek national health system in transition', *Health Policy* 62(1): 15–29.

Tountas, Y., Stenannson, H. and Fryssiras, S. (1995) 'Health reform in Greece: Planning and implementation of a national health system', *International Journal of Health Planning and Management* 10: 283–304.

Tragakes, E. and Polyzos, N. (1998) 'The evolution of health care reforms in Greece: Charting a course of change', *International Journal of Health Planning and Management* 13(2): 107–30.

Tsoukas, H. and Papoulias, D. (2005) 'Managing third-order change: The case of the public power corporation in Greece', *Long Range Planning* 38: 79–95.

Waitzberg, R., Hernández-Quevedo, C., Bernal-Delgado, E., et al. (2021) 'Early health system responses to the COVID-19 pandemic in Mediterranean countries: A tale of successes and challenges', *Health Policy* 126(5): 465–75.

Part II

Comparative analyses

10 The changing role of the state in a neo-liberal healthcare policy arena

Guido Giarelli

Introduction

In this chapter I shall first define the healthcare arena as a contested sphere of social actors from a neo-Weberian and neo-institutionalist perspective (Saks, 2016). This can be examined through the three key concepts of healthcare policy, politics and polity to understand the role the state plays in healthcare. Second, I shall operationalise these concepts by elaborating a multidimensional framework for analysing the role of the state in healthcare reforms. Third, I shall apply this framework to analysing the three Western European health macro-regions with National Health Services (NHSs) building on the first part of this volume, taking into account their inter-regional and intra-regional differences, and the impact of the Covid-19 pandemic on the role of the state. Finally, in conclusion, I shall assess to what extent the role of the state has changed or not (and if so, in what direction) after the last four decades of healthcare reforms, raising questions about their neo-liberal character.

Healthcare policy, politics and polity in a contested arena of social actors

In the first part of this volume, we have examined in detail healthcare reforms in national case studies of the three Western European macro-regions – Britain, Scandinavia and the Mediterranean – as characterised by different versions of the Beveridge model of healthcare system, the NHS. In the second part, a comparative analysis of the above case studies will be given by focusing on the roles of key social actors in shaping such reforms. Here in accord with the neo-Weberian approach: 'Actors, or stakeholders, are those with a vested interest, however large or small, in the policy process, and who have the ability to affect either positively or negatively the implementation of policy' (Rathwell, 1998:389). The centrality of social actors and their inter-relations as determinants of policy change is fundamental to understanding the reforms and their success or failure. According to Light (1995), there are four main social actors in the healthcare arena – the state, the medical and health professions, the patient and the medical–industrial complex. Since

DOI: 10.4324/9781003139799-16

these actors have their own interests and values, healthcare is a contested arena of conflicts and negotiations between them, often resulting in a compromise that defines policy choice.

I shall start in this chapter by considering the role of the state, since it is historically the main actor in healthcare policy. Even though healthcare *policy* usually 'refers to those courses of actions taken by governments that deal with the financing, provision or governance of health services' (Blank and Burau, 2007:2), other actors also play a more or less crucial role in framing health policy. Therefore, according to a neo-Weberian theoretical approach, healthcare policies are the outcome of *politics*, the conflict-ridden processes in which both divergent and common interests and political strategies of the key stakeholders develop through negotiation to achieve political goals. This is the reason why to understand the role of the state in healthcare reforms, we must consider the complex interplay of interactions of social actors and institutions representing healthcare politics in each country.

Walt (1998) in her framework for health policy analysis also indicates the relevance of the *context* in which policy is introduced. Although the context of healthcare can include such factors as the political and legal system, mass media, social structures, and public expectations and demands (Blank and Burau, 2007), from a neo-institutionalist viewpoint the political structures, institutions and cultures are the most relevant contextual factors framing political action. They consist of what is defined as the *polity* (Lawson, 2003): the institutional system comprising both the normative (laws), and structural (constitutional shape of the state) and informal (unwritten rules and political culture) elements in the political sphere.

For the analysis of the role of the state, the polity is particular significant because it can create 'path dependence', the reproductive mechanism that can explain continuities in health policy and politics (Greener, 2005), accounting for the difficulties of implementing a new health policy. Path dependence makes it increasingly difficult to leave historical pathways over time, leading to 'lock-in' until a new event occurs to disrupt the continuity. As Pierson (2004:21) says, 'the crucial feature of a historical process that generates path dependence is positive feedback or self-reinforcement . . . each step in a particular direction make it more difficult to reverse'. Social institutions are hard to change, and this is especially true of the state, where usually bureaucrats and civil servants once they have adapted to certain rules are unlikely to change, thereby making institutions self-sustaining.

Historical institutionalism has offered some interesting explanations for this 'stickiness'. Pierson (2000), for example, puts forward three factors for the particular susceptibility of politics and policy to path dependence: first, public institutions are durable, partly because of their legal basis, and partly because they shape the expectations of actors towards other actors, and thus become self-reinforcing; second, the long-term open exercise of power tends to be transformed into less open forms, reinforcing power asymmetries and limiting behaviour and aspirations for change; and, third, the complexity and opacity of politics means that actors have to simplify matters in cognitive terms by applying existing mental maps, which both frame how a given situation is perceived and filter out disconfirming information. All these factors can be applied to the analysis of the state in order to explain the difficulty of radical policy change – or, at best, of incremental change. Although, as Kay (2005:554) says, path dependence is 'neither a framework nor theory nor model' but 'an empirical category, an organising concept which can be used to label a certain type of temporal process', this concept can usefully explain the problems of reforms in certain polity contexts.

It is therefore argued that *policy, politics* and *polity* are the main elements to be taken into account in analysing the healthcare arena as a contested domain of social actors. However, to operationalise these concepts, it is necessary to define them more specifically and delineate the possible different interplay among them as a framework for analysing the role of the state in healthcare reforms.

A multidimensional framework for the analysis of the role of the state in the reforms

The starting point for the analysis of the role of the state in healthcare reforms is a comprehensive examination of the key social actors involved and their interactions. The state is one of these in the NHSs, and this marks a first difference compared with other types of healthcare systems. The classic tripartite typology of ideal-typical healthcare systems in fact considers the role of the state as fundamental in the genesis and rule of NHSs – to the point that Rothgang and colleagues (2010) define them as 'state healthcare systems', as distinct from 'societal healthcare systems' such as in Germany and France, where the main actors are health and social insurance schemes, and 'private healthcare systems' such as in the United States (US), where the key stakeholder until the 1980s was the medical profession, before it was corporatised by private health insurance bodies (Starr, 1982).

According to the tetrahedron model of Light (1995), healthcare can be considered as a multi-dimensional field of countervailing powers represented by the four main social actors indicated earlier. The concept of 'countervailing powers', inspired by the Montesquieu's idea of counterbalancing centres of power to check potential abuses of absolute power, has been sociologically elaborated by Light (1995:26) to focus

> on the interactions of powerful actors in a field where they are inherently interdependent yet distinct. If one party is dominant, as the American medical profession has long been, its dominance is contextual and eventually elicits counter-moves by other powerful actors, not to destroy it but to redress an imbalance of power.

This dynamic consideration of the *interactions* that develop among the actors in healthcare makes dominance by one of them always precarious due to the imbalances, excesses and neglects produced. It is also an important first factor in the analysis of the role of the state, as outlined in Figure 10.1. Sometimes, it can be the internal differentiation and expansion that weakens the dominant institution; in other cases, it could be ignorance of the concerns and interests of other actors or an expansion of control that are the main reasons affecting their dominant position and relationship with other countervailing powers.

What is important, though, in this structure which is elaborated later is the interplay of alliances and conflicts among actors in the healthcare arena. From this viewpoint, a useful tool is the distinction proposed by Peterson (1993) about 'representational communities' of organised interests and government institutions between *stakeholders* (who generally benefit from the *status quo* or are threatened by social change) and *stake challengers* (who wish to change the *status quo* because they do not benefit from it or are harmed by it). Their interconnections can create four distinct ideal-typical situations in healthcare – *block, dyad, amalgam* and *network* depending on the characteristics of stakeholders and the presence of stake challengers – where politics is either thwarted or translated into action (Walt, 1998), as set out in Figure 10.2.

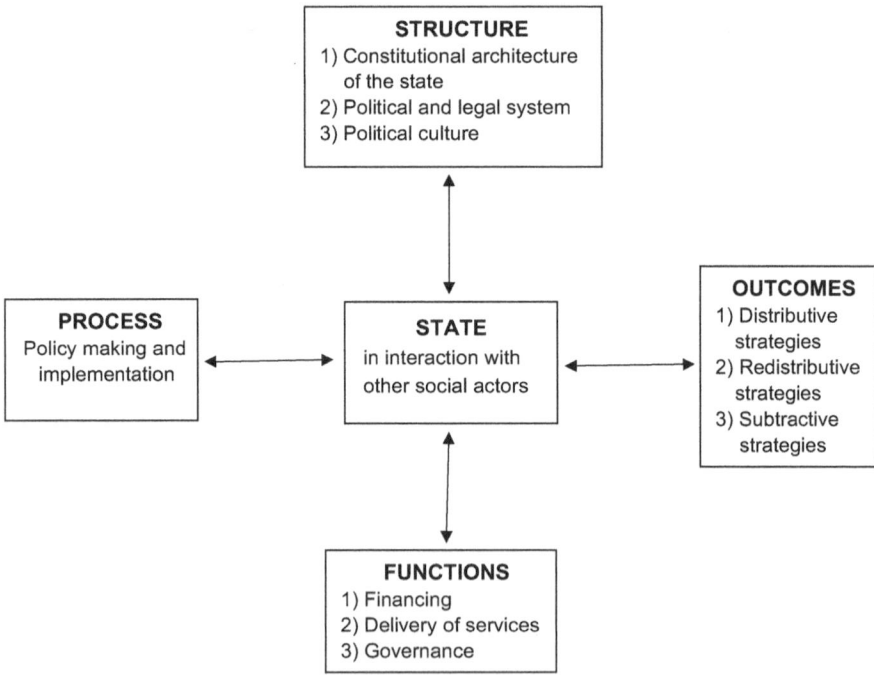

Figure 10.1 A multidimensional framework for analysing the role of the state in healthcare reforms

Source: Own elaboration.

Characteristics of the stakeholders	Presence of the stake challengers	
	No	Yes
Allied	*Block* (homogeneous)	*Dyad* (polarized)
Competitive	*Amalgam* (differentiated)	*Network* (heterogeneous)

Figure 10.2 Four possible situations in the healthcare arena

Source: Peterson (1993) modified.

As we have seen, these intertwinings of political conflicts and alliances do not takes place in a vacuum: the *polity* represents the historical and institutional environment of these social dynamics. This is what is defined as the structure in Figure 10.1, the backstage of the interactions taking place in the healthcare arena. As seen earlier, this includes (1) the *constitutional architecture of the state*, (2) the *political and legal system*, and (3) the *political culture*.

The first element refers to the state as an ensemble of institutions, procedures, authorities and agencies whose harmonious integration should not be taken for granted. As far as healthcare reforms are concerned, what assumes particular relevance is the *constitutional architecture of the state* in terms of centralisation or decentralisation of powers among different levels of government, and the consequent unitary or federal character of the state. As Terlizzi (2019:974) notes, since the end of World War II, decentralisation in Europe has been 'considered as a normatively superior mode of allocation of authority . . . the main argument for advocates of decentralization is that the shift of authority towards lower levels brings government closer to citizens, enhancing accountability and responsiveness'. However, since the 2000s, in several European countries with NHSs the role of central governments in steering healthcare systems has increased, reflecting concerns about the disadvantages of decentralisation (such as inequalities, inconsistencies and conflicts). This has produced a new trend towards re-centralisation (Saltman, 2008). Moreover, the different dimensions of the decentralisation/re-centralisation (politico-legislative, administrative and fiscal) issue need to be assessed to define which pattern has actually been adopted.

The second element of the polity structure is the *political and legal system*, including laws relevant to healthcare. The objectives of any reform policy have to confront the existing institutional structure of the healthcare system based on previous laws. This requires an understanding of the key characteristics of the government system in term of stability and strength: a single-party government, for example, is usually more stable and stronger than a coalition government, whose majority may be at risk. Moreover, a frequent change of governments of different political orientations does not guarantee the stability to ensure the proper implementation of reform. The third element of the polity structure is the dominant *political culture* of a country, its ideological orientation and the unwritten and informal rules of conduct implied. Setting the policy agenda for reform is an essentially value-laden process that often implies value conflicts between key actors. This can become a serious obstacle to reforms if there are no prior adequate mechanisms (unwritten procedures) to resolve the conflict and achieve a compromise. These three elements may also be complemented in the polity by the macroeconomic situation, shaped from the 1980s onwards by a series of cyclical economic crises culminating in the financial crisis of global capitalism in 2008. This was characterised as a time of scarce resources and low growth in all the European countries considered by Pierson (2001) as 'permanent austerity', with the notable exception of Norway with its oil revenue.

In terms of the *process of policymaking and implementation* in Figure 10.1, this is a crucial aspect that can explain the failure even of a well-designed reform when the potential difficulties created by decision-making are ignored. A widespread rational choice model considering policymaking just as a top-down linear process neglects the problem of how policymaking is implemented in practice, which can be of radical change (*big-bang approach*) or partial and gradual change (*incrementalism*). Politics, with its interplay of conflicts and alliances between different actors, therefore plays a significant role in the implementation of reforms. The public process of policymaking can be theoretically subdivided into four often overlapping and non-linear phases (Walt, 1998): (1) *problem identification*, with the policy agenda defined as a result of ideological values; (2) *policy formulation*, centred around the interaction between social actors in policy formulation; (3) *policy implementation*, including the role played by actors involved in influencing policy outcomes; and (4) *policy evaluation*, where a balanced consideration of positive and negative results of the reform takes place. What often happens is an iterative process whereby the original identification of problem and policy formulation are continuously redefined, and evaluation becomes part of implementation.

The implementation process is also related to the constitutional architecture of the state and the level of centralisation/decentralisation of political authority: a centralised system can favour a top-down policy approach more than a decentralised one, where a bottom-up approach may work better. Furthermore,

> implementation of policy is clearly dependent on the extent to which the centre can expect lower-level authorities to follow its guidelines. This will depend on how much political authority is vested in the system of government, and what mechanisms the centre can use to influence sub-national authorities: mechanisms may be through regulations or legislation (whether discretionary or mandatory) or financing inducements or sanctions.
>
> (Walt, 1998)

As regards the *functions* assigned to the state in Figure 10.1, the first element is *financing and expenditures*, as *provider* of services, and in the *governance* of the healthcare system. Traditionally, during the 'Golden Age' of the post-World War II expansion of the welfare state, in NHSs the state has played a central role. What is interesting is whether in the last four decades there were major changes in the *role of the state* in terms of both level and type of involvement (Rothgang et al., 2005). In relation to the first element, the involvement of the state can be assessed in terms of change in the ratio of public to total health expenditure. A similar question can be asked about the second element of the functions – the *delivery of services* in terms of whether the share of public healthcare services has increased or decreased. Here a difficulty arises from the fact that 'OECD heathcare data provide very limited information on the public-private dichotomy of *healthcare provision*' (Rothgang et al., 2005:207) which means we need to consider whether other sources are available. The third element of *governance* is more complex qualitatively, and shifts the focus to the type of governance adopted by the state to rule the NHS – a traditional hierarchical mechanism of direct command and control, or the regulatory role of the public–private internal market. In recent decades, the role of the state has generally changed from a more *dirigiste* involvement, related to the almost total public ownership of services and tightly controlled centralised planning, to a new *regulatory* role relying mainly on using this instrument in the newly introduced internal market in the NHS (Helderman, Bevan and France, 2012).

The last factor in the framework outlined in Figure 10.1 is the *outcomes* that the strategies of healthcare reforms produced – in terms of change of population coverage (access of patients to services), benefit packages (more or less comprehensive services) and population health (improved or worsened). By adopting a modified version of the classification of policy outcomes proposed by Lowi (1966), three different types of strategies exist according to their outcomes: *distributive, redistributive* and *subtractive*. While redistributive and distributive policies characterised the 'Golden Age' of the welfare systems from the post-war period to the 1970s, the austerity measures and retrenchement policies of many governments especially after the financial crisis of 2008 can be characterised in their outcomes as subtractive strategies (Pavolini and Guillén, 2013). A subtractive policy implies a reduction of public entitlements negatively affecting the most disadvantaged groups. Assessing whether this has happened with the healthcare reforms of the NHSs is the last task in our framework. The state interactions with other social actors, the structure of the polity, the process of policy implementation, the functions of the state in the healthcare system, and the outcomes produced will now be applied in the multidimensional model in examining the role of the state in the healthcare reforms to the NHSs in the three European health macro-regions, including the impact of the Covid-19 pandemic.

Four decades of neo-liberal health policies reforms in the three Western European macro-regions

The British macro-region

We cannot fail to start from the British macro-region and its NHS since this is the pioneering model of a comprehensive NHS. Undoubtedly, the state has historically played a strong and central role in British healthcare since the founding of the NHS in 1948. The fact that Aneurin Bevan, the minister of health, was at that time able to nationalise all the private and local authority hospitals demonstrates this. However, establishing alliances and compromises with other social actors to gain their support for the changes introduced was a fundamental strategic task, especially when vested interests were affected. In this way, the Labour government was able to win over the opposition of the medical profession, in particular influential hospital consultants, who were made into public employees while maintaining a high degree of control over their conditions of employment and clinical decision-making and continuing to undertake private work. On the other hand, general practitioners (GPs), represented by the British Medical Association, were assured of continuing their independence, even if paid on *per capita* basis, while acting as gatekeepers in the NHS. Moreover, the government gained legitimacy and support of the public on the promise of a more equal, universal, comprehensive and free at the point of service healthcare system (Gabe, 1997).

This configuration of the social actors in British healthcare substantially corresponds to the fourth case described by Peterson (1993) of competitive stakeholders (GPs and hospital consultants) and a stake challenger (the government) strong enough to create a 'heterogeneous network' capable of fostering radical social change through public support without a substantial medical–industrial complex. This scheme has been replicated, with different content, in subsequent neo-liberal reforms over the last four decades. Initially, the introduction of managerialism and the internal market by the Thatcher government

> were strongly opposed by the medical and nursing professions as well as opposition parties who argued that they would undermine the principles on which the NHS was established. Criticism focused particularly on plans to introduce competition between health care providers. It was argued that this would threaten achievement of equity and access in the NHS and result in the commercialization of health care.
>
> (Ham, 1997:47)

Notwithstanding the strength of this opposition, the Thatcher government passed proposals altering the previous balance of power in the NHS in favour of managers and at the expenses of professionals, especially hospital doctors who 'were to be more accountable to managers who had stricter control over professional and labour costs through a system of management budgets which related workload objectives to the resources available' (Ham, 1997:16–17). At the same time, hospital doctors were encouraged to participate in the new micro-management techniques for monitoring efficiency of performance and some were appointed as general managers, while largely retaining their clinical autonomy and power.

Meanwhile, the introduction of fundholding represented considerable enhancement for GPs, who were given budgets to negotiate services for their patients from provider units. This change in the balance of power between the different interests of hospital doctors and GPs was functional in dividing and widening competition between them, reinforcing the government position, which was sold to the public as a patient-based reform model. The rhetoric of consumerism adopted by the Conservative government, emphasising individual empowerment and free choice, ideologically legitimated a reform policy based on a management-led approach (Hughes, 1991). The emergence of a new class of public and private managers as a key social actor in healthcare – even as a consequence of the contemporary strong promotion of the private hospital and outpatient sector – was the result of the new mixed economy set up by the Thatcher reforms of 'privatising from within' (Ranade and Haywood, 1989). Moreover,

> it could be argued that the UK government successfully implemented radical reform by creating a situation whereby one set of actors (managers) perceived for themselves particular advantages in supporting change in terms of enhanced prestige and influence, such that they chose to discount the concern of other actors.
>
> (Rathwell, 1998:390)

The 'heterogeneous network' of stakeholder interests remained broadly stable during the New Labour governments of Blair and Brown since the internal market and managerialism remained untouched, and the role of the private sector was strengthened with the transformation of NHS providers into Foundation Trusts with their own regulatory body (Monitor), followed by the replacement of Primary Care Groups with Primary Care Trusts (PCTs) and the abolition of District Health Authorities. The substitution of public commissioning by Health Authorities with private practice-based commissioning of PCTs marked a retrenchment of the role of the state, but this was balanced by its increased control of medical and health professionals in assessing the costs and benefits of healthcare interventions through the National Institute for Clinical Excellence (NICE) in 1999 (later the National Institute for Health and Care Excellence) and its role as clinical governance regulator through the Commission for Health Improvement in 1999 (replaced by first the Healthcare Commission and then the Care Quality Commission in 2009). Therefore, while the government's ability to implement systemwide reforms was blocked by the interests of Foundation Trusts, the withdrawal of the state from direct public commissioning and ownership of many healthcare services in favour of private commissioning and new regulatory agencies was a significant step towards the rise of the 'regulatory state' in the NHS (Moran, 2003).

However, this trend cannot be generalised to the British NHS as a whole given the devolution of certain legislative matters including health to the newly established Scottish Parliament and the Welsh Senedd (as well as to Northern Ireland) by devolution acts in 1998. This ended half-a-century of centralised rule by the British government, significantly modifying the structure of the British polity: while the United Kingdom (UK) has remained a unitary state, each of the four countries thereafter developed their own NHS system. From this point, the roads diverged – and, especially since 2010, NHS England has continued to follow the neo-liberal path taken by previous governments with the Coalition and then Conservative governments. In contrast, NHS Scotland and NHS Wales have followed divergent policies exploring alternatives to the English approach. In England, the Conservative-Liberal Democrat Coalition dismantled the remaining bureaucratic hierarchical arrangements of the NHS in 2010. Despite opposition by medical and health professionals, a further privatisation policy abolished PCTs and replaced them with local Clinical Commissioning Groups (CCGs) led by practitioners, and greater leeway was given to Foundation Trusts to draw on private income. As such, government's responsibilities were resized to setting health strategies and allocating the overall NHS budget, while the provision of services was entrusted to market competition between public and private providers, with less central planning. In parallel, private spending as a proportion of total health expenditures rose significantly, and the provision of private NHS services almost doubled from 2010 to 2015 (Full Fact, 2017).

Subsequent Conservative governments since 2013 have had to contend with market failures marked by serious shortcomings and scandals in care quality in Foundation Trusts, providing them with support, further regulation and standards, tighter control and supervision in the interests of patient safety. The recent Covid-19 pandemic has prompted more central planning and integration, with the prospect in the 2021 government White Paper of a reorganised NHS with the abolition of CCGs and greater central control. Furthermore, the pandemic has brought prevention and public health to the fore, leading to structural changes in the governance with the establishment of a new national agency. However, because of the funding gap and a narrow focus on individual responsibility rather than environmental and structural factors in public health, the results of these commitments were limited, as one of the highest levels of excess deaths in Western Europe during the pandemic show (World Health Organization, 2021).

To summarise, the role of the state in English healthcare has changed significantly during the past four decades of neo-liberal healthcare reforms. As Helderman, Bevan and France say (2012:103):

> [W]hereas the former 'dirigiste' state used to be closely related to public ownership (e.g. hospitals), planning (volume and capacity planning) and centralised administration (e.g. fixed prices and budgets), the new regulatory state relies mainly on the instrument of regulation to achieve its objectives.

As already argued, it is a paradox that neo-liberal privatisation and marketisation policies have not led to deregulation but, instead, to such an increase in regulation as the main instrument of governance that England can be viewed as a new 'regulatory state' (Majone, 1994). Even though one of the consequences of Covid-19 pandemic has been strengthening central planning and weakening or suspending some neo-liberal reforms, it is yet to be seen how far this countertrend will be reflected in a new policy orientation.

In Scotland, following devolution in 1999, the government – first a Labour-led coalition and then the Scottish National Party (SNP) – dismantled the internal market and abolished Trusts with the 2004 NHS Reform Act – transferring their functions to 15 (later 14) integrated Regional Health Boards with an integrated public system. This was possible given the changed constitution of the state and the strong support of Scottish nationalist political culture, where the ideology emphasised the value of identity and unity of the local community as an alternative to neo-liberal market values. This implied building a new culture of partnership, co-ownership, mutuality and involvement between NHS professionals and the public, stressing cooperation and collaboration in a 'mutual NHS'. To support this process, the Health Boards were empowered to create Community Health Partnerships (CHPs) – as networks where NHS staff operated closely with local authorities and voluntary agency staff to improve the quality of health services. Moreover, the promotion of integrated health and social services and the strengthening of primary care were considered key to the new policy vision, as evidenced by the replacement of the CHPs with Health and Social Care Partnerships in 2014. Additionally, Public Health Scotland, founded in 2020, aimed to respond more effectively to the Covid-19 outbreak by unifying the functions of previously separate agencies.

A similar, less marked, path was pursued by the Welsh Labour–nationalists coalition governments following devolution: after initially continuing with a soft version of the internal market inclined towards greater system integration and cooperation by Local Health Boards with NHS Trusts. In 2009, they abolished the internal market, establishing seven unified health authorities, replacing the previous Local Health Boards and NHS Trusts, which were responsible for health services, including primary and specialised care, with a shared responsibility with Public Health Wales and local authorities. Since then, there has been a health policy focused on improved population health, the reduction of health inequalities, health promotion and disease prevention, and the integration of health and social care similar to Scotland – albeit more concerned with efficiency, as the idea of 'prudent healthcare' conveys, with a strong emphasis on 'co-production' of patients and public with professionals/managers in treatment and policy decision-making (Welsh NHS Confederation, 2017).

In Wales, as in Scotland, the Covid-19 pandemic has been an occasion for conflict with the UK central government. After an initial phase of centralised management of the pandemic without consultation, both the devolved administrations decided to pursue a divergent approach, establishing their own advisory boards – further evidencing their attempts to follow alternatives to the English policy. In our multidimensional model, the configuration of social actors in the healthcare arena was significantly different from England: the state in Scotland and Wales was not a stake challenger but acted as a partner with other stakeholders, involving health professionals and citizens in a homogeneous block of co-owners of the NHS as in Figure 10.2. This was facilitated by the strong ideological support of their nationalist political cultures for 'mutuality' and 'co-production', respectively, which have made policy implementation smooth and incremental, without the need for any 'big bang' approach like that in England. In terms of functions, this approach has translated into a return to a significant role of the state in public financing and ownership of services, minimising the part played by private providers and third payers. Meanwhile, recent changes in NHS England after the Covid-19 pandemic put it back in the direction of a planned, mainly publicly delivered service, although many common linkages between these NHS systems remain. Nonetheless, the type of governance in Scotland and Wales is far from both the 'regulatory state' of England and the *dirigiste* state of the past – as Guthrie and colleagues (2010) suggest, with a blend of control through group processes and government oversight.

This combination of continued hierarchical control and partnership with health professionals and local communities can best be described as a form of 'stewardship', where 'a function of governments responsible for the welfare of populations and concerned about the trust and legitimacy with which its activities are viewed by the general public' (Saltman and Ferroussier-Davies, 2000:735). This definition, emphasising trust and legitimacy of governments, highlights the ethical and responsible dimension of the policy strategies as key factors in their success. It transcends both the traditional Weberian concept of state institutions as bureaucracies – structures of authority based on impersonal norms and offices ruled by command and control – and the minimalist notion of a regulatory state based on control of the opportunistic behaviour of self-interested social actors in neo-liberal economic theories. The notions of trust, ethical behaviour and sound decision-making are inherent in the concept of stewardship in public administration (Kass, 1990). In Scotland and Wales, as we have seen, this ethical and accountable dimension of governance has been supported by their political cultures based on a strong nationalist and communitarian commitment of health professionals and citizenry to 'partnership', 'co-ownership' and 'mutuality' in their NHSs. It is still too early to assess, in terms of outcomes, whether this stewardship governance strategy has avoided ending up in a substantial subtractive policy like that of the regulatory state in England. However, the extreme attention to health inequalities in their policies (Forbes and Evans, 2008; Hughes and Vincent-Jones, 2008) implies a more direct orientation towards a redistributive policy unlike the English neo-liberal reforms. The future of this strategy, though, will largely depend for Scotland on the result of a possible second referendum on independence and for Wales on the government's ability to improve centre–periphery connections and relationships with the UK government.

The Scandinavian macro-region

It is well known that Scandinavian countries have historically been characterised by the central role of the state in healthcare. The long legacy of statism in the Swedish healthcare system goes back to the early establishment of the monarchic unitary state in the sixteenth century, which immediately entered the healthcare arena by establishing the first royal hospital and then organised outpatient care through a national system of provincial doctors. Since 1862 – with the institution of the elective County Council at provincial level in charge of, first, hospital care and then, with the Health and Medical Services Act of 1982, of outpatient and social care integration along with municipalities – the main characteristic of the structure of the Swedish state in healthcare has been decentralisation with shared governmental responsibilities among national, regional and municipal governments (Saltman, 1999). The decentralised character of the Swedish polity structure has also survived the neo-liberal reforms of the last four decades, showing a high level of path dependence in Swedish policy in spite of attempts to merge County Councils into wider regional units during the 1990s and 2000s – and the trend towards centralisation in terms of quality control and performance monitoring, reinforced during the Covid-19 pandemic. As a result, it has a well-established governance structure at three levels – national government and agencies, 21 County Councils and 290 municipalities – albeit with inevitable problems of coordination and integration.

However, according to Immergut (1999), this long-standing tradition of public provision of healthcare services cannot alone explain the nature of the Swedish healthcare system, which she believes is the result of a 'politics of compromise' not based on a pre-existing consensus or absence of conflicts, but

forged by political institutions that did not provide opportunity for minority interests to override the executive level consensus. The result of the pattern of executive-induced conciliation was a health system that represents the public extreme of government financing and delivery of health services.

(Immergut, 1999:201)

This tradition of 'soft governance' is a conciliatory mechanism for reaching consensus based on agreement between different class-based interest groups and political representatives at the three levels of the governance structure to draft, approve and implement legislative proposals that is still very much present. This politics of compromise has made the Swedish healthcare arena very close to 'amalgam' as set out in Figure 10.2: the competitive interests of various stakeholders are conciliated by the state, which, instead of acting as stake challenger as in the English case, amalgamates the differentiated interests. The result is that only incremental change is allowed for any reform policy.

The process of professionalisation of Swedish doctors is an example of this. As Garpenby (1989) argues, it was accomplished through the state, and this explains why Swedish physicians have maintained an orientation to the public sector. The *Collegium Medicum*, established in 1663, was replaced by the *Sundhetskollegiet* (Health Council) in 1813, which became the *Medicilanstyrelsen* (National Board of Health) in 1877, gradually assuming the role and functions of a government institution empowered to control professional licensing and work. Different from the British Royal Colleges which remained independent bodies licensed by the state, therefore, the Swedish Medical Association has gradually become an integral part of the state. This explains why, despite its organisational strength, the medical profession up to the 1980s was not in a veto position as in 1947

the Swedish government introduced national health insurance and controls on doctors' fees and finally placed all doctors on full-time salary in conjunction with severe restrictions on the ability of doctors to practice privately, thereby converting the system to a de facto national health service.

(Immergut, 1999:201)

The weak role of patients and the public in the healthcare arena, jointly recognised by right and left-wing parties since the 1980, is similarly the result of the mediation of their interests by the elected political representatives at various levels of governance. This explains why instead of a direct involvement and participation in the decision-making process of the healthcare system, as in the British case, it has been simply translated into a patient-free choice of providers, either private (right-wing parties) or public (left-wing parties). The role of the private sector in publicly mediated healthcare has traditionally been rather marginal, in terms of clinical practice and health insurance. Popular political culture imbued egalitarian and solidaristic values supporting the dominant political ideology of social democracy has represented a strong barrier to privatisation policies (Blomqvist and Winblad, 2021).

The neo-liberal reforms carried out by Conservative governments during the 1990s and 2000s are the result of the partial erosion of this political consensus due to the increasing social stratification of Swedish society related to the growing arrival of foreign immigrants and refugees (Immergut, 1999). However, the problematic implementation of reform shows that the legacy of the policy of compromise still had traction. Furthermore, the decentralised structure of the state limited the implementation of the internal market and privatisation of healthcare services mostly to right-wing County Councils and more profitable urban locations. While these reforms have gradually led to an increase of private providers delivering primary and specialised care (but not in hospitals), the tax-based financing system has never been questioned, and the governance function based on the multi-level system of planning and steerage has remained untouched. However, the subtractive outcomes of privatisation policies in terms of private providers and worse health outcomes among disadvantaged social and ethnic groups have increased inequalities in the system – even if its universalistic character and predominantly public nature are still evident. During the Covid-19 pandemic, though, Sweden had one of the highest contagion and mortality rates in Europe among the elderly in domiciliary settings and nursing homes. This indicates a significant failure of the primary care and preventive system, while the planned shift of resources to primary care and the government's efforts to improve coordination and integration with social care indicates that planning still occurs to avoid market failure (Valeriani et al., 2020).

The fact that a less egalitarian but still solid NHS system has survived after the wave of neo-liberal reforms in recent decades suggests that the amalgamation strategy of Swedish healthcare policy, while weakened, is still working. It also shows the continuance of a strong level of path dependence, confirming the view of Wilsford (1994:276–8) that, in highly decentralised systems based on non-hierarchical networks of autonomous decision-agents, it is difficult to implement major changes because 'the path dependency model characterizes especially the collective decision outcome of decentralized and independent decision-agents'. In consequence, 'establishing a new trajectory subsequently is extremely difficult and unlikely, except in the presence of an immensely powerful and compelling conjuncture'. The absence of such a conjuncture in the Swedish context – apart from dissatisfaction with the rigidities and inefficiencies of the healthcare system – helps to explain the difficult, fragmented, patchy and reversible character of the neo-liberal reforms in that country.

The amalgamation strategy and the policy of compromise on which it is based inform the shape the stewardship strategy of the state has taken in the Swedish context. This is apparent if we assess the existence of the five core attributes of stewardship (Kapoor, Kumar and Thakur, 2014). The first, the existence of a political will as a requirement for the strong role of the state in healthcare, is inscribed in the historical and political heritage of the country. The second, an explicitly normative and ethical dimension of this role, can be traced to the egalitarian and solidaristic values supporting the choice of the public system and the state responsibility to reduce health inequalities. The third, a balanced interventionist approach by the state in healthcare, characterises the Keynesian policy of the Social Democratic government as compared to the *laissez-faire* orientation of neo-liberalism. The fourth attribute, the need for responsible management of the functioning of the system and, ultimately, population health, mirrors the socially responsible management culture of Sweden. Finally, the last core attribute of stewardship is good governance; as the World Health Organization (WHO) (2000) says, '[W]hile governance more closely deals with the management arrangements of increasingly complex health systems, the stewardship forms the bedrock of underlying values and principles which in itself will guide those arrangement'. In other words, 'if governance is body, stewardship is its soul' (Kapoor, Kumar and Thakur, 2014:6). In Sweden, this bedrock is well inscribed in the polity structure and particularly in the political culture and behaviour of the country supporting management.

If the Swedish case is now compared with Denmark, we find strong similarities. Here political compromises have gradually created a state-regulated system, largely funded by taxation and dominated by the public ownership of hospitals. The polity structure of the Danish system also has an originally decentralised constitution very similar to the Swedish one. The national government just had responsibility for overall coordination by framework legislation and the funding of the healthcare system. However, since the 1971 reform that established the tax-based universal system, the counties were the decentralised authorities responsible for hospital ownership and primary care service delivery, while the municipalities were in charge of social care, care for the elderly, non-clinical long-term care, and child and maternity care. With the structural reform of 2007, the 13 counties were merged into five larger regions, and the number of municipalities reduced from 271 to 98 in a partial re-centralisation aimed at improving the overall efficiency of the system to address the long-term sustainability of county and municipal welfare governance (Christiansen and Vrangbæk, 2018).

The implementation of the above reforms was also gradual and incremental like the Swedish one, following a tradition of wider political compromise at national level on welfare reforms, based on shared principles of universality and equity. This long tradition of pragmatic collaboration, centred on well-established Danish political norms that major societal reforms are based on broad agreements across the three levels of multi-level governance, is due to the institutionalised structure of broad-based committees, and the existence of many small parties and often-shifting coalitions of left-wing and right-wing factions. In terms of functions, the Danish healthcare system has remained financially tax-based and universal. The delivery of services is still totally public for the hospitals by regions, whereas the outpatient general and specialist practices are privately owned and delivered – even if they are tightly integrated into public planning and regulation and mainly funded by public means. This does not make for easy governance of the coordination, tensions and conflicts of this complex, hybrid, semi-decentralised, multi-level system based on regulation, economic incentives and softer governance measures, but it resonates with the institutional principles of decentralised political management, universal coverage and public funding in terms of the steward-ship strategy (Brinkerhoff et al., 2019).

In terms of outcomes, this strategy has allowed for high levels of popula-tion coverage and health on the basis of comprehensive benefit packages. In relation to health inequalities, since there are no out-of-pocket payments for regional hospital or private GPs, there are restrictions as regards access – even if the increasing diffusion of voluntary health insurance may expand inequality in the near future. Danish healthcare therefore has a high degree of continuity and path dependence in the role of the state, although the gradual incorporation of New Public Management (NPM), New Public Governance and Digital Era Governance principles may gradually erode this continuity from within. Much will depend on the political support of the citizens for incremental reforms based on public governance control, and balancing cost containment and efficiency with high levels of quality and equity in public services. The development of new mechanisms of democratic involvement will greatly help here in fostering this support. On the other hand, much will ride on the ability of the state to carry out the policy of compromise and mediation given the interests of citizens, medical and health professionals and health insurance schemes – and to amalgamate them. The strong histori-cal alliance of the medical profession with the state and its integration into national and regional governance structures may offer a strong guarantee in this regard. Nonetheless, private health insurance schemes will become more threatening if they continue to grow and are supported by the Liberal/Con-servative parties (Vrangbæk, 2021).

In the Scandinavian macro-region, Norway – despite having been united with Sweden from 1814 to 1905 – has developed quite a different healthcare system from the second post-war period onwards that is defined by Saunes, Karanikolos and Sagan (2020) as semi-centralistic or semi-decentralised. Between the Hospital Act of 1969 to 2002, the 19 County Councils were in charge of the hospital sector and municipalities of primary healthcare and of nursing homes. However, this originally decentralised model has significantly changed since that time, after a long process of centralisation initiated in 1974 with the grouping of the counties in five (later four) healthcare regions. This transferred ownership of the 20 hospitals from the County Councils to the government, which became responsible for their funding, even though their management and delivery was entrusted with regional health authori-ties. Moreover, since 1997, hospitals were transformed into public enterprises funded by performance on the basis of activity-based financing, according to NPM principles (Martinussen and Magnussen, 2009).

These latter two trends have transformed the polity structure of the Norwegian healthcare system; it has moved from decentralisation to centralisation – even if the municipalities have remained in charge of primary healthcare and their role was strengthened through the 2012 Public Health Act. This assigned them greater responsibility for prevention, giving the system a more semi-centralised character despite the NPM-inspired shift from traditional bureaucratic management to enterprise organisation and business management. Both these trends have largely resulted from a different evolution of political culture from Sweden. While they have shared a common long post-war period of social democratic hegemony, the Norwegian Labour governments have adopted a more neo-liberal orientation following an NPM market ideology and de-politicising the issue of hospital management – considered as a pure 'technical' problem to be left in the hands of managers at arm's length from politicians. The implementation process of the hospital reform has also meant a completely different approach from the politics of compromise practised in the multi-level governance system by the Swedish government. The big-bang approach makes the Norwegian case more similar to the English one, without prior discussion and involvement of citizens, health professionals and other interest groups (Martinussen and Magnussen, 2009).

This picture of healthcare in Norway is different from Sweden and Denmark. Here the state, in the centralised version of government, has acted forcefully as a stake challenger towards the heterogeneous network of interests of other social actors, who have been strong enough to promote radical social change in spite of opposition, especially by the medical and health professions. The result is more similar to a 'regulatory state' model where health policy governance takes the form of grants, laws and regulation by the government instead of central planning – even though Parliament has tried to challenge the neo-liberal order of the state by claiming its own political role, and the new Labour-Centre government has announced its intention to soften the current market-oriented model. Overall, in the case of Norway, the replacement of the original decentralised model of healthcare with a centralised system and the big bang implementation strategy of the government demonstrate that path dependence can be eroded in the Scandinavian context once there is a more centralised and hierarchical structure of the state, again confirming Wilsford's (1994:278) view that 'centralization of decision process and hierarchical ordering of decision-agents render a system amenable to leveraging from the top and typically provide the top-most decision-agents with the means of decision and authority of enforcement down through the hierarchy'.

The Mediterranean macro-region

When we consider the role of the state in the healthcare arena of the European Mediterranean countries (Italy, Spain, Portugal and Greece), the problem of the so-called 'Mediterranean paradigm' is posed: that is, of a series of similar traits consisting of 'a distinctive pattern of health and disease, a common historical evolution of NHSs, shared principles, limited implementation, similar patterns of organization and delivery, and, in recent years, a common crisis and responses to it' (Figueras et al., 1994:143). With regard to the state, there are some historical similarities: all these countries experienced long periods of fascist authoritarian rule, and only after its overthrow and the restoration of democratic regimes with new constitutions, were NHSs enacted – first in Italy (1978) and then in Portugal (1979), Greece (1983) and Spain (1986). However, the legacy of the previous healthcare systems based on the Bismarckian model of health and social insurance has taken a different form in the four countries – while in Spain and Italy, it was abandoned, in Portugal and Greece, it continued to play a limited or dominant role.

A second point is the peculiar historical character of the state in these countries. Defining 'stateness' in terms of the degree of decision-making autonomy of public bureaucracies with respect to external political and social groups and their ability to implement their own decisions, Ferrera (1996) spoke of 'a double deficit'. On the one hand, there was the low degree of state penetration into the sphere of welfare in general and healthcare in particular, leaving ample room for manoeuvre to private institutions, which have benefited from using public funds through agreements. On the other hand, the low degree of state power meant that the administrative apparatus was highly open to external pressures from political and social groups, with the consequent frequent risk of political clientelism and corruption. As a result of this double deficit, Ferrera described the welfare systems of these countries as 'particularistic-clientelist', such that the NHSs have not promoted a significant strengthening of the public sphere, but rather peculiar forms of collusion between the public and private sectors. However, if we look at the scale of private healthcare expenditure on total healthcare expenditure, we can see that, while in two countries, it remained relatively low (Italy: 24.4% in 2021; Spain: 26.7% in 2020), in the others, it has increased significantly during the last decade (Portugal: 36% in 2021; Greece: 38.2% in 2020) (Organization for Economic Cooperation and Development, 2022).

Third, the constitutional architecture of the state and, consequently of their NHSs, shows that, while Spain has become a federal state with 17 regions (*Comunidades Autónomas*) and Italy a unitary but decentralised state divided into five autonomous and 15 ordinary regions, Portugal and Greece have remained unitary centralised states. The consequences of these different polity structures on the governance and management of the NHSs are quite evident in terms of different problems and conflicts and mechanisms for dealing with them (Giarelli, 2021).

For the above three reasons – despite the common historical legacy and formal establishment of NHSs – there is no unitary 'Mediterranean paradigm' (Petmesidou and Guillén, 2008). Starting with Italy and Spain, based on the polity structure and political culture, both countries founded NHSs during the 1970s and 1980s following a period of hegemony by a strong democratic culture in the wake of social movements, which led to the state taking responsibility for the health of citizens. The difference between the two countries is that, while in Italy the system of corporatist health insurance funds inherited from fascism has been heavily discredited due to enormous disparities in conditions of access and benefit packages and the level of debt to be paid, in Spain the organisation of the *Asistencia Sanitaria de la Seguridad Social* into a single health fund for all workers was much more efficient and homogeneous, and has provided the infrastructure facilitating a gradual, rather than instantaneous, transition to the NHS.

However, support for the democratisation of the healthcare system in both countries was not given by other actors in the healthcare arena, including the majority of doctors, who have traditionally taken a conservative stance. Their anti-reformist position, though, was not strong enough to hinder the approval and implementation of reforms given that they were supported by the majority of citizens and civil society. This shows that when the state gains such support, their alliance can overcome the resistance of other interest groups such as the middle and upper classes, doctors, health insurance schemes and private healthcare. This leads to a healthcare configuration approximating to the polarised dyad of opposite coalitions as set out in Figure 10.2, the two alliances of stakeholders versus stake challengers. The outcome will depend on the veto power of the alliance of stakeholders – and this explains the troubled implementation of the Italian reforms of the NHS, which in 1978, 1992/93 and 1999 were the result of the struggles of the two coalitions. The veto power of the medical profession was particularly evident after the third reform, when it forced the minister of health to resign (Vicarelli, 2005).

As regards the contents of the neo-liberal reforms adopted from the 1990s onwards, in both countries their implementation has only been partial. In Spain, the reforms tended to affect more the supply side than the demand side at management level – with measures aimed at controlling costs and at boosting performance and efficiency, with less impact on equity. The only exception was the Royal Decree 16/2012 of the Conservative government re-establishing the social insurance principle as the basis of entitlement to healthcare, restricting access for irregular immigrants and introducing new co-payments. This was subsequently either not applied or attenuated because of strong opposition from citizens, civil society associations and the health trade unions. In Italy, a soft form of internal market or quasi-market was introduced with the Decree 502/1992, which took the form of a partial purchaser–provider split and corporatisation with the transformation of the Local Health Authorities into Trusts that manage the system based on a form of administrative cooperation. In summary, health financing has remained predominantly public in both countries, and the share of private ownership of services and of private health insurance schemes, although increasing, is still limited (Vicarelli, 2005).

In terms of governance, this has in both cases become much more complex with the regional decentralisation of systems. However, while in Spain the devolution of power from the central state to the 17 *Comunidades Autónomas* has been implemented incrementally but completely (albeit with a partial re-centralisation during the last economic crisis and the Covid-19 pandemic), in Italy, the process of devolution has been partial especially in terms of financing and taxation. It has also been contradictory, with a substantial re-centralisation for the regions in budgetary default during the last decade. Furthermore, while in Spain, an institutional mechanism has been devised to regulate the inevitable problems of coordination and conflicts among the regions and between them and the state with the establishment of the Interterritorial Council of Health, in Italy, the State-Regions Conference has mainly remained an informal discussion forum about the criteria for subdividing the National Health Fund among the regions – without any real institutional power to coordinate them and their organisation and activities. Indeed, the split of the Conference between the centre-left and centre-right regions has often blocked its functioning. We can therefore define the two cases of governance, especially in Italy, as incomplete forms of decentralised stewardship, due largely to healthcare being based on a dyad of opposite coalitions that makes the approval and implementation of any reform complex and problematic (Giarelli and Giovannetti, 2019).

Moving to the second pair of countries – Portugal and Greece – they represent two cases of partial implementation of the NHS. Although the establishment of the NHSs in 1979 and 1983, respectively, in these countries was the outcome of a process of democratisation of the polity structure and political culture, the counteraction of internal and external actors hindered the implementation and the improvement of the NHS. The main internal stakeholders opposing reforms were the medical corporation, the private voluntary and the social and health insurance schemes, which through their strong interest-based veto powers stopped or delayed reforms. The previously existing occupational social and health insurance schemes have been able to survive by supplementing the NHS thanks to their superior provision of healthcare services. This has created a peculiar three-tier system based on the overlapping of public, social and private spheres of healthcare, with widespread inequalities between users who can access two or three spheres and those who can only access the public sphere (Barros, Machado and Simões, 2011; Economou, 2010).

However, the healthcare arena of these two countries was heavily hit by an even stronger pool of external actors – the so-called 'Troika', made up of the EU Commission, Central European Bank and International Monetary Fund – which forced them to accept bailout plans because of their budget deficits and to sign Memoranda of Understanding imposing, among other things, significant restrictions on public health spending. Both countries were heavily shaken by the 2008 financial crisis, and the austerity policies imposed by the Troika further reduced public financial resources for healthcare services, heavily affecting their delivery, efficiency, efficacy and quality. In this case, the Troika ousted the role of the national state, transforming the healthcare arena into a transnational governance structure of a more technocratic-managerial type. Given the negative effects both for the NHSs and for the health of the population, it is not surprising that, in both countries since 2015, left-wing governments have been elected which have largely rejected Troika austerity policies – and tried to revive public healthcare to improve the health of the public. This has had more efficacious and long-lasting effects in Portugal than in Greece, notwithstanding the further negative impact of the Covid-19 pandemic (Wainwright, n.d.).

Another key difference characterising these two countries compared to Italy and Spain is the weak centralised architecture of the state: in terms of polity structure, this has meant that, despite repeated attempts at decentralisation of the governance and management of the NHSs at regional and local levels, they have largely remained under the rule of the national Ministries of Health. This has had denigratory consequences, for example, in terms of limiting the capacity for implementing effective community-based primary care in Portugal. Even when some partial forms of decentralisation were implemented, they remained at the purely administrative level, without any substantial transfer of financial and legislative power. The same is true of Greece, where in the NHS a primary healthcare system of urban and rural health centres staffed by GPS and governed by a referral system was envisaged, but never implemented. The same fate befell legislation passed in 2014 and 2017 aiming to develop a nationwide primary healthcare service, where implementation has been slow and partial, not helped by the change of government in 2019 (Economou and Panteli, 2019).

The above features of healthcare and polity structure in Portugal and Greece have also had consequences in terms of the three other dimensions of our framework. In terms of process, as has been seen, the implementation of most of the reforms has been delayed, and partially or completely blocked. In Portugal, the WHO (2018) noted Portugal's strong record in developing health plans and strategies but weaknesses in local approaches to implementation. Moreover, in the law founding the Greek NHS, much was never or only partially implemented, and the neo-liberal reforms externally imposed by the Troika were *de facto* the only ones actually put into practice. The main reasons for this structural lack of implementation by the state in both countries were the outcome of the polity structure containing a centralised weak state and government instability, and the configuration of healthcare as a dyad of opposed coalitions with a strong veto power by stakeholders and an externally imposed logic of transnational governance (Giarelli, 2021).

In terms of functions, a fully tax-based NHS has never been implemented, since it is mostly still financed by the social security system through contributions. Moreover, the level of private expenditure (out-of-pocket user charges and co-payments) has always been very high and has increased during the last decade. Even the share of private providers is very significant and, as has been seen, has increased since the 2008 economic crisis. It is difficult to define the type of governance of this semi-public healthcare system: probably the best definition is a hybrid mix of persistent historical 'particularistic-clientelist' governance, new regulatory governance imposed by the Troika with neo-liberal reforms and some attempts at stewardship governance by recent left-wing governments (Giarelli, 2021).

Finally, in terms of outcomes, considering the last decade, the overall balance is clearly that of a subtractive strategy in both countries: previous positive trends in population coverage, comprehensivity of benefit packages and population health (based on mortality and life expectancy) have been progressively eroded by the impact of the austerity policies imposed by the Troika, with a significant increase in health inequalities. The Covid-19 pandemic has further contributed significantly to these worsening health outcomes, particularly affecting the weakest sections of the population (Economou et al., 2021).

Conclusion: has the role of the state in NHSs really changed?

On the basis of the above application of the multidimensional framework to the analysis of the three European health macro-regions with NHSs, we can now address in conclusion the crucial question for the future of NHSs in Western Europe – namely, to what extent has the role of the state in healthcare really changed (and if so, in what direction) after the last four decades of healthcare reforms? The relevance of this question is also linked to the distinct role played by the state in the NHS in comparison with other types of healthcare systems during the post-war period of economic expansion. Is this still the case after the advent of 'permanent austerity' and the neo-liberal reforms?

The first answer is that the role of the state has actually changed in the NHSs considered, not simply in the direction of replacing the previous *dirigiste* role with the rise of a new 'regulatory state' mainly relying on the philosophy and instruments of NPM (Helderman, Bevan and France, 2012). Instead of a single general trend, it appears that there are different, and even contradictory, trends in opposite directions. When, during the 1980s, the UK and Scandinavian NHSs were already struggling with neo-liberal efficiency issues and cost-containment measures, all four Mediterranean countries considered the main aim of reform was the founding of universal, tax-based, comprehensive, free-of-charge NHSs. This situation has been partially blurred since the 1990s, when some neo-liberal reforms were introduced in the Mediterranean NHSs too – such as internal markets, cost containment and the corporatisation of purchaser and providers. However, over the past two decades in some countries – Scotland and Wales after devolution, Greece with the Syria government and Portugal with the Costa government – the orientation of reform policies has been anything but neo-liberal. Scotland and Wales have abolished the internal market, and Greece and Portugal have struggled to mitigate the negative social effects of the austerity policy imposed by the Troika. In Italy and Spain, there has been an alternation between neo-liberal and progressive reforms depending on the politics of successive governments. Furthermore, the experience of the Covid-19 pandemic has highlighted in all these countries – including in England, the only country that has consistently followed an ever increasing neo-liberal orientation – the indispensable role of the state in guaranteeing adequate preventive and control measures, and coordinating efforts to address its social impact.

The second answer that emerges, beyond questioning the overall neo-liberal character of the reforms, concerns the marked differences between and within Western European health macro-regions in terms of the governance function attributed to the state. While for the other two functions, there are no significant differences – despite a generally decreasing share of expenditure on health and public provision of services, the highest proportion is still spent on the NHSs – the governance function has assumed particular characteristics in the various contexts. In England, for instance, market-oriented reforms have greatly reduced top-down hierarchical control but have created a growing need for regulation to avoid market failure in the most advanced example of a 'regulatory state' among the NHSs. As has been seen, the other two countries in the same macroregion – Scotland and Wales – have followed a rather different path after devolution. Over and above maintaining the significant role of the state in public financing and ownership of services, and downsizing the share of private suppliers and third-party payers, they have devised a mix of continuous hierarchical control and partnership with health professionals and local communities as a form of stewardship. This type of governance, instead of regulatory mechanisms of control, emphasises trust and legitimacy in policymaking, with the involvement of both professionals and citizens in the participatory governance of the NHS with state actors. Here, as Brinkerhoff and colleagues (2019:4) say:

> [T]he stewardship notion combines an ethical and moral dimension with managerial principles of efficiency and effectiveness directed toward addressing national health. State actors with responsibility for a population's health perform as stewards when they exercise authority and employ resources for the common good above and beyond narrow efficiency and effectiveness objectives.

This mobilisation of capacity and commitment of public actors in partnership with health professionals and civil society on the basis of a common heritage of ethical and political values is the hallmark of stewardship as defined by the WHO (2000).

In the Scandinavian region, as previously noted, there is a significant difference in terms of governance between the Swedish and Danish cases and that of Norway. In the former cases, the 'amalgamation strategy' among different interest groups and the 'policy of compromise' on which it is based can be considered the type of stewardship strategy taken by the state – albeit in partial form. As Saltman and Ferroussier-Davis (2000:736) state: 'There are positive elements of stewardship in the behaviour of certain states, e.g. the welfare states of northern Europe, but one cannot as yet point to a fully fledged embodiment of the stewardship model at national level'. However, these 'positive elements' are well rooted in the Scandinavian political culture and its state interventionist tradition, and could represent the basis on which to ground an overall rethinking of the role of state given that:

> Stewardship, an explicitly ethically-based, outcome-oriented policy approach, is substantially more interventionist than the economically driven agency approach to state regulation which some health economists have proposed. . . . The ability of stewardship to reassert a normative outcome-oriented focus in health sector policy-making through a relegitimized social contract model could conceivably become its greatest contribution to the future role of the state in this sector.

The case of Norway meanwhile, although culturally and politically very close to the previous Scandinavian countries in terms of governance, has taken a different path, with a partial difference based on its big bang centralisation policy, and the emergence of a more 'regulatory state' model where health policy governance outcomes take the form of grants, laws and regulation by the government instead of central planning.

In the Mediterranean region too, there is a significant difference between Italy, Spain, Portugal and Greece. With a common historical background of a 'particularistic-clientelist' state grounded in the dyadic configuration of their healthcare arenas, stewardship in Italy and Spain was able to overcome the veto power of particularistic interest groups during periods of left-wing governments. In Portugal and Greece, on the other hand, such groups have prevailed over the plans and legislation approved by governments, making rapid implementation impracticable. Moreover, the role played by an external supranational actor represented by the Troika has imposed an artificial form of regulatory governance, inadequate to the specific cultural and political context. In the case of the Mediterranean region, we can therefore define the cases of Italy and Spain as a hybrid mix of particularistic-clientelist governance and stewardship, variable according to different periods and governments, whereas in the case of Portugal and Greece, the same mix has been further complicated with the artificial imposition of a regulatory governance by the Troika modifying the balance of powers in national healthcare arenas and substituting the role played by the nation state.

The third answer to the question, giving due consideration to differences of space and time, lies in understanding the above divergencies in terms of path dependence or path deviance according to differential historical configurations of healthcare, of the polity structure and, consequently, of the implementation process of reform in the cases concerned. As we have seen, path dependency strongly characterises both Scandinavian and Mediterranean countries: in the first case positively, by favouring an incremental processes of reform, with the exception of Norway; in the second case negatively, in particular in the cases of Portugal and Greece, where the veto power of interest groups largely delayed or blocked reform. The decentralised polity structure and the policy of compromise amalgamating the actors of the healthcare arena have driven the successful reforms in the Scandinavian countries. On the other hand, the fragmented configuration of healthcare into two opposite dyads in Portugal and Greece has won over the centralised structure of their governments. Path deviance occurred, as Wilsford (1994) suggests, in the case of England and Norway, where a centralised, hierarchical order of less autonomous (dependent) decision-agents characterises the polity structure. As Wilsford (1994:278) notes, 'centralized hierarchies are better at leveraging a wholly new policy path'. For him, the other circumstance is 'the presence of an immensely powerful and compelling conjuncture'. In the cases of Scotland and Wales, this was represented by devolution, which made possible a different policy from England; in the cases of Italy and Spain, the democratisation of the state and changing political cultures led to the successful implementation of their NHSs.

In conclusion, if as Rothgang and colleagues (2005:192) state, 'the three types of healthcare system are characterized by a distinct role of the state' – namely, hierarchy in the NHSs, collective bargaining in the social insurance system and markets in the private insurance system – hierarchy is no longer the exclusive and distinctive mechanisms of governance of the NHSs in comparison with the other two types of systems. The picture we have drawn on the basis of our framework is much more complex and varied, with different forms of governance in the different macro-regions. This suggests a trend towards mixed models rather than convergence, because of 'a general tendency to introduce into each type of healthcare system such modes of coordination that are unfamiliar to that type', but this does not mean that 'these changes . . . lead to the conclusion that system-specific characteristics have disappeared' (Rothgang et al., 2005:207–9). Despite a slight reduction in public healthcare financing and public ownership of services, major differences in the role of the state remain as regards healthcare financing, delivery of services and governance between all the NHSs of Western Europe considered here (Wendt, Frisina and Rothgang, 2009).

References

Barros, P. P., Machado, S. R. and Simões, J. de A. (2011) 'Portugal: Health system review', *Health Systems in Transition* 13(4): 1–156.

Blank, R. H. and Burau, V. (2007) *Comparative Health Policy*, 2nd edition, New York: Palgrave Macmillan.

Blomqvist, P. and Winblad, U. (2021) 'Sweden', in Immergut, E. M., Anderson, K. M., Devitt, C. and Popic, T. (eds) *Health Politics in Europe: A Handbook*, Oxford: Oxford University Press.

Brinkerhoff, D. W., Cross, H. E., Sharma, S. and Williamson, T. (2019) 'Stewardship and health systems strengthening: An overview', *Public Administration and Development* 39: 4–10.

Christiansen, T. and Vrangbæk, K. (2018) 'Hospital centralization and performance in Denmark – Ten years on', *Health Policy* 122(4): 321–8.

Economou, C. (2010) 'Greece: Health system review', *Health Systems in Transition* 12(7): 1–177.

Economou, C., Kaitelidou, D., Konstantakopoulou, O. and Vildiridi, V. (2021) 'COVID-19 policy responses for Greece', *COVID-19 Health System Response Monitor*, Copenhagen: European Observatory on Health Systems and Policies. Available at: www.covid19healthsystem.org/countries/greece/countrypage.aspx

Economou, C. and Panteli, D. (2019) *Monitoring and Documenting Systemic and Health Effects of Health Reforms in Greece*, Copenhagen: WHO Regional Office for Europe. Available at: www.euro.who.int/__data/assets/pdf_file/0011/394526/Monitoring-Documenting_Greece_eng.pdf

Ferrera, M. (1996) 'The "Southern model" of welfare in social Europe', *Journal of European Social Policy* 6(1): 17–37.

Figueras, J., Mossialos, E., McKee, M. and Sassi, F. (1994) 'Health care systems in Southern Europe: Is there a Mediterranean paradigm?', *International Journal of Health Sciences* 5(4): 135–46.

Forbes, T. and Evans, D. (2008) 'Health and social care partnerships in Scotland', *Scottish Affairs* 65(1): 87–106.

Full Fact (2017) *How Much More Is the NHS Spending on the Private Sector?* Available at: ww.fullfact.org

Gabe, J. (1997) *The Americanization of British Health Care?*, Occasional Papers of the Department of Social Policy and Social Studies, Royal Holloway University of London.

Garpenby, P. (1989) *The State and the Medical Profession. A Cross-national Comparison of the Health Policy Arena in the United Kingdom and Sweden 1945–1985*, Linköping: Linköping Studies in Arts and Sciences.

Giarelli, G. (2021) 'A Mediterranean paradigm? Convergence and divergence in the Southern European health care systems', *Interface (Botucatu)* 25: e210116. Available at: https://doi.org/10.1590/interface.210116

Giarelli, G. and Giovannetti, V. (eds) (2019) *Il Servizio sanitario nazionale italiano in prospettiva europea. Una analisi comparata*, Milan: Franco Angeli.

Greener, I. (2005) 'The potential of path dependence in political studies', *Politics* 25(1): 62–72.

Guthrie, B., Davies, H., Greig, G., et al. (2010) *Delivering Health Care Through Managed Clinical Networks (MCNS): Lessons From the North*, Report for NIHR SDO Programme, London: HMSO.

Ham, C. (ed) (1997) *Health Care Reform. Learning From International Experience*, Buckingham: Open University Press.

Helderman, J.-K., Bevan, G. and France, G. (2012) 'The rise of the regulatory state in health care: A comparative analysis of the Netherlands, England and Italy', *Health Economics, Policy and Law* 7: 103–24.

Hughes, D. (1991) 'The reorganization of the National Health Service: The rhetoric and reality of the internal market', *The Modern Law Review* 54: 88–103.

Hughes, D. and Vincent-Jones, P. (2008) 'Schisms in the church: NHS systems and institutional divergence in England and Wales', *Journal of Health and Social Behavior* 49(4): 400–16.

Immergut, E. (1999) 'Historical and institutional foundations of the Swedish health care system', in Powell, F. D. and Wessen A. F. (eds) *Health Care Systems in Transition. An International Perspective*, Thousand Oaks, CA: Sage.

Kapoor, N., Kumar, D. and Thakur, N. (2014) 'Core attributes of stewardship: Foundation of sound health system', *International Journal of Health Policy and Management* 3(1): 5–6.

Kass, H. D. (1990) 'Stewardship as a fundamental element in images of public administration', in Kass, H. D. and Catron, B. (eds) *Images and Identities in Public Administration*, London: Sage.

Kay, A. (2005) 'A critique of the use of path dependency in policy studies', *Public Administration* 83(3): 553–71.

Lawson, K. (2003) *The Human Polity. A Comparative Introduction to Political Science*, Boston, MA: Houghton Mifflin.

Light, D. (1995) 'Countervailing powers: A framework for professions in transition', in Johnson, T., Larkin, G. and Saks, M. (eds) *Health Professions and the State in Europe*, London: Routledge.

Lowi, T. J. (1966) 'Distribution, regulation, redistribution: The functions of government', in Ripley, R. B. (ed) *Public Policies and their Politics: Techniques of Government Control*, New York: W. W. Norton.

Majone, G. (1994) 'The rise of the regulatory state', *West European Politics* 17(3): 77–101.

Martinussen, P. E. and Magnussen, J. (2009) 'Healthcare reform: The Nordic experience', in Magnussen, J., Saltman, R. B. and Vrangbæk, K. (eds) *Nordic Health Care Systems: Recent Reforms and Current Policy Challenges*, Buckingham: Open University Press.

Moran, M. (2003) *The British Regulatory State. High Modernism and Hyper-Innovation*, Oxford: Oxford University Press.

Organization for Economic Cooperation and Development (2022) *Health Stat*, Geneva: OECD. Available at: https://stats.oecd.org/

Pavolini, E. and Guillén, A. M. (eds) (2013) *Health Care Systems in Europe Under Austerity. Institutional Reforms and Performance*, Basingstoke: Palgrave Macmillan.

Peterson, M. A. (1993) 'Political influence in the 1990s: From iron triangles to policy networks', *Journal of Health Politics, Policy and Law* 18: 395–438.

Petmesidou, M. and Guillén, A. M. (2008) '"Southern-style" National Health Services? Recent reforms and trends in Spain and Greece', *Social Policy and Administration* 42(2): 106–24.

Pierson, P. (2000) 'Increasing returns, path dependence and the study of politics', *American Political Science Review* 94(2): 251–67.

Pierson, P. (2001) 'Coping with permanent austerity: Welfare state restructuring in affluent democracies', in Pierson, P. (ed) *The New Politics of Welfare State*, Oxford: Oxford University Press.

Pierson, P. (2004) *Politics in Time: History, Institution and Socialò Amalysys*, Princeton, NJ: Princeton University Press.

Ranade, W. and Haywood, S. (1989) 'Privatizing from within: The national health service under Thatcher', *Local Government Studies* 15: 19–34.

Rathwell, T. (1998) 'Implementing health care reforms: A review of current experience', in Saltman, R. B., Figueras, J. and Sakellarides, C. (eds) *Critical Challenges for Health Care Reform in Europe*, Buckingham: Open University Press.

Rothgang, H., Cacace, M., Frisina, L., et al. (2010) *The State and Healthcare: Comparing OECD Countries*, Berlin: Springer.

Rothgang, H., Cacace, M., Grimmesein, S. and Wendt, C. (2005) 'The changing role of the state in healthcare systems', *European Review* 13(1): 187–212.

Saks, M. (2016) 'Review of theories of professions, organizations and society: Neo-Weberianism, neo-institutionalism and eclecticism', *Journal of Professions and Organization* 3(2): 170–87.

Saltman, R. B. (1999) 'Evolving roles of the national and regional governments in the Swedish health care system', in Powell, F. D. and Wessen, A. F. (eds) *Health Care Systems in Transition. An International Perspective*, Thousand Oaks, CA: Sage.

Saltman, R. B. (2008) 'Decentralization, re-centralization and future European health policy', *European Journal of Public Health* 18: 104–6.

Saltman, R. B. and Ferroussier-Davis, O. (2000) 'The concept of stewardship in health policy', *Bulletin of the World Health Organization* 78(6): 732–9.

Saunes, I. P., Karanikolos, M. and Sagan, A. (2020) 'Norway. Health system review 2000', *Health Systems in Transition* 22(1), Copenhagen: WHO Regional Office for Europe.

Starr, P. (1982) *The Social Transformation of American Medicine*, Cambridge, MA: Basic Books.

Terlizzi, A. (2019) 'Health system decentralization and recentralization in Italy: Ideas, discourse, and institutions', *Social Policy and Administration* 53: 974–88.

Valeriani, G., Sarajlic Vukovic, I., Lindegaard, T., Felizia, R., Mollica, R. and Andersson, G. (2020) 'Addressing healthcare gaps in Sweden during the COVID-19 outbreak: On community outreach and empowering ethnic minority groups in a digitalized context', *Healthcare* 8(4): 445.

Vicarelli, G. (2005) 'Control, competition and cooperation in European health systems: Points of contact between health policy and industrial policy', in Di Tommaso, M. and Schweitzer, S. (eds) *Health Policy and High-Tech Industrial Development*, Cheltenham: Edward Elgar.

Vrangbæk, K. (2021) 'Denmark', in Immergut, E., Anderson, K., Dewitt, C. and Popic, T. *Health Politics in Europe: A Handbook*, Oxford: Oxford University Press.

Wainwright, H. (n.d.) 'Remain and reform: The Portuguese experience of being "in and against" the European Union', Transnational Institute, London School of Economics. Available at: portugal-report.pdf (europeforthemany.com).

Walt, G. (1998) 'Implementing health care reform: A framework for discussion', in Saltman, R. B., Figueras, J. and Sakellarides, C. (eds) *Critical Challenges for Health Care Reform in Europe*, Buckingham: Open University Press.

Welsh NHS Confederation (2017) *Finance and the NHS in Wales*. Available at: www.nhsconfed.org/-/media/Confederation/Files/public-access/Welsh-NHS-Confederation-Finance-Briefing.pdf

Wendt, C., Frisina, L. and Rothgang, H. (2009) 'Healthcare system types: A conceptual framework for comparison', *Social Policy and Administration* 43(1): 70–90.

Wilsford, D. (1994) 'Path dependency, or why history makes it difficult but not impossible to reform health care systems in a big way', *Journal of Public Policy* 14(3): 251–83.

World Health Organization (2000) *Health Systems. Improving Performance. The World Health Report*, Geneva: WHO.

World Health Organization (2018) *Health System Review: Portugal*, Geneva: WHO.

World Health Organization (2021) *Coronavirus (COVID-19) Dashboard. Situation by Country, Territory and Area*. Available at: https://covid19.who.int/table

11 The evolution of the medical and health professions in the National Health Services

Mike Saks

Introduction: defining a profession

There are many different ways of defining professionals, such as accountants, doctors, and lawyers. In everyday usage, these range from being in a highly skilled occupation to simply earning an income from work – with this belief deriving from the traditional distinction between amateurs and professionals in sport and other areas (Saks, 2021). Others see professions as having a religious spin – manifested in healthcare in the contemporary context by the Hippocratic Oath still sworn by many doctors to the health gods, testifying to their formal adherence to high ethical standards (Miles, 2005). With reference to the Western European national contexts in this book, this chapter focuses on health professions as collective groups opposed to individual professionals – even if the two are interconnected.

From a theoretical perspective, the analysis of health and other professions has involved much debate. In the Anglo-American context, taxonomic writers up to the 1950s and 1960s generally took a very deferential approach to the professions in which their positive self-presentation was taken largely at face value. Key attributes of medicine and other mainstream professions were therefore features like an altruistic orientation, systematic knowledge and formal education and training (Millerson, 1964). As such, professions were typically seen as possessing unique characteristics separating them from other occupations and playing a positive role in the wider society. Indeed, functionalist contributors felt that their higher socio-economic rewards derived from such groups using their esoteric knowledge of high importance to society in a non-exploitative manner (for example, Barber, 1963). Semi-professions like nursing were seen as not possessing these characteristics to such a high degree, hence their lower position in the professional pecking order (Etzioni, 1969).

Symbolic interactionists were among the first critics, along with free market economists like Milton Friedman (1962), who saw the monopoly of the medical profession as stifling innovation, limiting opportunities for new recruits and driving up costs. The interactionists argued from a more micro-perspective that there were actually no substantive distinctions between professional

DOI: 10.4324/9781003139799-17

groups like physicians and other occupations, even those in more marginalised spheres of 'dirty work' (Hughes, 1963). Instead, the term was simply seen as a symbol deployed to varying effect to gain political advantage in the work sphere (Becker, 1962). This perspective, however, was not based any more on systematic research evidence than earlier sycophantic approaches to professions and tended to ignore the historical role of wider structures of power in making such definitions stick. This was certainly not the case in terms of the more dynamic structural neo-Marxist and Foucauldian theories of professions that emerged during the 1960s/70s counter culture.

The Marxist approach covered a range of views, but mainly saw professions as part of the petty bourgeoisie involving the ideological inculcation and political repression of lower classes (Poulantzas, 1975). Thus Esland (1980) regarded doctors as well-rewarded agents of the capitalist class individualising health problems caused by system dynamics in order to preserve the capitalist *status quo*. Moreover, in terms of the labour process, writers like Braverman (1998) viewed professional groups like nurses as being increasingly deskilled and proletarianised over time as work was degraded under capitalism. Nonetheless, in terms of health and other professions, the more critical Marxist analyses also often suffer from a lack of empirical evidence. Indeed, many are centred on the self-fulfilling assumption that states in the West necessarily function in the long-run interests of capital (Saks, 2012).

Much the same is true of the now more in vogue, but no less critical, Foucauldian perspective based on the critical work of the French philosopher Michel Foucault. His prolific work on the archaeology of knowledge includes historical studies on the development of clinical medicine and the origins of psychiatry (Foucault, 1989, 2001). He applied the concept of governmentality to professions, in which they are conceived as being increasingly and dispiritingly incorporated into state governance in Western Europe, to the prejudice of the public. This enabled Foucault and his followers to question the ideology of scientific progress linked to health and other professions – whether in dentistry (Nettleton, 1992) or general practice (Pickard, 2009). However, aside from its high-level abstraction, Foucauldianism has been accused of making unsubstantiated generalisations and ignoring historical detail (Macdonald, 1995) – which brings us to the neo-Weberian approach underpinning this book.

The neo-Weberian approach to health professions

While these conflicting theoretical interpretations of what it means to be a profession in general and health professions in particular each have some merits (Saks, 2016), the preference here is to define professions in neo-Weberian terms. The key aspect of the neo-Weberian approach to professions is centred on Weber's original notion of social closure, which he ironically did not himself apply to groups like doctors and lawyers (Swedberg and Agevall, 2016). More specifically, professions are seen here in terms of exclusionary social closure in which such groups establish self-regulatory monopolies – thereby creating a group of legally privileged insiders and disenfranchised outsiders in relation to income, status and power. As outlined by writers like Parkin (1979) in the Anglo-American context, this process is viewed as typically being based on the strategic exercise of interests through credentialism in a competitive marketplace.

The reason why this approach to health and other professional groups is favoured over the other perspectives previously set out is briefly summarised by Saks (2021) as follows. First, it enables professions to be analysed in more open fashion as compared to the reflexively deferential taxonomic perspective. Second, it goes beyond symbolic interactionism by addressing the historical and structural dimensions of professionalism. Third, neo-Weberianism is not restricted by the rigid and self-fulfilling notion of the capitalist state enshrined in many Marxist approaches. Fourth, it allows the systematic empirical examination of professions outside the blinkers of Marxism and Foucauldianism. Although there are interlinkages with competing perspectives, therefore, as Freidson (1970:187) notes, such an approach liberates us from 'the confusion and special pleading which permeates most discussions of professions'.

This applies in all of the wide range of forms that neo-Weberianism social closure takes from market control of services through self-governing associations (Parry and Parry, 2019) to more derivative market-based interpretations, including where the producer defines the needs of the consumer and how these are satisfied (Johnson, 2016). Typically, in its strongest form, more fully fledged professions have statutory registers of qualified practitioners in the Anglo-American context. In medicine in Britain, in contrast to the United States (US), this supplanted the previous localised controls of the guilds in the eighteenth and nineteenth centuries – where physicians, surgeons and apothecaries operating at a local level held sway up to the time of their national unification through the 1858 Medical Act (Krause, 1996).

Neo-Weberians also acknowledge the contemporary hierarchical relationships of power and dominance enacted by doctors and other leading professional groups based on differential levels of state legitimation. Thus, more subordinated groups are defined by Parkin (1979) as characterised by the concept of 'dual closure', which combines the benefits of exclusionary closure with usurpationary closure based on the defensive and sometimes illegal tactics of working class unionism. Their intermediary position can be illustrated by a number of groups that defend their positions in this manner both above and below, including the allied health professions in Britain (Nancarrow and Borthwick, 2021). This more conflictual politicised narrative is held to underpin the location of the 'semi-professions', whose subordinated position is explained by the functionalist variant of taxonomy largely in terms of the needs of the social system (Etzioni, 1969).

It should finally be added that this neo-Weberian approach is complemented theoretically in this volume and chapter by neo-institutionalism which locates professions in the context of institutional logics in organisational and other settings. More specifically, Suddaby and Muzio (2015) argue that neo-institutionalism expresses the notion of one institution vying with others for survival in an ecological system. This places the professions in a wider process and collection of actors, including the state, in a manner very resonant with a neo-Weberian perspective – in which professional groups compete politically for jurisdiction and position in the marketplace in their own interests. We shall now critically highlight the application of the neo-Weberian perspective further in the Western European context, after first analysing its strengths and weaknesses.

An evaluation of the neo-Weberian approach to professions

The neo-Weberian framework has been widely applied to professions, including the evolution of the medical and health professions. Freidson (1970), for instance, drew attention to the variation in the extent to which independent diagnosis and prescribing was legally sanctioned for optometrists and pharmacists in American states – despite the same minimum training period and parallel levels of specialisation and abstract knowledge. This highlights the importance of the trademark neo-Weberian emphasis on the socio-political dynamics of healthcare. The application of this approach can be further exemplified by the study by Whiting, May and Saks (2020) on the interplay between professional self-interests and the public interest in the historical pattern of professionalisation of veterinary medicine. Similarly, Kuhlmann and Annandale (2012) have used the Weberian concept of social closure to map gender issues in the evolution of the health professions internationally.

Having said this, the neo-Weberian approach to understanding the evolution of medicine and the health professions – as well as professionalisation in other spheres – is certainly not above criticism. While Saks (2010) considers himself to be a neo-Weberian, he has made three major criticisms of the application of neo-Weberianism in Britain and the US. The first is that it has frequently been implemented without sufficient empirical scrutiny – in part because of its advocates being swept along by the wave of the anti-professional counter culture that developed on both sides of the Atlantic in the 1960s and 1970s (Saks, 1983). This is exemplified by Johnson (2016) who fails to provide evidence for his argument that the emergence of the professions auxiliary to medicine in Britain was related to the manner in which doctors delineated their own roles, thereby leading to 'irrational' resource utilisation. Such contributors do not go far beyond the reflexive thinking of earlier writers on the professions, simply substituting negativity for positivity.

The second interlinked criticism of the neo-Weberian study of professions in health and other areas is that its claims tend too often to lean in an adversarial rather than supportive direction (Saks, 1998). Thus, Beattie (1995), for example, without systematic evidence, highlights the negative implications of professional tribalism in the evolution of British healthcare. As such, while hitting the mark in certain ways, he does not sufficiently recognise that health professions can be just as much a humanising as a destructive influence in this field – as Borsay and Hunter (2012) indicate in their analysis of the development of nursing and midwifery since the eighteenth century in Britain. In analysing the evolution of health professions, therefore, we need to be open to the need to reconstruct as well as deconstruct their role in proceedings depending on available research data in the cases concerned.

The third criticism of the neo-Weberian approach to the professions is that its proponents have not fully linked their work to the broader occupational division of labour (Saks, 2003). In the health field, this has meant that there has been rather too much emphasis on medicine which has gained full exclusionary social closure in the British context. In consequence, the relationship of doctors to newly professionalising groups like complementary and alternative medicine (CAM) practitioners has been given too little attention (Saks, 2015). This is also true of their links to support workers who form the largest proportion of the healthcare workforce both nationally and internationally (Saks, 2020). Aside from the need for greater inclusivity, more appreciation is needed of the light that the success or failure of such groups in professionalising can shed on the dynamics of more established and dominant health professional groups.

However, it should be stressed that these more generalisable issues that affect the analysis of professions relate more to the operationalisation of neo-Weberianism than the approach itself. Its frailties can be readily addressed in considering the evolution of the health professions within a more balanced, evidence-based framework (Saks, 2021). This is no more evident than in the case of the British National Health Service (NHS) to which the neo-Weberian concept of social closure particularly applies – albeit with the previously noted caveats, including the need to situate the development of professions within the wider healthcare division of labour. In factoring neo-institutionalism into the equation, moreover, we must also be very clear that the ecological premises of this approach relating to animals and plants are simply a metaphor which should not cloud the neo-Weberian analysis based on politics and power (Perreault, Bridge and McCarthy, 2015).

The earlier evolution of the medical and health professions in Britain

In considering the development of the health professions in Britain in the context of an NHS introduced in 1948, the contemporary focus will be on England given the varying paths in health policy that have recently been taken with devolution in Scotland and Wales – not to mention in Northern Ireland in the wider United Kingdom (UK) where there has, for instance, been greater integration of health and social care (Hudson, 2000). In this setting, the medical profession has historically been dominant since the 1858 Medical Act which – following extensive medical lobbying – established a legally independent and self-regulating medical profession, with a register and codes of ethics overseen by the General Medical Council (GMC) (Stacey, 1992). This body still exists today, albeit – as we shall see – in rather different form as it has changed aspects of its defining template over time (Saks, 2015).

The effective monopoly by doctors initially created followed a period of medical pluralism from the eighteenth to mid-nineteenth centuries in Britain, in which practitioners from herbalists to homoeopaths competed with each other for custom on a level playing field (Cant and Sharma, 1999). Although they were able to practice under the Common Law in Britain, such CAM therapists were subsequently increasingly marginalised and fell into a low point by the 1960s and 1970s, after which their fortunes were revived by the counter culture in which all things alternative, from drugs to fashion, came to the fore (Roszak, 1995). As a result of increasing demand in the market and positive evaluations of the outcomes of their practice, chiropractors and osteopaths were statutorily regulated – albeit on less favourable terms to medicine – in the 1990s (Saks, 2002). As such, they followed in the footsteps of the allied health professions such as occupational therapy and physiotherapy which were regulated by the Council for the Professions Supplementary to Medicine from 1960 onwards and now hold their registration with the less hierarchically named Health and Care Professions Council (Saks, 2015).

Nurses and midwives had achieved their subordinated statutory regulation in Britain in 1902 and 1919, respectively – from a neo-Weberian perspective in face of gender-based issues in a patriarchal society (Witz, 1992). Their regulatory functions were taken over in 2002 by the Nursing and Midwifery Council (NMC) which had greater lay membership. The regulation of nurses and midwives paralleled that of groups like dentists and opticians underpinned by the 1957 Dentists Act and the 1958 Opticians Act. In the professional regulatory framework, their professional standing can best be characterised by limitation as opposed to subordination. This means that, while having exclusionary closure based on title, they are in effect trapped within their own boundaries – in the cases concerned, the terrain of the mouth and the eye (Saks, 2015). However, whether as subordinated or limited professions, each of the aforementioned health professional groups has attained social closure with the associated higher-level income, status and power – in contrast to the vast majority of health workers in support roles which are largely unregulated (Saks and Zagrodney, 2020).

Crucially, as Nancarrow and Borthwick (2021) indicate in the case of the allied professions, the monopolistic positions of a wide range of health professions were won in the interest-based politics of work against competitors. This has also been the case with doctors who – while differentiated by a growing range of specialisms (Le Fanu, 2011) – occupy the pinnacle of the health professional hierarchy. Saks and Adams (2019) underline this by highlighting the importance in neo-Weberian terms of understanding the role of the state as well as the medical profession in gaining, maintaining and extending its position of exclusionary social closure up to the 1950s and 1960s. What happened thereafter in a more neo-liberal climate is fascinating in light of the subsequent growing criticism of professions in general – from clients and citizens, the state and corporate organisations (Saks, 2021).

The attack on the medical profession in Britain from the late 1970s onwards

The shift that occurred was partly brought about by a questioning of how far the profession was serving the wider public. As Saks (2015) notes, this was accentuated in Britain by a number of scandals involving doctors and other health professions culminating in the inquiry in 2004 into the general practitioner, Dr Harold Shipman, who was legally found to have murdered over 200 patients over a period of some 30 years without detection by the GMC. At the same time, from 1979 to 1997, the Conservative government was seeking greater control of doctors as a result of its unease at the impact of the autonomous self-regulation of the profession which interrupted the flow of market forces. It was not surprising that during this period, the government introduced first general managers into the NHS to improve effectiveness and efficiency, then the internal market based on a purchaser–provider split, followed by a Patients' Charter setting out patient rights and standards for the health professions.

None of these measures proved particularly helpful, as they proved unworkable, were too formalistic or were undermined by the actions of the medical profession (Klein, 2013). They were also complemented by an attempt to apply organisational logic more locally in the public and private sector to bring doctors more fully to heel under the New Public Management (NPM) (Dent, Chandler and Barry, 2004). This had the effect not just of growing bureaucratisation of medical services but also of increasing hybridisation in which professional and organisational logics both came to bear (Kirkpatrick, 2016). Rising corporatisation therefore has not led to the crushing of professional autonomy for doctors and other health professions as Evetts (2013) suggests in charting their move from occupational to organisational professionalism. As Noordegraaf (2018) observes, the logics may co-exist, combine or become merged in some fashion so professions behave in new ways.

The modernising Labour government from 1997 posed an even greater challenge to the medical profession. When New Labour came to power, Tony Blair was determined to modernise the state health service including by forging new methods of health governance, driving service improvements and building stronger relationships with private providers – in the interests of patients and the wider public. This led to some professional restratification, in which general practitioners (GPs) moved up the hierarchy at the expense of hospital specialists with the advent of multiprofessional primary care commissioning (Calnan and Gabe, 2009). But the largest impact under Labour was in increasing the proportion of lay members on the GMC and the establishment of the Council for Healthcare Regulatory Excellence to oversee the public interest in relation to the health professions – as well as commissioning the

Donaldson Review aimed at further enhancing patient safety through service functionality (Chamberlain, 2012).

With first the Conservative-Liberal Democratic Coalition in 2010 and then the Conservative governments from 2015 onwards, these measures were intensified. As a result, the profession further lost influence over government and patient choice was increased with the provision of more medical performance data in an active market approach, in which Primary Care Trusts were replaced by more localised Clinical Commissioning Groups chaired by GPs. This period also saw the implementation of some of the reforms seeded under Labour – such as the independent adjudication of disciplinary cases and the requirement for the periodic revalidation of doctors to help ensure continuing fitness-to-practice (Roche, 2018). Although there are issues about how far these reforms have been effectively carried through, this challenged the interests of the medical profession in terms of income, status and power – together with the reduction of the GMC to 12 members with 50% lay representation, and the rise of the Professional Standards Authority with enhanced health professional oversight across the UK (Allsop and Jones, 2018).

As such, even if this does not amount to deprofessionalisation (Saks, 2015), these changes represented a shift from professional self-regulation to what has been termed 'regulated self-regulation' (Chamberlain, 2015). Metaphorically, as Saks (2014) has pointed out – in a move which has since cascaded to other health professions – this can be seen as a transition from zoos to circuses. In this imagery, the former involved the profession building its own exclusive cages as a form of self-protective regulatory closure from the public, while the latter saw the emergence of the state as the ringmaster, generating new hoops through which the human animals in the circus were encouraged to jump in terms of performance. Most recently, though, the shift has been towards the safari park in which certain animals at least are encouraged to wander free and commune with each other – albeit while endeavouring to ensure that there are sufficient numbers to serve the public, whether through recruitment from abroad or internal means. This mirrors the trend over the past two decades to increase the integration of health and social care in Britain, alongside efforts, as in other Western societies, to maintain a sustainable healthcare workforce (Walton-Roberts, 2022).

Here it should be stressed that, in terms of health professional regulation *per se*, the devolution of healthcare in Britain from the late 1990s to Scotland and Wales has not had a great impact. There are of course significant variations in the form of these NHSs linked to different political preferences that have developed since that time – including in the dissolution of many trusts and in the creation of separate inspectorates for health and social care services, as compared to the Care Quality Commission in England (Klein, 2013). Scope has been provided in the devolved administrations for specific national regulation of new health professions. However, the professional regulatory mechanisms for mainstream, longer-standing healthcare professions, such as medicine and nursing, have remained centralised in core professional bodies like the GMC and the NMC with unified oversight regulation of these regulators across the UK (Allsop and Jones, 2018). This, together with devolved decision-making in Scotland and Wales, also aided the management of Covid-19 across the three nations, in face of some questionable decision-making in England (Calnan and Douglass, 2022).

This said, there is a current UK-wide consultation by the Department and Health and Social Care (2022) on what the appropriate balance might be between voluntary and statutory regulation of the health professions, which is still to be concluded. An early resolution of this and other related issues is awaited as there are a number of known gaps in the current health regulatory framework in light of more recent scandals involving patient care such as those thrown up by the recent Cumberlege medicines safety review in what was seen as a disjointed, still largely siloed, unresponsive and defensive healthcare system (Haskell, 2020). What, though, of the evolution of medical and other health professions in other areas of Western Europe? Having analysed the evolution of the medical and health professions in Britain from a neo-Weberian perspective, we now turn to examine the development of such groups in the NHSs of continental Europe – which is seen to encompass, among other countries, both the Scandinavian and Mediterranean macro-regions.

The development of the health professions in continental Europe

Before considering developments in parts of the aforementioned regions, the claim by Sciulli (2005) that the neo-Weberian approach to professions based on social closure is restricted to the Anglo-American context should be addressed. It is of course true that there are fewer professions based in the same way on exclusionary social closure in continental Europe (Collins, 1990), not least since they are often more strongly embedded in government and other public-sector bureaucracies (Evetts, 2000). But there are many professions so constituted in countries ranging from Australia and Canada to Western Europe (Allsop and Jones, 2008). In the latter, indeed, such occupations can be seen to lie on a spectrum on a sliding scale up to full social closure. While not all approach the self-regulatory heights of the classic British medical profession, there are contemporary deviations from the Weberian ideal type which – as elsewhere – can be productively examined within this framework (Saks, 2018).

Schepers and Casparie (1999), for instance, have drawn parallels between the medical profession in Belgium, The Netherlands and Britain. They argue that, in all three countries, the medical profession was very powerful by the 1960s and 1970s – even if its organisation and position in the health system differed. The Dutch medical professional was involved in regulation and representation, as well as trade union activities, with independent specialist scientific and GP societies, and indirect statutory links with the bodies that establish educational requirements and register medical practitioners. In Belgium meanwhile, the medical profession has a predominant trade union identity, mainly because divisions – between medical specialists and GPs and regionally – adversely affect its political influence. However, they note that in all three societies there were interest-based confrontations of doctors with other actors in the health system, together with profession-driven improvements in medical quality assurance based on peer review and audit as a result of external and internal pressures.

Since then, there have been a growing number of health scandals in the first two decades of the twenty-first century in Western Europe which have not just been restricted to Britain. The NPM has also emerged on the horizon. In consequence, Dent (2018) notes that there has been an even stronger move towards introducing new systems of governance in medical and other health professions. Although there are differences in the contested scope of practice of such professions as in the case of community care in Germany (Burau, 1999), where there is institutionalised medical authority (Burau and Vrangbæk, 2008), this is exemplified by the establishment of compulsory medical revalidation in countries such as Belgium, France and Germany aimed at ensuring that doctors are up-to-date with best practice and fit for practice (Dent, 2018). There have also been reforms in health support work that challenge conventional patterns of health professional governance in societies like The Netherlands – such as the recent innovative recruitment of paid peer support workers in Dutch mental health settings to improve service delivery (Leemeijer and Noordegraaf, 2020).

The apparent dilution of medical authority that these initiatives represent, as in Britain, has been paralleled in other Western European countries with an NHS. Drawing primarily on Denmark from the Scandinavian macro-region and Italy from the Mediterranean macro-region as illustrative cases, Dent (2018), for instance, argues that co-production with clients and the enhancement of patient choice have increasingly been taken up in healthcare. However, as we shall see, there is not a monolithic approach to the regulation of health professions across such societies related to such factors as politics and culture. This can be highlighted by the particular emphasis on patients' rights and the citizens' voice in Denmark (Vrangbæk, 2015), as against a greater stress on self-help and mutual aid in Italy (Giarelli and Spina, 2014). This leads us to examine in more detail the evolution of medical and health professions in Western European countries outside Britain which possess a national health system in the macro-regions examined in this volume.

The Scandinavian macro-region

Brante (1999) argues that, as states have sought to develop effective bureaucratic machinery for governance, skilled modern professions like medicine in Scandinavia in general and Sweden in particular have developed from what were primarily scholarly rather than practical professions in pre-industrial times. Drawing on a Foucauldian approach, he says that health professions like physicians – alongside less powerful, but increasingly scientifically based semi-professions such as nurses, physiotherapists and X-ray technicians (Elzinga, 1990) – became both the 'guardians of normality' and the 'backbone of the welfare state'. As such, they were based on a looser and more tiered form of state-engendered neo-Weberian social closure, as Hellberg (1990) argues is also classically exemplified by Swedish veterinarians who based their professional project on the indispensability of their services in protecting the interests of the state.

In these terms, medical professionalisation in Sweden was effected through the state. Here, distinctively, the profession became a government institution controlling licensing, as well as the organisation of work – even if physicians lacked the autonomy gained by British doctors from the mid-nineteenth century onwards (Garpenby, 1989). However, from the 1940s to the 1970s, the ever-increasing university education of physicians in Sweden helped to make them the most successful profession in terms of power, with substantially growing numbers and influence. Moreover, after the early 1970s, the transition from participatory to corporate capitalism meant that health professions took on more complex responsibilities and dominated politics in terms of institutional logics, along with other middle class professions (Brante, 1999). This resulted in them being better positioned to exercise veto powers over government decision-making from the 1980s to the mid-1990s (Immergut, 1999).

Nonetheless, as Castro (1999) observes, welfare state professions in Sweden were faced with a wave of deregulation and austerity by the end of the 1990s – prompting serial resignations by groups such as surgeons and anaesthetists in face of attacks by politicians and administrators. He claims from a neo-Weberian perspective that this represented a challenge to their self-interests at a time when they had relatively high-level positions and rewards in the division of labour. As such, medicine constituted a profession that was far from being subjugated in a relational interplay with clients, the market, the state and other institutions (Bertilsson, 1990). Such health professions, moreover, rode out subsequent challenges from support workers and others in the first two decades of the twenty-first century given their centrality to the welfare state and the emerging NPM (Kuhlmann, Agartan and Von Knorring, 2016). They did so mainly by continuing to adopt a collectivistic professional identity along with other public-sector professions like economists and lawyers, in face of the challenge of gender divisions based on social closure across Scandinavia, including in Finland (Einarsdottir, 1999; Wrede, 2008).

In the contemporary neo-liberal Scandinavian political context, Vrangbæk (2018) points out that the NHSs of Denmark, Norway and Sweden remain closely linked by extensive welfare provision and a commitment to patient and public involvement, based on this cultural and historical lineage. In line with their commitment to improving the partnership between the wide range of health professionals and the patient, they are now restructuring their hospital infrastructure as a result of the pressure of increased demand, new medical technology, ageing populations and a desire for greater coordination.

However, there are also variations between these countries because – while they all have institutionalised forums for negotiation between decentralised authorities and the government – the economic power of the state is stronger in Denmark and Norway than in Sweden, where counties have greater autonomy in dealing with health professional issues, as in the case of the organisation of midwifery and maternity care (Benoit, 1999).

As Olejaz and colleagues (2012) note, landlords and artisan masters in Denmark were responsible for providing healthcare for their charges in the pre-industrial era. This was supplanted in the eighteenth century by public welfare and decentralised welfare management in towns and counties – funded mainly by local authority taxes within the guiding principles established by the central state. From the mid-1940s to 1970, there was political agreement that access to healthcare should be independent of economic resources and shaped by the technical judgement of medical professionals. However, since the 1980s – as in other societies under the influence of the NPM (Dent, Chandler and Barry, 2004) – the ascendance of clinical practitioners has been contested, at a time when hospitals increasingly became run by other university-educated managers with a greater focus on cost containment and performance management. This resulted in 2007 in a greater swing towards re-centralisation, with a reduction in the number of municipalities and the establishment of five regions to provide a more efficient and egalitarian standards of care across the country. This was driven by economic incentives, funding based on diagnostic related groups and accreditation to promote quality – in a system where the number of hospital beds was falling and outpatient visits to health professionals, such as GPs, were rising (Olejaz et al., 2012).

A similar position as regards the shifting role of health professions in Norway is outlined by Erichsen (1995). From the early nineteenth century until the early 1980s, there was a particularly close relationship between the state and the medical profession. In this period, medicine was integrated into the state at all levels of government, and the profession carried out an important role in health policy. Here, interestingly, health policy had tended to be formulated and implemented in relative isolation from other policy sectors in the welfare state. However, with a broadening of the policy agenda and the emergence of NPM, in parallel with the rest of Scandinavia, health reforms in the 1980s and 1990s led to other professions replacing physicians as experts at local and central levels, with an associated waning of the 'profession state'. This erosion of health professional power was paralleled by the common aim of increasing the level of primary care – notwithstanding variations in remuneration systems and certain aspects of organisational structure that may be explained by economic, political and cultural factors, and differences in political potency (Lian, 2003).

As Vrangbæk (2018) relates, GPs in Denmark and Norway are currently largely paid on nationally negotiated tariffs in a fee-for-service system, with the majority of hospital doctors in Scandinavia, as in Britain, salaried in public hospitals. As a result, public managers can influence professional practices because employers are externally overseen by the national authorities responsible for the licensing of health professionals and addressing malpractice breaches, not least through the revocation of licences. While there is publicly embedded medical authority in which doctors are highly involved in negotiations with the state (Burau and Vrangbæk, 2008), clinical performance and the patient experience involve administrative and political accountability through the internet and other mechanisms. Similar to Britain, though, medical associations overtly support this form of quality assessment and change as long as it delivers health benefits, is not overly burdensome for individual doctors, and does not greatly threaten the income, status and power of the professional body. This approach generally appears to have stood countries like Denmark and Norway in good stead in addressing Covid-19 and other crises.

However, there are sometimes circumstances where the health professions have acted to defend their own parochial interests. A case in point relates to the goal of promoting integration in healthcare in Denmark. Here, as Seemann and Gustafsson (2016) point out, there has historically been silo-based resistance to integration, in part centred on existing power constellations in conflicts over professional jurisdictions and boundaries. Although the situation has not been helped by the lack of overall hierarchical management of, and collaborative leadership in, the healthcare system, this has impeded change despite government administrative restructuring. A successful backlash from Danish health professionals has also since occurred over the periodic assessment of such practitioners because standards were regarded as being too inflexible, too removed from quality considerations and too resource intensive (Vrangbæk, 2018). These cases indicate that, while the Danish medical profession does not have the classic self-regulatory position of its British counterpart, it is far from powerless in terms of the neo-Weberian concept of social closure. We now turn to consider the Mediterranean macro-region.

The Mediterranean macro-region

Of most comparative interest, here are the health professions as they have developed in the Italian NHS, as this is one of the closest models in Western Europe to the British self-regulatory model linked to the neo-Weberian concept of social closure. Historically, physicians practised in Italy from the early Renaissance in the city-states, with a focus on university-based training as opposed to the apprenticeship model which dominated in Britain. As Krause (1996) observes, though, a state regulated medical professional monopoly, though, did not come into existence until the early twentieth century and this continued through the Fascist period under Mussolini because of the special need for their services. The biggest issue up to the founding of the Italian NHS in 1978 was dealing with one of the highest ratios of physicians to patients in the world – which ran at almost three times that of Britain. Despite this, patients suffered because of the lack of bedside clinical training at medical school and the absence of a requirement for a year-long internship. This situation continued, according to Krause, because it was not in the interests of those at the top of the medical hierarchy to use their power to correct given the adverse effect on their earnings.

In contemporary Italy, Krause (1996) notes that these issues to some degree persist, but in terms of the regulation of health professionals the state remains key. However, it is directly controlled by political parties, which – although they regularly disagree, causing governments to frequently fall – also have formal control of professions through policymaking. This historic context is based on the state regulation of independent professional bodies. At the hub of this system – as in Scandinavian macro-region – is the university, which has added significance in Italy because of the greater emphasis on classroom learning as distinct from supervised practice. State-regulated exclusionary professional closure in neo-Weberian terms is based on *ordini* with licensing functions which heavily define the healthcare division of labour – even if paramedics have demanded an ever greater voice. Here the dominant faction is the smaller group of elite hospital specialists, in contrast to the vast majority of generalist physicians.

As Krause (1996) says, since the establishment of the Italian NHS, the medical profession has increased its power and solidarity from the viewpoint of its interests, as professional groups need to contract collectively with the state over fees and payments. Like other professions, it is affected by intense regionalism with relatively weak central government, which results in what can be described as a vertically decentralised and insecure command and control system (Burau and Vrangbæk, 2008). This is reflected in the lack of a uniform health system, as well as major health inequalities between the more affluent North and comparatively impoverished South (Pavolini and Vicarelli, 2012). It is testimony to the level of medical power in a system which combines professional self-regulation with a limited amount of hierarchical control based on negotiation, that physicians have come to have strong representation on regional and national decision-making boards. Nonetheless, as in Britain, the dominance of the medical profession in a neo-liberal era began to be challenged from the 1990s onwards by pressures on the state to engage in more cost control with rising health expenses, increasing patient power and lobbying by allied health professions which led to greater modernisation and rationalisation of the health system (Tousjin, 1999).

Pavolini and Vicarelli (2013) note the subsequent tension between cost containment and innovation and between the public nature of the NHS and growing privatisation of provision in relation to the health professions. These tensions have been addressed, among other things, through the employment of diagnostic related groups by government to set the level of reimbursements and the introduction of top managers to run healthcare institutions. This has been complemented by measures like the accreditation of healthcare to better control performance in an era of growing austerity. Such change resulted in a far smaller percentage of the labour force working in health and care in Italy as compared to Britain and Scandinavia, which has been under increasing pressure. This in turn has adversely affected the income, autonomy and political influence of doctors. According to Vicarelli and Pavolini (2017), the outcome of managerialism has been complex and dynamic including the restratification of self-employed doctors in general practice in the national health system. As such, it has followed the pattern of GPs taking on enhanced roles as gatekeepers of demand – as in countries such as Britain, Denmark, Norway, Spain and Portugal.

As a result of the above reforms in Italy, a small group of NHS physicians have been co-opted, while most others have developed resistance to managers (Vicarelli and Pavolini, 2017). This latter pattern of hybrid professionalism was underlined by the medical response to Covid-19 in Italy where physicians have greater room for manoeuvre and collaborative relations with nurses have emerged, albeit with a highly stressful workload (Vicarelli, 2022). This form of adaption has also been apparent in Portugal where nurses have not only suffered burn out but also taken a similar hybrid position in face of managerial and organisational logics (Carvalho, 2014). While there have been strikes against medical dominance in the Mediterranean sub-region, the strong position of the orthodox health professions in the market has therefore been largely retained. This is despite such cases as the Portuguese government recently granting several CAM therapies like homeopathy and phytotherapy independent statutory regulation, which is likely to enhance the position of competitor groups in terms of social closure relative to medicine and other health professions (Almeida, Siegel and Barros, 2018).

In Portugal itself, the NHS was established in 1979 following the earlier transition in 1974 from a military regime to a democracy. Here public health and hospital physicians and nurses were the main professional deliverers of healthcare in the first-contact Health Centres founded in the period immediately beforehand – with GPs only recognised as a specialty in the early 1980s (Biscaia and Heleno, 2017). Thereafter, the regulatory role of the state was strengthened in partnership with other bodies – including the health professions. This positively included, among other things, such measures as developing and coordinating long-term care. As in other countries, a period of austerity occurred after the 2008 financial crisis, in which the resulting reduction in resources heavily impacted efficiency and quality. Among other things, this meant Portuguese doctors were only able to prescribe cheaper generic medicines within an enhanced monitoring system (European Commission and Directorate-General for Economic and Financial Affairs, 2011) – thus highlighting some degree of reduction of their independence, following that of other health professionals in relation to the state with the emergence of the NPM, in step with wider trends in Western Europe (Saks, 2021).

In Spain, the health professions have also had a measure of exclusionary social closure linked to state power. For Rodriguez (1995), the monopoly existed before the creation of the national health system in 1986, during both the Franco period from 1939 to 1975 and the consolidation of a more democratic regime. He notes in particular the dominance of the medical profession in defining and controlling medical work at this time, following which it needed to share with government regulators and corporate interests its influence and power – including its oversight of nurses (Olejaz, 2012). However, in this process, it has largely escaped bureaucratising and proletarianising influences, despite healthcare mainly being in the organised public sector with consequent difficulties in maintaining jurisdictional control (Rodriguez, 1995). The current form of social closure in medicine and other health professions in neo-Weberian terms is enshrined in the national Registry of Healthcare Professions which collects information on them from workforce registries in the Spanish autonomous communities (Olejaz, 2012). Nonetheless, with the end of the Official Medical Association's representational monopoly under Franco, the medical profession has polarised into an elite in prestigious private practices and specialties, and generalists in the public sector with lesser esteem.

In Greece, there are many similarities in health professional development with Spain – not least given the relatively recent background of dictatorship from 1967 to 1974 which preceded the introduction of the Greek NHS in 1983, as well as the growing representation of women in the health professions, including medicine, and the increased role of primary care (Economou et al., 2017). Greece also shares with Spain, and indeed Italy, an apparent oversupply of physicians which has resulted in substantial medical unemployment and a net migration of doctors to other Western European countries. This has been matched by one of the lowest proportions of nurses in Europe, such that this group is outnumbered by doctors – a position for which Spain, where generalist and specialist physicians, nurses, midwives, dentists and pharmacists are regulated under the Sectoral Directive system, runs Greece quite close (Kuhlmann et al., 2015). However, there are differences associated with the health professions in Greece, including those based on its especially poor financial controls, large-scale inequalities in health resources and widespread inefficiencies (Economou et al., 2017).

None of this was helped by the deep fiscal crisis the Greece experienced from 2010 onwards which led to severe economic measures that heavily impacted health professional agendas leading to severe cuts in hospital departments and units (Economou et al., 2015). Nonetheless, according to Nikolentzos and Mays (2016), the Greek medical profession critically played a vital role in establishing the NHS and has since used its power and influence to bring about key health reforms. Hospital doctors in particular have consequently been able to protect their interests by resisting most reforms affecting their dominant position because of the particularities of the Greek state and society. Although the power of the medical profession was critiqued in the wake of the financial crisis, they believe change is by no means inevitable, notwithstanding the emergency measures adopted during the recent Covid-19 pandemic. This underlines, that for all the parallels in changes affecting health professions in the Mediterranean macro-region, there is also considerable diversity in the evolution of medical and health professions in the NHSs concerned. Such variations exist despite the similarities forged by common membership of the European Union, including free movement of health professionals – which Britain of course no longer shares after Brexit (Hopkins, 2020).

Conclusion: the value of the neo-Weberian approach

The brief overview in this chapter has hopefully highlighted the utility of the neo-Weberian perspective in analysing the development of the medical and other health professions in the NHSs of Western Europe. The significance of this approach is accentuated when we turn to consider the case of Russian medicine in Eastern Europe. While in Western European societies, including Britain, the ideal typical model of exclusionary closure has generally been eroded by substantially increased state involvement, growing corporatisation and moves to provide greater public protection, nowhere does this approach the levels of depletion extant in Russia. Here there has never been a fully independently regulated profession of medicine, with the income, status and power that has gone hand in hand with this in Britain and other countries in the West (Saks, 2015). This is not to deny that the position of groups like doctors has shifted over time, but Russia certainly lies at the other end of the spectrum from Britain in terms of exclusionary social closure in a wider European context.

As Saks (2018) outlines, such a state of affairs in Russia largely goes back to the late nineteenth century under Tsardom when physicians formed the oppositional Pirogov Society, which sought socio-political reform – including establishing a self-regulatory medical regime. When Tsarism was overthrown, the Pirogov Society was given the brief to lead such medical professional reform, but once the Bolsheviks took over after the Russia Revolution in 1917, this Society was regarded as bourgeois and counter revolutionary and medical care was put under the control of the Communist Party. The Party imposed state bureaucratic controls on medicine and literally flooded the market with physicians, such that by the 1960s as many as one in four doctors globally was a Soviet doctor – which had the effect of eroding their income, status and power (Field, 1967). Little has changed in the post-Soviet era where medical self-regulation has still not been established as efforts to create an independent profession have generally been thwarted because this has remained too challenging to the state (Moskovskaya et al., 2013).

In Russia, issues such as medical entry, licensing, medical examinations and codes of ethics remain primarily under state control unlike in Britain – and to a far greater degree than in other societies in Western Europe with an

NHS (Saks, 2015). This has led to very significantly lower financial and other rewards for doctors and has helped to bring about serious gender imbalances, with a much higher female proportion of Russian physicians than in Western societies (Harden, 2001). While an elite group of doctors exercise some political influence through the Russian Academy of Sciences in Moscow and the state has supported medical personnel through the Ministry of Health in facing the challenge from CAM therapies by restricting most of these practices such as acupuncture and osteopathy to doctors (Yurchenko and Saks, 2006), the general situation of physicians is the inverse of the exclusionary social closure model (Saks, 2015). As such, it is not possible in neo-Weberian terms to class medicine as a profession in Russia.

However, as witnessed in the helicopter view provided in this chapter, the neo-Weberian exclusionary social closure model clearly acts as a helpful ideal type in understanding the broad spectrum of less extreme arrangements that we find in studying the evolution of the medical and other health professions in the NHSs of Western Europe. While there is some differentiation in this respect between such societies, it is also very useful to examine them, as has been seen, from the perspective of a neo-institutionalist perspective as doctors and related groups vie with other actors for their place in the sun in a fast-changing milieu, including in hybrid forms. In this context, across the range of countries considered here, the interest-based agendas of health professions have recently been increasingly challenged by the emergence of the NPM. This has been linked to the rise of managerialist, corporatist and consumerist logics which have often been pitched – with health workforce consequences – against professional logics in Western European countries with an NHS. For all this, the evolution of health professions in the societies considered here remains dynamic with both convergent and divergent trends. In all this, it is to be hoped that going forward, health professions and other influential actors exercise responsible leadership in accord with broader notions of the public interest (Saks, 2023)

References

Allsop, J. and Jones, K. (2008) 'Protecting patients: International trends in medical governance', in Kuhlmann, E. and Saks, M. (eds) *Rethinking Professional Governance: International Directions in Health Care*, Bristol: Policy Press.

Allsop, J. and Jones, K. (2018) 'Regulating the regulators: The rise of the United Kingdom Professional Standards Authority', in Chamberlain, J. M., Dent, M. and Saks, M. (eds) *Professional Health Regulation in the Public Interest: International Perspectives*, Bristol: Policy Press.

Almeida, J., Siegel, P. and Barros, N. (2018) 'Governing complementary and alternative medicine (CAM) in Brazil and Portugal: Implications for CAM professionals and the public', in Chamberlain, J. M., Dent, M. and Saks, M. (eds) *Professional Health Regulation in the Public Interest: International Perspectives*, Bristol: Policy Press.

Barber, B. (1963) 'Some problems in the sociology of professions', *Daedalus* 92: 669–88.

Beattie, A. (1995) 'War and peace among the health tribes', in Soothill, K., Mackay, L. and Webb, C. (eds) *Interprofessional Relations in Health Care*, London: Edward Arnold.

Becker, H. (1962) 'The nature of a profession', in National Society for the Study of Education (ed) *Education for the Professions*, Chicago, IL: University of Chicago Press.

Benoit, C. (1999) 'Midwifery and health policy: Equity, workers' rights and consumer choice in Canada and Sweden', in Hellberg, I., Saks, M. and Benoit, C. (eds) *Professional Identities in Transition: Cross-cultural Dimensions*, Södertälje: Almqvist & Wiksell.

Bertilsson, A. (1990) 'The knowledge aspect of professionalization: The case of science-based nursing education in Sweden', in Torstendahl, R. and Burrage, M. (eds) *The Formation of Professions: Knowledge, State and Strategy*, London: Sage.

Biscaia, A. R. and Heleno, L. C. (2017) 'Primary health care reform in Portugal: Portuguese, modern and innovative', *Ciência e Saúde Coletiva* 22(3): 701–12.

Borsay, A. and Hunter, B. (eds) (2012) *Nursing and Midwifery in Britain Since 1700*, Basingstoke: Palgrave Macmillan.

Brante, T. (1999) 'Professional waves and state objectives: A macro-sociological model of the origin and development of continental professions, illustrated by the case of Sweden', in Hellberg, I., Saks, M. and Benoit, C. (eds) *Professional Identities in Transition: Cross-cultural Dimensions*, Södertälje: Almqvist & Wiksell.

Braverman, H. (1998) *Labor and Monopoly Capital: The Degradation of Work in the Twentieth Century*, New edition, New York: Monthly Review Press.

Burau, V. (1999) 'The politics of internal boundaries: A comparative analysis of community nursing in Britain and Germany', in Hellberg, I., Saks, M. and Benoit, C. (eds) *Professional Identities in Transition: Cross-cultural Dimensions*, Södertälje: Almqvist & Wiksell.

Burau, V. and Vrangbæk, K (2008) 'Global markets and national pathways of medical re-regulation', in Kuhlmann, E. and Saks, M. (eds) *Rethinking Professional Governance: International Directions in Health Care*, Bristol: Policy Press.

Calnan, M. and Douglass, T. (2022) *Power, Policy and the Pandemic: A Sociological Analysis of COVID-19 Policy in England*, Bingley: Emerald Publishing.

Calnan, M. and Gabe, J. (2009) 'The restratification of primary care in England? A sociological analysis', in Gabe, J. and Calnan, M. (eds) *The New Sociology of the Health Service*, Abingdon: Routledge.

Cant, S. and Sharma, U. (1999) *A New Medical Pluralism? Alternative Medicine, Doctors, Patients and the State*, London: UCL Press.

Carvalho, T. (2014) 'Changing connections between professionalism and managerialism: A case study of nursing in Portugal', *Journal of Professions and Organization* 1(2): 176–90.

Castro, F. W. (1999) 'After the wave: The welfare state professionals in Sweden', in Hellberg, I., Saks, M. and Benoit, C. (eds) *Professional Identities in Transition: Cross-cultural Dimensions*, Södertälje: Almqvist & Wiksell.

Chamberlain, J. M. (2012) *The Sociology of Medical Regulation*, London: Springer.

Chamberlain, J. M. (2015) *Medical Regulation, Fitness to Practice and Medical Revalidation: A Critical Introduction*, Bristol: Policy Press.

Collins, R. (1990) 'Market closure and the conflict theory of the professions', in Burrage, M. and Torstendahl, R. (eds) *Professions in Theory and History: Rethinking the Study of the Professions*, London: Sage.

Dent, M. (2018) 'Health care governance, user involvement and medical regulation in Europe', in Chamberlain, J. M., Dent, M. and Saks, M. (eds) *Professional Health Regulation in the Public Interest: International Perspectives*, Bristol: Policy Press.

Dent, M., Chandler, J. and Barry, J. (eds) (2004) *Questioning the New Public Management*, Aldershot: Ashgate.

Department and Health and Social Care (2022) *Healthcare Regulation: Deciding Where Statutory Regulation Is Appropriate*, London: DHSC.

Economou, C., Kaitelidou, D., Karankolos, M. and Maresso, A. (2017) 'Greece: Health system review', *Health Systems in Transition* 19(5): 1–166.

Economou, C., Kaitelidou, D., Kentikelenis, A., Maresso, A. and Sissouras, A. (2015) 'The impact of the crisis on the health system and health in Greece', in Maresso, A., Mladovsky, P., Thomson, S., et al. (eds) *Economic Crisis, Health Systems and Health in Europe: Country Experience*, Copenhagen: European Observatory on Health Systems and Policies. Available at: https://eurohealthobservatory.who.int/publications/i/economic-crisis-health-systems-and-health-in-europe-country-experience-study

Einarsdottir, G. (1999) 'The gendering of status and the status of gender: The case of the Swedish medical profession', in Hellberg, I., Saks, M. and Benoit, C. (eds) *Professional Identities in Transition: Cross-cultural Dimensions*, Södertälje: Almqvist & Wiksell.

Elzinga, A. (1990) 'The knowledge aspect of professionalization: The case of science-based nursing education in Sweden', in Torstendahl, R. and Burrage, M. (eds) *The Formation of Professions: Knowledge, State and Strategy*, London: Sage.

Erichsen, V. (1995) 'Health care reform in Norway: The end of the "profession state"?', *Journal of Health Politics, Policy and Law* 20(3): 719–37.

Esland, G. (1980) 'Diagnosis and therapy', in Esland, G. and Salaman, G. (eds) *The Politics of Work and Occupations*, Milton Keynes: Open University Press.

Etzioni, A. (ed) (1969) *The Semi-professions and Their Organization*, New York: Free Press.

European Commission and Directorate-General for Economic and Financial Affairs (2011) *Portugal: Memorandum of Understanding on Specific Economic Policy Conditionality*, 17 May.

Evetts, J. (2000) 'Professions in European and UK markets: The European professional federations', *International Journal of Sociology and Social Policy* 18: 395–415.

Evetts, J. (2013) 'Professionalism: Value and ideology', *Current Sociology* 61(5/6): 778–96.

Field, M. G. (1967) *Soviet Socialized Medicine: An Introduction*, New York: Free Press.

Foucault, M. (1989) *The Birth of the Clinic*, London: Routledge.

Foucault, M. (2001) *Madness and Civilization: A History of Madness in the Age of Reason*, London: Routledge Classics.

Freidson, E. (1970) *Profession of Medicine: A Study in the Sociology of Applied Knowledge*, New York: Dodd, Mead & Co.

Friedman, M. (1962) *Capitalism and Freedom*, Chicago, IL: University of Chicago Press.

Garpenby, P. (1989) *The State and the Medical Profession. A Cross-National Comparison of the Health Policy Arena in the United Kingdom and Sweden 1945–1985*, Linköping: Linköping Studies in Arts and Sciences.

Giarelli, G. and Spina, E. (2014) 'Self-help/Mutual aid as active citizenship associations: A case-study of the chronically ill in Italy', *Social Science and Medicine* 123: 242–9.

Harden, J. (2001) '"Mother Russia" at work: Gender divisions in the medical profession', *European Journal of Women's Studies* 8(2): 181–99.

Haskell, H. (2020) 'Cumberlege review exposes stubborn and dangerous flaws in healthcare', *British Medical Journal* 370: m3099. Available at: https://doi.org/10.1136/bmj.m3099

Hellberg, I. (1990) 'The Swedish veterinary profession and the Swedish state', in Torstendahl, R. and Burrage, M. (eds) *The Formation of Professions: Knowledge, State and Strategy*, London: Sage.

Hopkins, M. (2020) *Brrrexit! Why England Will Be Left Out in the Cold*, London: Amazon UK.

Hudson, B. (2000) 'Inrer-agency collaboration: A sceptical view', in Brechin, A., Brown, H. and Eby, M. A. (eds) *Critical Practice in Health and Social Care*, London: Sage.

Hughes, E. (1963) 'Professions', *Daedalus* 92: 655–68.

Immergut, E. (1999) 'Historical and institutional foundations of the Swedish health care system', in Powell, F. D. and Wessen, A. F. (eds) *Health Care Systems in Transition. An International Perspective*, Thousand Oaks, CA: Sage.

Johnson, T. (2016) *Professions and Power*, Abingdon: Routledge Revivals.

Kirkpatrick, I. (2016) 'Hybrid managers and professional leadership', in Dent, M., Bourgeault, I., Dennis, J. and Kuhlmann, E. (eds) *The Routledge Companion on Professions and Professionalism*, Abingdon: Routledge.

Klein, R. (2013) *The New Politics of the NHS: From Creation to Reinvention*, 7th edition, London: Radcliffe Publishing.

Krause, E. (1996) *Death of the Guilds: Professions, States and the Advance of Capitalism, 1930 to the Present*, New Haven: Yale University Press.

Kuhlmann, E., Agartan, T. and Von Knorring, M. (2016) 'Governance and professions', in Dent, M., Bourgeault, I. L., Denis, J.-L. and Kuhlmann, E. (2016) *The Routledge Companion to the Professions and Professionalism*, Abingdon: Routledge.

Kuhlmann, E. and Annandale, E. (eds) (2012) *The Palgrave Handbook of Gender and Healthcare*, 2nd edition, Basingstoke: Palgrave Macmillan.

Kuhlmann, E., Groenewegen, P. P., Batenburg, R. and Larsen, C. (2015) Health human resources policy in Europe', in Kuhlmann, E., Blank, R. H., Bourgeault, I. L. and Wendt, C. (eds) *The Palgrave International Handbook of Health Policy and Governance*, Basingstoke: Palgrave Macmillan.

Leemeijer, A. and Noordegraaf, M. (2020) 'Health professionals and peer support workers in mental health settings', in Saks, M. (ed) *Support Workers and the Health Professions in International Perspective: The Invisible Providers of Health Care*, Bristol: Policy Press.

Le Fanu, J. (2011) *The Rise and Fall of Modern Medicine*, 2nd edition, London: Abacus.

Lian, O. S. (2003) 'Convergence or divergence? Reforming primary care in Norway and Britain', *Milbank Quarterly* 81(2): 305–30.

Macdonald, K. (1995) *The Sociology of the Professions*, London: Sage.

Miles, S. H. (2005) *The Hippocratic Oath and the Ethics of Medicine*, Oxford: Oxford University Press.

Millerson, G. (1964) *The Qualifying Associations*, London: Routledge & Kegan Paul.

Moskovskaya, A., Oberemko, O., Silaeva, V., Popova, I., Nazarova, I., Peshkova, O. and Chemysheva, M. (2013) 'Development of professional associations in Russia: Research into institutional framework, self-regulation activity and barriers to professionalization', *Working Paper BRP 26/SOC/2013*, Moscow: Higher School of Economics.

Nancarrow, S. and Borthwick, A. (2021) *The Allied Health Professions: A Sociological Perspective*, Bristol: Policy Press.

Nettleton, S. (1992) *Power, Pain and Dentistry*, Buckingham: Open University Press.

Nikolentzos, A. and Mays, N. (2016) 'Explaining the persistent dominance of the Greek medical profession across successive health care system reforms from 1983 to the present', *Health Systems and Reform* 2(2): 135–46.

Noordegraaf, M. (2018) 'Enterprise, hybrid professionalism and the public sector', in Saks, M. and Muzio, D. (eds) *Professions and Professional Service Firms: Private and Public Sector Enterprises in the Global Economy*, Abingdon: Routledge.

Olejaz, M., Juul Nielsen, A., Rudkjøbing, A., Okkels Birk, H., Krasnik, A. and Hernández-Quevedo, C. (2012) 'Denmark: Health system review', *Health Systems in Transition* 14(2): 1–192.

Parkin, F. (1979) *Marxism and Class Theory: A Bourgeois Critique*, London: Tavistock.

Parry, N. and Parry, J. (2019) *The Rise of the Medical Profession: A Study of Collective Social Mobility*, Abingdon: Routledge.

Pavolini, E. and Vicarelli, G. (2012) 'Is decentralization good for your health? Transformations in the Italian NHS', *Current Sociology* 60(4): 472–88.

Pavolini, E. and Vicarelli, G. (2013) 'Italy: A strange NHS with its paradoxes', in Pavolini, E. and Guillén, A. M. (eds) *Health Care Systems in Europe Under Austerity: Institutional Reforms and Performance*, Basingstoke: Palgrave Macmillan.

Perreault, T., Bridge, G. and McCarthy, J. P. (eds) (2015) *The Routledge Handbook of Political Ecology*, Abingdon: Routledge.

Pickard, S. (2009) 'The professionalization of general practitioners with a special interest: Rationalization, restratification and governmentality', *Sociology* 43: 250–67.

Poulantzas, N. (1975) *Political Power and Social Classes*, London: New Left Books.

Roche, W. (2018) 'Medical regulation for the public interest in the United Kingdom', in Chamberlain, J. M., Dent, M. and Saks, M. (eds) *Professional Health Regulation in the Public Interest: International Perspectives*, Bristol: Policy Press.

Rodriguez, J. (1995) 'The politics of the Spanish medical profession: Democratization and the construction of the national health system', in Johnson, T., Larkin, G. and Saks, M. (eds) *Health Professions and the State in Europe*, London: Routledge.

Roszak, T. (1995) *The Making of a Counter Culture*, Berkeley, CA: University of California Press.

Saks, M. (1983) 'Removing the blinkers? A critique of recent contributions to the sociology of professions', *Sociological Review* 31(1): 1–21.

Saks, M. (1998) 'Deconstructing or reconstructing professions? Interpreting the role of professional groups in society', in Olgiati, V., Orzack, L. and Saks, M. (eds) *Professions, Identity and Order in Comparative Perspective*, Onati: Onati International Institute for the Sociology of Law.

Saks, M. (2002) 'Professionalization, regulation and alternative medicine', in Allsop, J. and Saks, M. (eds) *Regulating the Health Professions*, London: Sage.

Saks, M. (2003) 'The limitations of the Anglo-American sociology of the professions: A critique of the current neo-Weberian orthodoxy', *Knowledge, Work and Society* 1: 11–31.

Saks, M. (2010) 'Analyzing the professions: The case for a neo-Weberian approach', *Comparative Sociology* 9(6): 887–915.

Saks, M. (2012) 'Defining a profession: The role of knowledge and expertise', *Professions and Professionalism* 2: 1–10.

Saks, M. (2014) 'The regulation of the English health professions: Zoos, circuses or safari parks?', *Journal of Professions and Organization* 1(1): 84–98.

Saks, M. (2015) *The Professions, State and the Market: Medicine in Britain, the United States and Russia*, Abingdon: Routledge.

Saks, M. (2016) 'Review of theories of professions, organizations and society: Neo-Weberianism, neo-institutionalism and eclecticism', *Journal of Professions and Organization* 3(2): 170–87.

Saks, M. (2018) 'Regulation and Russian medicine: Whither medical professionalisation?', in Chamberlain, J. M., Dent, M. and Saks, M. (eds) *Professional Health Regulation in the Public Interest: International Perspectives*, Bristol: Policy Press.

Saks, M. (2020) 'Introduction: Support workers and the health professions', in Saks, M. (ed) *Support Workers and Health Professions in International Perspective: The Invisible Providers of Health Care*, Bristol: Policy Press.

Saks, M. (2021) *Professions: A Key Idea for Business and Society*, Abingdon: Routledge.

Saks, M. (2023) 'Professions and responsible leadership', in Saks, M. (ed) *Responsible Leadership: Essential to the Achievement of the UN Sustainable Development Goals*, Abingdon: Routledge.

Saks, M. and Adams, T. (2019) 'Neo-Weberianism, professional formation and the state: Inside the black box', *Professions and Professionalism* 9(2): 1–14.

Saks, M. and Zagrodney, K. (2020) 'Health professions, support workers and the precariat', in Saks, M. (ed) *Support Workers and the Health Professions in International Perspective: The Invisible Providers of Health Care*, Bristol: Policy Press.

Schepers, R. M. J. and Casparie, A. F. (1999) 'Medical quality assurance and professional identity in Belgium, the Netherlands and England', in Hellberg, I., Saks, M. and Benoit, C. (eds) *Professional Identities in Transition: Cross-cultural Dimensions*, Södertälje: Almqvist & Wiksell.

Sciulli, D. (2005) 'Continental sociology of professions today: Conceptual contributions', *Current Sociology* 53(6): 915–42.

Seemann, J. and Gustafsson, J. (2016) 'Integration in the spotlight: Fighting silo barriers and fragmented healthcare in Denmark', in Giarelli, G., Jacobsen, B., Nielsen, M. and Reinbacher, G. S. (eds) *Future Challenges for Health and Healthcare in Europe*, Aalborg: Aalborg University Press.

Stacey, M. (1992) *Regulating British Medicine: The General Medical Council*, Chichester: Wiley & Sons.

Suddaby, R. and Muzio, D. (2015) 'Theoretical perspectives of the professions', in Empson, L., Muzio, D., Broschak, J. and Hinings, B. (eds) *The Oxford Handbook of Professional Service Firms*, Oxford: Oxford University Press.

Swedberg, R. and Agevall, O. (2016) *The Max Weber Dictionary: Key Words and Central Concepts*, 2nd edition, Stanford, CA: Stanford University Press.

Tousjin, W. (1999) 'Medical professionalisation in Italy: A comparative perspective', in Hellberg, I., Saks, M. and Benoit, C. (eds) *Professional Identities in Transition: Cross-cultural Dimensions*, Södertälje: Almqvist & Wiksell.

Vicarelli, G. (2022) 'The non-existent knights? Doctors in the age of Covid-19', Paper given at Conference on Pandemics, Globalisation, Society and Politics Between Crisis and Catastrophe, University of Florence, September.

Vicarelli, G. and Pavolini, E. (2017) 'Dynamics between doctors and managers in the Italian national health care system', *Sociology of Health and Illness* 39(8): 1381–97.

Vrangbæk, K. (2015) 'Patient involvement in Danish health care', *Journal of Health Organization and Management* 29(5): 611–24.

Vrangbæk, K. (2018) 'The regulation of health care in Scandinavia: Professionals, the public interest and trust', in Chamberlain, J. M., Dent, M. and Saks, M. (eds) *Professional Health Regulation in the Public Interest: International Perspectives*, Bristol: Policy Press.

Walton-Roberts, M. (2022) *Global Migration, Gender and Health Professional Credentials: Transnational Value Transfers and Losses*, Toronto: Toronto University Press.

Whiting, M., May, S. and Saks, M. (2020) 'Exclusionary social closure and the professionalization of veterinary medicine in the UK: A self-interested or public interested endeavour?', *Professions and Professionalism* 10(1).

Witz, A. (1992) *Professions and Patriarchy*, London: Routledge.

Wrede, S. (2008) 'Educating generalists: Flexibility and identity in auxiliary nursing in Finland', in Kuhlmann, E. and Saks, M. (eds) *Rethinking Professional Governance: International Directions in Health Care*, Bristol: Policy Press.

Yurchenko, O. and Saks, M. (2006) 'The social integration of complementary and alternative medicine in official health care in Russia', *Knowledge, Work and Society* 4: 107–27.

12 The participation of patients and the public in National Health Services

Mauro Serapioni

Introduction

In the neo-Weberian and neo-institutionalist approaches adopted in this book, different stakeholder groups are competing in the health arena, in particular physicians and other health professions, the state, local governments, managers, medical–industrial complex, as well as citizens and civil society associations (Saks, 2010). In the last two decades, the greater involvement of the public in the monitoring and quality assurance of healthcare work has led to a revision of the social closure model of professional work (Chamberlain, 2018). According to Saks (2016:10), 'the framework of regulation of professions is fast changing at the macro level, with increasing demand for more accountability and inclusivity'. In fact, among the characteristics of the neo-Weberian state model it is important to mention the following two elements as highlighted by Pollitt (2008:15): (1) shifting external orientations towards 'meeting citizens' needs and wishes' and (2) complementing representative democracy with an array of mechanisms 'for consultation and direct representation of citizens' opinions'. Thus, expectations that users and citizens play a significant role in health governance processes have been increasing. However, it is worth asking, as Dent (2018:17) points out, whether 'user involvement impacts on medical regulation and governance in any significant way'.

How best to involve the public in local health policy development and decision-making is an ongoing challenge for National Health Services (NHSs). The potential benefits of public participation (PP) have been widely discussed in the literature. To date, several initiatives have been put forward and substantial resources have been invested in the design and implementation of PP exercises. However, the degree of institutionalisation of PP is still far from satisfactory. Results of different studies have highlighted many critical points that affect PP in NHSs. Some of the most noteworthy are the lack of representativeness and the failure to prioritise the involvement of vulnerable groups (Freer, 2021); the need for more mechanisms to produce collective decisions to increase the legitimacy of decisions (Bobbio, 2018); and the need to assess properly the effectiveness of PP (Fredriksson and Tritter, 2017).

DOI: 10.4324/9781003139799-18

This chapter provides an overview of the state of the art of PP in the NHSs of the three macro-regions (Britain, Scandinavia and the Mediterranean), outlining its evolution over recent decades and the characteristics of the main participation mechanisms and approaches implemented in each country of the three macro-regions. Then, adapting the theoretical approach based on Hirschman (1970) to the field of participation, the chapter proceeds with the discussion of the main results that emerged from the analysis of PP in the three macro-regions, highlighting the main critical aspects and some insights into possible reforms.

The British macro-region

The British NHS, which was established in 1948 under the auspices of the Ministry of Health, has been subject to constant tension since its inception between accountability to the central authority or the local community (Klein, 1990). Successive reorganisations of the NHS were intended to reduce this tension, which grew during the 1960s as a result of protests by women's movements and self-help groups that questioned the way in which services were being managed. As a result of such dysfunctions and complaints in 1974, Community Health Councils (CHCs) were established as means of promoting and defending citizens' interests. CHCs were independent, funded, and empowered to direct disagreements about changes in local health services to the minister of health (Freer, 2021). When the Conservative Party came to power, a process of reform of the NHS began at the beginning of the 1980s, associated with the increased importance given to the role of the market and patients as consumers of health services. The National Health Service and Community Care Act introduced by the Conservative government in 1990 brought about radical structural change.

The rise of the consumerist approach was accompanied, as Lupton, Peckham and Taylor (1998) point out, by an attitude of 'suspicion' towards traditional forms of citizen participation. The new Labour government, elected in 1997 to restore citizens' confidence in the NHS after 18 years of rule by the Conservative Party, re-launched the 'third way' model, between centralist and neo-liberal models. In 2001, the second Labour government launched a new reform titled *Involving Patients and the Public in Healthcare* and proposed ending CHCs. This took place in 2003, which led to CHCs being replaced with four distinct bodies to represent the interests of citizens: the Patient Advice and Liaison Service, the Independent Complaints Advocacy Service, the Patient's Forum, and Overview and Scrutiny Committees. This was viewed as a 'fragmented and unstable' public representation structure (Hogg, 2007). The adversarial and demanding approach of CHCs was no longer suitable in the new Labour Party philosophy, which was centred on partnership and local authority accountability. In the opinion of Freer (2021), the abolition of CHCs was related to the beginning of the fragmentation of the NHS and marketising reforms.

Unlike England, Scotland and Wales maintained parallel organisations to CHCs in the wake of the 1999 legislation that established national parliaments in both countries and transferred government powers in areas such as health and social care (Bevan et al., 2014). In England, though, in the five years after its creation, the new participation system was strongly criticised due to its fragmentation, scarcity of resources and ineffectiveness (Baggott and Jones, 2014) and was replaced with 151 local involvement networks (LINKs), which started operation in 2008. The explanation for this rapid change in participation policy in the opinion of Hughes, Mullen and Vincent-Jones (2009:242) was 'complicated and contested'. Among the various problematic aspects identified, the inability of this forum to represent local communities probably carried great weight. It was a model of participation based on interaction between a diverse range of agencies and actors, including voluntary organisations, stakeholders and local communities (Tritter, 2011). Like CHCs, LINKs operated within defined local authority areas.

A little later, the Health and Social Care Act of 2012 replaced the local involvement networks (LINKs) with local healthwatch organisations, which from 2013 became advocates for patients, service users and the public in the field of health and social assistance. A network of 150 local Healthwatch bodies was instituted across England, in liaison with local authorities, and was coordinated and supported by a national body, Healthwatch England. This is the current system of patient and public participation in England. However, research has indicated some difficulties and fragilities in the Healthwatch bodies. Gilbert, Dunn and Foot (2015), for example, pointed out a significant variation in the way in which they are organised, how they conduct activities and their effectiveness in carrying out their statutory activities. For Zoccatelli and colleagues (2020), the degree of autonomy of the host organisations, the quality and quantity of the relationship with stakeholders, and the different financing arrangements contribute to this high level of variability in performance.

In practice, since the 2001 reform Involving Patients and the Public in Healthcare, which phased out CHCs in the UK, market mechanisms have become increasingly prominent in the provision of health services – resulting in the promotion of policies oriented towards patient choice and a consumerist approach. In the words of Carter and Martin (2016:259), defining Healthwatch as 'a new consumer champion' – as it was presented by the Department of Health (2012) – is 'a description that seemingly endorses a market orientation'. In this respect, it is important to point out how changes in health policies, particularly the excessive emphasis on patient choice, the market and competition, has weakened the actions of patient associations, reducing their independence from the government and other actors and their ability to influence policymakers. Baggott and Jones (2014:9) summed up this situation as follows: 'Too strong a focus on individuals can undermine the role of health consumer and patients' organizations'.

As already mentioned, Scotland and Wales, unlike England, followed a different path regarding PP. In Scotland, local health councils were created in 1974 – similar to the CHCs in England and Wales – to assist patients in the complaints process, and were also consulted in case of reorganising and closing services (Steel and Cylus, 2012). In 2005, they were replaced by the Scottish Health Council (SHC), created as part of the NHS and composed of local advisory councils in each health board area (Longley, Llewellyn and Simpson, 2012a). They were constituted by around ten volunteer members and met regularly to discuss relevant issues of public engagement with the aim of promoting a focus on patients and public participation in the NHS. The aim was to ensure that NHS boards listened to people's views and took them into account. In 2007 the Scottish government published the *Better Health, Better Care: Action Plan*, with the aim of developing a more inclusive relationship, in order to recognise patients and the public as partners and not just recipients of care (Scottish Health Council, 2014). This plan introduced the concept of the participation standard to collect systematic information on participation across the Scottish NHS, and to measure the extent to which NHS boards ensured that people were involved in decisions about their care and in the development of local health services. Along these lines, in 2010 the Scottish government published guidelines for NHS boards on 'informing, engaging and consulting people in developing health services and community care services' (Scottish Health Council, 2014:13). The SHC meets four times a year and has a network of 14 local offices across Scotland (one in each NHS board area) and a national office in Glasgow.

Among the structures that support public involvement in Scotland, the following can be highlighted: public partnership forums, networks of patients, caregivers, community groups, and voluntary organisations and individuals interested in the development and design of local health services and social assistance services, which represent the main link between services and local communities; patient participation groups, linked to the primary care service (general practice); and a body called Visioning Outcomes in Community Engagement, with a planning and recording software tool that assists individuals and associations in promoting effective community engagement.

In Wales in 2003, unlike England, CHCs were confirmed and 22 Local Health Boards (LHBs) were created to strengthen the voice of local communities in decision-making processes (Hughes, Mullen and Vincent-Jones, 2009). CHCs, supported by their Board, have had an important role to play in influencing the way health services are designed and delivered, to ensure the best possible health and well-being outcomes for all. CHCs have been in operation since their inception in 1974, although they have been subject to a series of revisions and reorganisations. In 2000, the National Assembly of Wales introduced a new structure and the CHCs were grouped into nine federations. However, an assessment found that the work of CHCs was very heterogeneous across the country (Longley,

Llewellyn and Simpson, 2012a). In 2010, the Community Health Council (Establishment, Transfer of Functions and Abolition) (Wales) Order 2010 reduced the CHCs from 19 to 8, one in each of the new areas of the LHB. In 2015, the merger of two CHCs led to the current seven CHCs. These cover larger geographic areas and are largely co-terminous with the lower number of LHBs. Each of the seven new CHCs is made up of local committees (LCs), which correspond to the number of local authorities in the CHC area. Each LC is composed of 12 members, who are also members of the CHC. The board of CHCs meets at least four times a year and works at a strategic and national level, advising and assisting all CHCs in Wales. CHCs have the statutory power to be consulted on major service changes and are empowered to inspect NHS facilities, including those of primary care providers and agencies providing services to the NHS (Longley et al., 2012b). CHCs also provide free, independent and confidential advocacy activities to patients seeking advice and in support of the process of filing complaints against the NHS. The CHCs are composed of: representatives of local authorities; members nominated by third sector organisations; and those appointed by the Ministry of Health.

In 2017, the Welsh government published a White Paper *Services Fit for the Future* that proposed the establishment of a new body to represent citizens' voices: the Citizen Voice Body for Health and Social Care. This proposal was incorporated into Health and Social Care (Quality and Engagement) Wales Bill, which was approved by the National Assembly for Wales, and will enter into force in April 2023. The abolition of CHCs, after 50 years of existence, is justified by the 'significant disadvantages of its legislative model that limit the exercise of its functions only to the health services within its district', and by the need to guarantee its 'independence and a stronger organisation' (Welsh Government, 2022:1).

Devolution therefore implied divergences in PP strategies. In fact, the changes were evident in the continuous evolution of the national system for surveying and managing patient dissatisfaction and complaints, as well as the increasing emphasis placed on promoting individual choice, which has, according to Tritter (2011), reinforced the process of individualisation of PP. Patient choice was implemented mainly in England and to a limited extent in Scotland and Wales. In the latter countries, it was introduced as an option to reduce long waiting times in surgical procedures and not as a patient choice policy in and of itself, as was the case in England, which went down a 'choose and book' route, which allowed NHS patients to choose available hospitals. In Scotland and Wales, the biggest concern has been promoting the voice of patients and greater engagement of local communities. However, the changes and reforms implemented in recent years have contributed to reducing the difference between England and other countries in the UK. In fact, in the Scottish and Welsh NHSs, the hiring of private health service providers has increased and, of course, private health expenditure has also increased to meet waiting-time targets.

The Scandinavian macro-region

Scandinavian healthcare systems were built on the principle of universalism and have several characteristics in common: universal coverage for all residents, predominantly financed by taxes; public provision through hospitals and general practitioners (GPs); decentralised management at regional and local level; and the reduced role of household expenditure in health services (out-of-pocket payments for health services) (Terkel, 2018). However, due to external factors (the influence of the doctrine of New Public Management (NPM) and also internal pressures (increasing financial constraints and public dissatisfaction with long waiting lists and rigidities of the system), the Scandinavian health model has undergone important changes, and it is no longer possible to think of a single model of public health policies (Vallgårda, 2007). Indeed, in the three countries of Norway, Denmark and Sweden, the private market for supplementary voluntary health insurance has increased in recent decades, as has the number of private health services and professionals (Tynkkynen et al., 2018) as a result of reforms that supported market expansion and patient choice (Fredriksson and Tritter, 2019). However, these changes did not shake the basic foundations of the welfare state in this European region, based on the principles of equal opportunities, social solidarity and security for all (Magnussen et al., 2009; Torjesen et al., 2017).

In this context, improving the quality and safety of social and health services has always been the prime policy objective for health systems in Nordic countries, thus making patient-centredness a priority (Storm and Coulter, 2017). Strengthening the role of patients in health services has been a government priority in Norway in recent decades, where the main model of citizen involvement in health and social care has been based on permanent consultative bodies called 'user councils' (Andreassen, 2017), which have been successfully implemented at the regional level. The promotion of quality assurance programmes at the national level has led the Danish Ministry of Health to develop strategies to enhance public involvement and patient-centred care (Knudsen, Engel and Eriksen, 2015). Similarly, in Sweden, public health policy has emphasised participation as an important resource in improving social life, introducing citizen councils, panels and forums (Fredriksson and Tritter, 2019).

Public participation through democratically elected political bodies such as municipal and county councils has historically been a central pillar of the Scandinavian welfare states (Winblad and Ringard, 2009). Councils are also responsible for health service policy and planning. This type of governance is based on the idea that those responsible for organising and delivering welfare services, including healthcare, 'should be held accountable by citizens in elections' (Vrangbaek, 2015:612). However, this participatory practice has been challenged by the NPM and by the alleged providential qualities attributed to the market during the health system reform processes which began in the 1990s. The governance structure has been complemented by other mechanisms of public involvement. Here the two most widespread approaches to patient and citizen involvement in the three Nordic countries should be presented, summarised from the seminal work of Hirschman (1970), as 'Exit' (patient choice) and 'Voice' (active involvement) (Dent et al., 2011).

Concerning 'Choice', according to the Patients' Rights Act (1999) in Norway, which was amended several times in order to strengthen rights, patients can choose any hospital, including private hospitals. Patients are also free to choose their GP and be part of treatment decisions. In Denmark, free choice of public hospitals, diagnosis and treatment has been recognised since 1990, and, in 2002, free choice was extended to private hospitals if health authorities fail to provide a diagnosis within 30 days (Vrangbæk, 2015). In Sweden, during the 1990s and early 2000s, a series of reforms was carried out which aimed to offer patients greater opportunities for choosing health services. The Primary Care Choice Reform, in force since 2010, required regions to introduce the so-called 'choice system', to give all citizens the right to choose public or private primary healthcare providers anywhere in the country.

Finally, in all three countries, various rules and legal arrangements were introduced to expand patients' right to choose, in both primary and hospital care (Winblad and Ringard, 2009). However, several scholars have questioned whether the right to choose and individual involvement in decision-making can really be configured as a public involvement strategy. As Fredriksson, Eriksson and Tritter (2018:475) commented in their analysis of the situation in Norway: 'Defining patient choice as a form of involvement is contested and distinct from active involvement in decision-making'. The critical analysis by Dent and Pahor (2015:549) is along these same lines: 'In general, patient choice and the other variants are presented by governments as empowering citizens, but scratch the surface and one finds that cost containment is a key concern behind much of the policy innovations'. As such, the 'choice system' adopted in Sweden in the early 2000s, which was centred on the principles of free enterprise by private actors and consumer choice, may be seen as a new form of privatisation of social and health services.

In addition to the modes of involvement centred on patient choice, the significant presence of the other approach to public participation in the three Nordic countries should be noted. Hirschman defined this as 'Voice', a set of mechanisms and channels – both individual and collective – based on dialogue and negotiation with other actors, including in decision-making processes. In this field, it is worth highlighting both the mechanisms of individual involvement (individual voice) – adopted to present patient complaints and the levels of satisfaction with the services (regional and national surveys) – as well as the channels of collective participation (collective voice). Here, it is important to highlight the role played by voluntary patient organisations (VPOs), which have represented a noteworthy channel for the involvement of citizens in the formulation of policies at the national, regional and municipal levels. In each of the Nordic countries, there are a large, growing number of VPOs, usually created around specific diseases or health issues. VPOs vary in size and in the way they are administered. The most structured of these participate in parliamentary hearings and aim to influence health policy (Storm and Coulter, 2017). They provide information for members, help and support patients, collaborate in research, interact and have dialogue with health authorities, and even in some cases, collaborate in the provision of services (co-production). VPOs have also taken on a lobbying and advocacy role, participating in assemblies, and acting as members of advisory boards and committees. In addition, the largest associations in Norway, Sweden and Denmark act as an advisory body for new legislation on health and healthcare.

In Norway, VPOs are closely linked to user committees, legal entities which are present in regional health authorities and local committees, and which play an important role in setting the health policy agenda, particularly in favour of people with disabilities and chronic diseases (Saunes, Karanikolos and Sagan, 2020). The Norwegian Federation of Organizations of Persons with Disabilities is an umbrella organisation comprising 80 bodies (Storm and Coulter, 2017). In Denmark, there are between 200 and 300 patient groups; many of them work to defend the health rights of patients and contribute to debates on care, ensuring that patients' opinions are not neglected (Olejaz et al., 2012). In Sweden, there are more than 200 patient and consumer organisations representing different social groups, the main objective of which is to defend the interests of their members and influence decision makers (Storm and Coulter, 2017).

Over the past 20 years, VPOs have acquired an increasingly important role in the health systems of the three Nordic countries; they show significant potential both to strengthen the voice of patients and users and to exert influence over health policymakers (Magnussen et al., 2009; Storm and Coulter, 2017). However, the result of research carried out in Sweden indicates that people believe more in the patient's individual activities than participating through collective actions and playing an active role as a citizen (Fredriksson, Eriksson and Tritter, 2018). This greater importance attributed to individual activities could be the result of the implementation of consumerist policies which in recent decades have emphasised the possibility for the patient to 'leave the service providers' (that is, opt for patient choice), rather than encouraging 'voice activities' (Fredriksson, Eriksson and Tritter, 2018:475).

The Nordic countries have pioneered the introduction and development of progressive health policies. There has been great progress in recognising such areas as patients' rights, options for choosing services, possibilities of expressing satisfaction and complaints. But it is still some way off being able to say that these health systems are truly patient centred, as the role of citizens as active participants needs to be strengthened and more channels of involvement need to be promoted.

The Mediterranean macro-region

Health systems in the Mediterranean countries – Greece, Spain, Italy and Portugal – have certain common socio-political elements. They include many similarities and shared challenges, especially financial, organisational and managerial (Giarelli, 2021), without underestimating the difficulties of promoting and implementing mechanisms for PP (Serapioni and Matos, 2014). PP is a recurring theme in national agendas and can be found in the legal statutes that form the structure of the health systems of the different South European countries (SECs). Nevertheless, according to the literature, PP within the legislative framework has little correspondence in practice, despite the implementation of some successful experiences – with the exception of Greece, where there has been very little participation. Most initiatives still depend on the incentive of regional government, as shown by some very interesting experiments carried out in Spain (Aguilar Gil and Bleda, 2018) and Italy (Cervia, 2018).

Adopting the definition of Rowe and Frewer (2005:254) of public engagement and the three possible types of involvement (public communication, public consultation and public participation) in the case of the SECs, most involvement is based around public communication, in which information is transmitted from policymakers to citizens, who are passive recipients of information. This also occurs in public consultation, where information is transmitted from citizens to decision makers via a process initiated by the decision makers – for example, soliciting opinions and preferences through questionnaires and other types of surveys. Access to information in SECs has progressively improved in the last 20 years, by means of accessible institutional websites and interactive tools, including for patients. The information available on these websites usually encompasses the range of services provided, and the location and availability of contracted public and private providers. As regards public consultation, there are help desks in the various hospital and territorial health units and on the institutions' websites in all four countries, although with different types and levels of development. Here, patients and family members can be heard and suggestions, complaints and protests are collected. In all four countries, this role is shared with voluntary organisations and associations that defend the rights of patients and users, and are also able to give voice to vulnerable social groups (Bernal-Delgado et al., 2018; Economou et al., 2017; Ferré et al., 2014; Simões et al., 2017).

Far less developed are experiments with involvement based on the active participation of citizens' representatives in the decision-making process on health policies and the organisation of care. Italy, Portugal and Spain, in the first phase of the institution of their NHSs in 1978, 1979 and 1986, respectively, implemented experiments with community and local participation, to help democratise the health system. This was a result of the political and trade union struggles and social movements of the 1970s and also the influence of the International Conference on Primary Health Care in Alma-Ata.

Subsequently, in the early 1990s, a new cycle of neo-liberal reforms, which affected welfare states and all health systems, changed the conception of participation: from social and collective participation to individual participation, based on a consumer perspective (Calnan and Gabe, 2001). In Spain, Ruiz-Giménez and Irigoyen (2014) suggest that the 1991 report and 1997 law on new forms of management of the NHS enabled a counter-reform in health that hindered participation, which in the 1970s was considered to be leverage for the new democratic state. In Italy, the legislative decrees 502/1992 and 517/1993 introduced some forms of internal market and started the process of decentralisation, transferring state responsibilities to regional government. However, participation – considered an 'inspiring principle and a strategic theme' of the Italian NHS (Ardigò, 1979:10) – was not put into operation in organisational models; the decrees were limited to recommending that regions promote channels of participation to engage voluntary and user associations. In Portugal, although both the Basic Health Law of 1990 and the Health Statute of 1993 provided some forms of citizen involvement in different instances and levels of governance, participation has been influenced by the restructuring of health systems, oriented to the principles of the NPM. In Greece, when the NHS was created in 1983, the vision included the creation of Regional Health Councils, through which the perspectives of local communities on the planning and implementation of health programmes could be represented, but they were never established (Theodorou et al., 2010). Since then, as argued by Theodorou and colleagues (2010:201), community participation in defining health priorities 'has not been included in any subsequent legislation'.

In line with the health systems reform process of the 1990s – oriented towards managerialism, competition in the domestic market and a greater role attributed to the private sector – choice was also implemented in the NHSs of the SEC. This, however, was in a limited and differentiated way, with the aim of offering patients the possibility of choosing where to get treatment. There is obviously a wider choice of provider for those covered by a public health insurance system or by occupational-based health insurance funds – and by those who benefit from the voluntary health insurance present in all four countries, with the highest prevalence in Greece and Portugal (Hespanha, 2019; Petmesidou and Glatzer, 2015).

Despite the limited progress, it is of interest to briefly describe some PP initiatives that have flourished in the Mediterranean NHSs. With regard to Italy, it is important to highlight the mixed advisory committees of the Emilia-Romagna Region, which have operated since 1994 and are composed mainly of representatives of patient and user associations and a minority component indicated by the health authorities – as well as the participatory structure of the region of Tuscany, created in 2008 and formed by participation committees made up of representatives of the local community and third sector consultation groups, including voluntary organisations. These innovative experiences of citizen empowerment, initiated within the Italian socio-political tradition and context and characterised by the presence of a wide network of civic and voluntary associations, are particularly rich in the regions of Emilia-Romagna and Tuscany (Petrangolini et al., 2021). Despite the innovative nature of these initiatives, such as strengthening the role and power of local community representatives and introducing some approaches on deliberation, these experiences have also revealed some critical aspects. In the case of the Emilia-Romagna committees, research has highlighted the difficulties of representing all social groups in the population and the limited influence exerted on decisions around health (Serapioni and Duxbury, 2014). In Tuscany, studies have highlighted the insufficient definition of participation methods and decision-making processes and the inadequate resources for implementation (Cervia, 2018).

In Spain, the Health Councils, provided for in the *Ley General de Salud* of 1986, were implemented only in some autonomous communities (ACs), and were criticised for limitations in legal compliance. Their mission was limited to the transmission of information (Sáinz-Ruiz, Mínguez-Arias and Martínez-Riera, 2019). For Cassetti and colleagues (2018:4), these models of participation are 'merely informative, occasional and distant from decision-making'. However, in the last 15 years, some ACs, such as Castilla-La Mancha, Aragon, Catalonia, Extremadura, among others, have introduced other mechanisms of participation in their respective health systems. Nonetheless, some of these experiences ended with change in the political framework and the replacement of regional governments – as in the innovative deliberative experience between 2007 and 2011 promoted by the government of the AC of Castilla-La Mancha in the city of Puertollano and the dismantling of the new governance model in the AC of Catalonia between 2006 and 2010, based on 37 territorial health governments, each including a health council (see, for example, Aguilar Gil and Bleda, 2018). But some significant experiences of participation within the scope of community health and primary care programmes did occur namely, in *Barcelona Saúde no Bairro*, which aimed to reduce social inequalities in the health of vulnerable groups (Daban et al., 2021) and in *Comunidad, Participación y Salud* for the development of comprehensive primary care in the city of Badajoz (Cassetti et al., 2018). In both programmes, community participation is seen as essential for achieving the expected results, albeit both of these cases are too recent for any assessment to be carried out.

In Portugal, it is important to mention the 2017 implementation and full functioning of the National Health Council (CNS), already provided for by the Basic Law of 1990, but never established. The CNS is made up of patient representatives (6/30), health professionals, delegates from municipal councils, universities and other entities in the territory and constitutes an important impulse in the democratisation of the NHS and in the participation of civil society in planning and evaluating health policies. Less active are both the Community Councils of the Health Centre Group, many of which do not include representatives of user associations and the NHS hospital consultative councils, that have an insufficient level of involvement in planning, assessment and consultation, as provided for in national regulations. However, in recent years, patient associations have begun to gain importance as social actors in terms of participation in health, exerting increasing pressure on national health institutions and demanding new channels of engagement. In this regard, it is worth mentioning the approval of the *Charter for Public Participation* by the Assembly of the Republic in 2019, More Participation, Better Health, promoted by the network of patient associations (Crisóstomo and Santos, 2018). The Charter aims to encourage patients, users and citizens to participate in decisions that affect the health of the population at national, regional and municipal levels (Assembleia da República Portugal, 2019).

In Greece, as previously mentioned, there has traditionally been little PP in health services (Theodorou et al., 2010). For Boudioni, McLaren and Lister (2017), the focus of policy and the legislature has been on patient rights bodies to protect rights to health and the quality of services, with concern about citizen empowerment being very recent. Due to the lack of independent local organisations or mediating bodies, the independent health ombudsman has taken on vital importance. However, the difficulties faced by the Greeks during the severe economic crisis gave prominence to social movements and collective actions which promoted many social solidarity initiatives, as illustrated by the people's clinics in Athens and other cities.

In the Mediterranean macro-region in the last two decades, there was a prevalent political discourse that extolled the importance of PP in the NHS, but it has not been accompanied by the adequate implementation of experiments which could make this participation effective. Participatory practices are still limited and the debate about the quality and effectiveness of different methods of user involvement is still in its early stages. However, nowadays, there is a need to establish conditions to promote active participation in health decision-making, and no longer to understand involvement only as open channels of information, communication and consultation, as it is also about essential interactions between health systems and citizens.

Conclusion

Returning to Hirschman's options, adapted to the field of participation in health with the three approaches of choice, voice and co-production (Dent et al., 2011), it can be seen that patient choice – that is, the possibility of choosing physicians, hospitals and health insurance – is a widespread PP typology, particularly in the macro-regions of the UK and Scandinavia. It is obviously a minimal form of involvement, which many scholars define as consumerist participation, where patients and users of health services are considered as simple individuals and not holders of a collective vision (Beresford, 2019). The growing importance attributed to patient choice in the last two decades has implied a concomitant weakening of collective participation in the decision-making processes of health institutions. However, the continued relevant role of patient associations should be highlighted; thanks to their collective and organised action (voice), they have contributed to checking the drift of patient choice towards individualism. Indeed, associations, which are increasing in number in all the countries under analysis, are highly active and carry out important functions in terms of representation, defence, advocacy and promoting the rights of patients and users of public health services. It should not be forgotten, of course, that the reform process of health systems, focused as is it on privatisation and competition, has reduced associations' capacity for influence and financial autonomy, as noted by Baggott and Jones (2014) in the case of England.

The role of associations is even more significant where institutionalised spaces and channels for public participation are scarce, as is the case in Mediterranean countries (Serapioni, 2018). It is noteworthy that analysis of public participation has enabled some similarities and approximations to be identified between SHI systems and NHS systems. Indeed, reinforced patients' individual rights and expanded patient choice can be observed in both types of systems, as can the increasing influence exerted by patient organisations on decision-making processes (Baggott and Jones, 2014; Fredriksson and Tritter, 2019). Is a collapse or blurring of the boundaries between the Beveridge and Bismarck models imminent?

The third approach to participation, also inspired by the model of Hirschman (1970), is 'co-production', which requires citizens to play an active role in the production of healthcare. Co-production settings vary. In the literature analysed – most of which came from the macro-regions of the UK and Scandinavia – co-production is understood as the individual participation of the patient in the provision of their own care, as well as the collective involvement of users in the provision of care services in partnership with healthcare professionals (Dent and Pahor, 2015; Holland-Hart et al., 2018). In this latter case, citizens become co-producers of services and make policy decisions about health. In the former case, especially in some diagnostic and rehabilitative activities, a certain degree of co-production is inherent in the care process and naturally involves the participation of patients (McMullin and Needham, 2018). However, co-production experiences are more common in terms of patients' involvement in decisions about their own care process than they are regarding involvement in the planning, delivery and improvement of health services (Holland-Hart et al., 2018). In this individual view of co-production, as pointed out by some authors (Fotaki, 2011; Pestoff, 2009), there is a risk that user involvement will be more oriented towards consumerism and individual choice than towards deliberative and collective participation.

In recent years, co-production has been promoted in the countries of the three health macro-regions at different levels and intensity; the aim is to seek new strategies for engaging citizens and the third sector in the provision of social care and healthcare, in order to meet key demographic, political and economic challenges. However, the question should be asked: Can the involvement of citizens as providers of health services – through third sector organisations and voluntary associations – be considered an adequate form of participation? Is confusion not being created between public participation and service delivery? The questions raised by De Leonardis (2011:131), as a result of analysis of the experiences of active citizenship promoted in the north of Italy, goes along the same lines: 'Does the definition of recipients and providers as partners in a contract change the asymmetry of power intrinsic to the service relationship?' These forms of hybrid governance, where the citizen is both recipient and provider of services, inevitably raise some critical issues about active citizenship.

Furthermore, analysis carried out in the countries of the three macro-regions also confirms other challenges and weaknesses highlighted by the international literature over the last two decades, in particular the complexity of representativeness and the problem of the effectiveness of PP (Fredriksson and Tritter, 2017; Serapioni, 2022). It has been observed in many studies that descriptive or statistical representation cannot be considered the only way to legitimise participation; the recognition of symbolic representation or representation based on experiential participation called for by patient associations has also been recommended. In terms of effectiveness, many studies have highlighted the lack of evaluation of the effects of PP on health systems and the urgent need to design solid and reliable models for assessment.

In short, and returning to the question posed at the beginning of this chapter, there appears, as Dent (2018:26) argues, that there has been little or no influence by users and patients in the field of medical regulation and health governance, with the exception of information rights. In this regard, the small amount of influence exercised by participatory practices is in part the result of the resistance of health professionals and decision-makers, who often question the representativeness of users and patient associations involved in participatory processes as a strategy to defend existing power relations and control of decision-making processes (Martin, 2008; Boivin et al., 2014).

Finally, this analysis cannot be concluded without addressing the impact of the Covid-19 pandemic on the systems and practices of participation in the three macro-regions, even if the research carried out on this subject is limited because the crisis is not yet over. During Covid-19, where urgent intervention was needed, policymakers only involved groups of public health experts, without valuing the experience and knowledge of patient and user associations, and without promoting consultation mechanisms with civil society. In Britain, for example, the suspension of citizen involvement in health decision-making was reported by an editorial in the *British Medical Journal* (2020) which highlighted the regrettable drop in public and patient involvement. In Portugal too, the emergency situation and the need quickly to implement the measures defined by the national task force limited public participation. In fact, none of the technical meetings included representatives of civil society, who 'felt relegated to mere recipients of health care' (Conselho Nacional de Saúde, 2020:29). These expert-only task forces were characteristic of the governments of several countries during the pandemic, resulting in the unfortunate suspension of participatory practices.

Acknowledgement

This publication is the result of work carried out with the support of the Foundation for Science and Technology of Portugal, under the Multiannual Financing of the R&D Unit (UIDP/50012/2020).

References

Aguilar Gil, M. and Bleda García, J. M. (2018) 'El modelo de participación ciudadana en salud en Puertollano (España): más allá de la voluntad política y del empoderamiento ciudadano', *Revista Crítica de Ciências Sociais* 117. Available at: http://journals.openedition.org/rccs/8293

Andreassen, T. A. (2017) 'From democratic consultation to user-employment: Shifting institutional embedding of citizen involvement in health and social care', *Journal of Social Policy* 47(1): 99–117.

Ardigò, A. (1979) 'La partecipazione nel servizio sanitario nazionale', *La Ricerca Sociale* 20: 7–43.

Assembleia da República Portugal (2019) *Carta para a Participação Pública em Saúde*. Available at: https://dre.pt/dre/detalhe/lei/108-2019-124539903

Baggott, R. and Jones, K. (2014) 'The big society in an age of austerity: Threats and opportunities for health consumer and patients' organizations in England', *Health Expectations* 18: 2164–73.

Beresford, P. (2019) 'Public participation in health and social care: Exploring the co-production of knowledge', *Frontiers in Sociology* 3: 41.

Bernal-Delgado, E., García-Armesto, S., Oliva, J., et al. (2018) 'Spain: Health system review', *Health Systems in Transition* 20(2): 1–179.

Bevan, G., Karanikolos, M., Exley, J., Nolte, E., Connolly, S. and May, N. (2014) *The Four Health Systems of the United Kingdom: How Do They Compare*, Research Report, The Health Foundation and Nuffield Trust. Available at: www.nuffieldtrust.org.uk/research/the-four-health-systems-of-the-uk-how-do-they-compare

Bobbio, L. (2018) 'Designing effective public participation', *Policy and Society* 38(1): 48–57.

Boivin, A., Lehoux, P., Burgers, J. and Grol, R. (2014) 'What are the key ingredients for effective public involvement in health care improvement and policy decisions? A randomized trial process evaluation', *The Milbank Quarterly* 92(2): 319–50.

Boudioni, M., McLaren, S., Lister, G. (2017) 'A critical analysis of national policies, systems, and structures of patient empowerment in England and Greece', *Patient Preference and Adherence* 11: 1657–69.

British Medical Journal (2020) 'Patient and public involvement in Covid-19 policy making', *British Medical Journal* 370. Available at: https://doi.org/10.1136/bmj.m2575

Calnan, M. and Gabe, J. (2001) 'From consumerism to partnership? Britain's national health service at the turn of the century', *International Journal of Health Services* 31(1): 119–31.

Carter, P. and Martin, G. (2016) 'Challenges facing Healthwatch, a new consumer champion in England', *International Journal of Health Policy Management* 5(4): 259–63.

Cassetti, V., Paredes-Carbonell, J., Riuz, V. L., García, A. M. and Bautista, P. S. (2018) 'Evidencia sobre la participación comunitaria en salud en el contexto español: Reflexiones y propuestas', *Gazeta Sanitária* 32(S1): 41–7.

Cervia, S. (2018) 'Citizen engagement and the challenge of democratizing health: An Italian case study', *Revista Crítica de Ciências Sociais* 117. Available at: http://journals.openedition.org/rccs/8309

Chamberlain, J. M. (2018) 'Introduction: Professional health regulation in the public interest', in Chamberlain, J. M., Dent, M. and Saks, M. (eds) *Professional Health Regulation in the Public Interest: International Perspectives*, Bristol: Policy Press.

Conselho Nacional de Saúde (2020) *Participação Pública em Saúde. Todas as Vozes contam*, Lisbon CNS. Available at: www.cns.min-saude.pt/2020/12/16/participacao-publica-em-saude-todas-as-vozes-contam/

Crisóstomo, S. and Santos, M. (2018) 'Participação pública na saúde: das ideias à ação em Portugal', *Revista Crítica de Ciências Sociais* 117. Available at: http://journals.openedition.org/rccs/8325

Daban, F., Pasarín, M. I., Borrell, C., Artazcoz, L., Pérez, A., Fernández, A., Porthé, V. and Díez, E. (2021) 'Barcelona Salut als Barris: Twelve years' experience of tackling social health inequalities through community-based interventions', *Gaceta Sanitária* 35(3): 282–8.

De Leonardis, O. (2011) 'Dividing or combining citizens. The politics of active citizenship in Italy', in Newman, J. and Tonkens, E. (eds) *Participation, Responsibility and Choice*, Amsterdam: Amsterdam University Press.

Dent, M. (2018) 'Health care governance, user involvement and medical regulation in Europe', in Chamberlain, J. M., Dent, M. and Saks, M. (eds) *Professional Health Regulation in the Public Interest: International Perspectives*, Bristol: Policy Press.

Dent, M., Fallon, C., Wendt, C., Vuori, J., Pahor, M., de Pietro, C. and Silva, S. (2011) 'Medicine and user involvement within European healthcare: A typology for European comparative research', *International Journal of Clinical Practice* 65(12): 1218–20.

Dent, M. and Pahor, M. (2015) 'Patient involvement in Europe – A comparative framework', *Journal of Health Organization and Management* 29(5): 546–55.

Department of Health (2012) *Local Healthwatch: A Strong Voice for People – The Policy Explained*, London: Department of Health. Available at: https://assets.publishing.service.gov.uk/government/uploads/system/uploads/attachment_data/file/215097/dh_133288.pdf

Economou, C., Kaitelidou, D., Karanikolos, M. and Maresso, A. (2017) 'Greece: Health system review', *Health Systems in Transition* 19(5): 1–192.

Ferré, F., de Belvis, A. G., Valerio, L., Longhi, S., Lazzari, A., Fattore, G., Ricciardi, W. and Maresso, A. (2014) 'Italy: Health system review', *Health Systems in Transition* 16(4): 1–168.

Fotaki, M. (2011) 'Towards developing new partnerships in public services: Users as consumers, citizens and/or co-producers in health and social care in England and Sweden', *Public Administration* 89(3): 933–55.

Fredriksson, M., Eriksson, M. and Tritter, J. (2018) 'Involvement that makes an impact on healthcare: Perceptions of the Swedish public', *Scandinavian Journal of Public Health* 46: 471–7.

Fredriksson, M. and Tritter, J. (2017) 'Disentangling patient and public involvement in healthcare decisions: Why the difference matters', *Sociology of Health and Illness* 39(1): 95–111.

Fredriksson, M. and Tritter, J. (2019) 'Getting involved: The extent and impact of patient and public involvement in the Swedish health system', *Health Economics, Policy and Law* 15(3): 325–40.

Freer, J. (2021) 'If I was minister of health: Democratising healthcare', *Journal of the Royal Society of Medicine* 114(3): 140–5.

Giarelli, G. (2021) 'A Mediterranean paradigm? Convergence and divergence in the Southern European health care systems', *Interface* 25: e210116.

Gilbert, H., Dunn, P. and Foot, C. (2015) *Local Healthwatch: Progress and Promise*, London: King's Fund.

Hespanha, P. (2019) 'The impact of austerity on the Portuguese National Health Service, citizens' well-being, and health inequalities', *e-cadernos CES* 31. Available at: https://doi.org/10.4000/eces.4187

Hirschman, A. O. (1970) *Exit, Voice and Loyalty*, Cambridge, MA: Harvard University Press.

Hogg, C. N. L. (2007) 'Patient and public involvement: What next for the NHS?' *Health Expectations* 10: 129–38.

Holland-Hart, D. M., Addis, S. M., Edwards, A., Kenkre, J. E. and Wood, F. (2018) 'Coproduction and health: Public and clinicians' perceptions of the barriers and facilitators', *Health Expectations* 22: 93–101.

Hughes, D., Mullen, C. and Vincent-Jones, P. (2009) 'Choice vs. voice? PPI policies and the re-positioning of the state in England and Wales', *Health Expectations* 12: 237–50.

Klein, R. (1990) 'Looking after consumers in the new NHS', *British Medical Journal* 6736: 1351–2.

Knudsen, J. L., Engel, C. and Eriksen, J. (2015) 'Denmark', in Braithwaite, J., Matsuyama, Y., Mannion, R. and Johnson, J. (eds) *Healthcare Reform, Quality and Safety. Perspectives, Participants, Partnerships and Prospects*, Farnham: Ashgate Publishing.

Longley, M., Llewellyn, M. and Simpson, A. (2012a) *Moving Towards World Class. A Review of Community Health Councils in Wales*, Cardiff: Welsh Government. Available at: https://pure.southwales.ac.uk/ws/portalfiles/portal/3035571/Review_of_CHCs_Final_report_2_.pdf

Longley, M., Riley, N., Davies, P. and Hernández-Quevedo, C. (2012b) 'United Kingdom (Wales): Health system review', *Health Systems in Transition* 14(11): 1–84.

Lupton, C., Peckham, S. and Taylor, P. (1998) *Managing Public Involvement in Healthcare Purchasing*, Buckingham: Open University Press.

Magnussen, J., Vrangbæk, K., Saltman, R. B. and Martinussen, P. E. (2009) 'Introduction: The Nordic model of healthcare', in Magnussen, J., Vrangbæk, K. and Saltman, R. B. (eds) *Nordic Health Care Systems. Recent Reforms and Current Policy Challenges*, Buckingham: Open University Press.

Martin, G. (2008) 'Representativeness, legitimacy and power in public involvement in health-service management', *Social Science and Medicine* 67: 1757–65

McMullin, C. and Needham, C. (2018) 'Co-production and healthcare', in Brandsen, T., Steen, T. and Verschuere, B. (eds) *Co-production and Co-creation: Engaging Citizens in Public Service Delivery*, New York: Routledge.

Olejaz, M., Juul Nielsen, A., Rudkjøbing, A., Okkels Birk, H., Krasnik, A. and Hernández-Quevedo, C. (2012) 'Denmark: Health system review', *Health Systems in Transition* 14(2): 1–192.

Pestoff, V. (2009) 'Towards a paradigm of democratic participation: Citizen participation and co-production of personal social services in Sweden', *Annals of Public and Cooperative Economics* 80(2): 197–224.

Petmesidou, M. and Glatzer, M. (2015) 'The crisis imperative, reform dynamics and rescaling in Greece and Portugal', *European Journal of Social Security* 17(2): 157–80.

Petrangolini, T., Morandi, F., Delle Monache, L., Moro, M., Di Brino, E. and Cicchetti, A. (2021) *La storia delle associazioni dei pazienti e dei cittadini impegnate in sanità in Italia: conquiste, ostacoli e trasformazioni*, Rome: KOS Editrice.

Pollitt, C. (2008) 'What is a Neo-Weberian state? Reflections on a concept and its implications', *The NISPAcee Journal of Public Administration and Policy*. Special Issue 1(3): 9–16.

Rowe, G. and Frewer, L. J. (2005) 'A typology of public engagement mechanisms', *Science, Technology and Human Values* 30(2): 251–90.

Ruiz-Giménez, J. L. and Irigoyen, J. (2014) 'Participação Comunitária na Saúde, Madrid', in Serapioni, M. and Matos, A. R. (eds) *Saúde, Participação e Cidadania Experiências do Sul da Europa*, Coimbra: Almedina.

Sáinz-Ruiz, P. A., Mínguez-Arias, J. and Martínez-Riera, J. (2019) 'Los consejos de salud como instrumento de participación comunitaria en La Rioja', *Gaceta Sanitária* 33(2): 134–40.

Saks, M. (2010) 'Analyzing the profession: The case for the neo-Weberian approach', *Comparative Sociology* 9(6): 887–915.

Saks, M. (2016) 'A review of theories of professions, organizations and society: The case for neo-Weberianism, neo-institutionalism and eclecticism', *Journal of Professions and Organization* 3(2): 1–18.

Saunes, I. S., Karanikolos, M. and Sagan, A. (2020) 'Norway: Health system review', *Health Systems in Transition* 22(1): 1–163.

Scottish Health Council (2014) *The Participation Toolkit. Supporting Patient Focus and Public Involvement in NHS Scotland*. Available at: www.scottishhealthcouncil. org/toolkit.aspx

Serapioni, M. (2018) 'Participação pública nos sistemas de saúde. Uma introdução', *Revista Crítica de Ciências Sociais* 117: 91–8.

Serapioni, M. (2022) 'Rappresentatività ed efficacia: due dimensioni critiche della partecipazione nei sistemi sanitari. Una revisione della letteratura', *Salute e Società* 1: 13–28.

Serapioni, M. and Duxbury, N. (2014) 'Citizens' participation in the Italian Healthcare System: The experience of the mixed advisory committees', *Health Expectations* 17: 488–99.

Serapioni, M. and Matos, A. R. (2014) 'Citizen participation and discontent in three Southern European health systems', *Social Science and Medicine* 123: 226–33.

Simões, J., Augusto, G. F., Fronteira, I. and Hernández-Quevedo, C. (2017) 'Portugal: Health system review', *Health Systems in Transition* 19(2): 1–184.

Steel, D. and Cylus, J. (2012) 'United Kingdom (Scotland): Health system review', *Health Systems in Transition* 14(9): 1–150.

Storm, M. and Coulter, A. (2017) 'Patient-centred care in the Nordic countries', in Aase, K. and Shibevarg, L. (eds) *Researching Patient Safety and Quality in Healthcare. A Nordic Perspective*, London: CRC Press.

Terkel, C. (2018) 'Healthcare, health and inequality in health in the Nordic countries', *Nordic Journal of Health Economics* 6(2): 10–28.

Theodorou, M., Samara, K., Pavlakis, A., Middleton, N., Polyzos, N. and Maniadakis, N. (2010) 'The public's and doctors' perceived role in participation in setting health care priorities in Greece', *Hellenic Journal of Cardiology* 51: 200–8.

Torjesen, D. O., Aarrevaara, T., Time, M. S. and Tynkkynen, L. K. (2017) 'The users' role in primary and secondary healthcare in Finland and Norway', *Scandinavian Journal of Public Administration* 21(1): 103–22.

Tritter, J. (2011) 'Policy digest', *Health Expectations* 14: 220–3.

Tynkkynen, L. K., Alexandersenb, N., Kaarbøe, O., Anell, A., Lehto, J. and Vrangbæk, K. (2018) 'Development of voluntary private health insurance in Nordic countries – An exploratory study on country-specific contextual factors', *Health Policy* 122: 485–92.

Vallgårda, S. (2007) 'Public health policies: A Scandinavian model?', *Scandinavian Journal of Public Health* 35: 205–11.

Vrangbæk, K. (2015) 'Patient involvement in Danish health care', *Journal of Health Organization and Management* 29(5): 611–24.

Welsh Government (2022) *Summary of Questions and Answers Raised at the Citizen Voice Body Online Information Events (January 2022)*. Available at: https://gov.wales/citizen-voice-body-information-sessions-questions-and-answers

Winblad, U. and Ringard, A. (2009) 'Meeting rising public expectations: The changing roles of patients and citizens', in Magnussen, J., Vrangbæk, K. and Saltman, R. B. (eds) *Nordic Health Care Systems. Recent Reforms and Current Policy Challenges*, Buckingham: Open University Press.

Zoccatelli, G., Desai, A., Martin, G., Brearley, S., Murrels, T. and Robert, G. (2020) 'Enabling "citizen voice" in the English health and social care system: A national survey of the organizational structures, relationships and impacts of local Healthwatch in England', *Health Expectations* 23(5): 1108–17.

13 The role of the medical–industrial complex in the National Health Services

Mike Dent

Introduction

The medical–industrial complex is a radical concept that originated in the United States (US) derived from the earlier concept of the military-industrial complex that was introduced into the political lexicon by President Eisenhower in the 1950s. The medical–industrial complex has played a crucial role in perpetuating that country's expensive, fragmented, and, for many, poor-quality health system (Light, 2004:2). Critics of the US healthcare system cite the European National Health Service (NHS) systems favourably, as good examples of cost-effective, integrated high quality health delivery systems (Gaffney and Muntaner, 2018; Light, 2003). However, with the encroachment of neo-liberalism, this is now under threat (Waitzkin and the Working Group on Health Beyond Capitalism, 2018; Gaffney and Muntaner, 2018) because over recent decades these NHS systems have adopted elements of the US health system. This can be dated from the 1980s onwards (Dent, 2003), with the introduction of the New Public Management (NPM) and later with policies encouraging the privatisation of NHS services. This raises the question as to the degree and extent this has meant the medical–industrial complex within the European context is now comparable to the US.

This chapter will examine the role and character and impact of the medical–industrial complex within the Western European NHS systems. It will do so by drawing particularly on the work of Light (2004, 2010) whose use of the term medical–industrial complex is closely linked to his elaboration of the theory of 'countervailing powers'. Riska (2001:149) commenting on Light's work, notes that by his references, he 'locates his work within the neo-Marxist tradition of professional theory . . . even though his own theoretical arguments suggest a pluralist perception of power'. This is an approach that is compatible with a neo-Weberian and neo-institutional approach. In this chapter, I shall, first, discuss the medical–industrial complex and the theory of countervailing powers and comparatively analyse the role of the medical profession within this matrix of relations. Second, I shall examine the impact of neo-liberalism on the selection of Western European NHS systems, highlighting the similarities and differences between them. Then, third, I shall

DOI: 10.4324/9781003139799-19

identify the changing relations between the principal actors in any health system, the state, the medical and health professions, patients and the public, together with the private industries that supply the health system. Fourth, I shall provide an answer to the question as to the extent and implications of the medical–industrial complex for the Western European NHS systems. This will form the basis of some informed speculation as to what the future may hold for such systems.

The medical–industrial complex and the theory of countervailing powers

The medical–industrial complex concept first appeared within American Marxist discourse in the 1970/80s (see, for example, Ehrenreich and Ehren-reich, 1970). Ehrenreich (2016:57) defines it as the 'tightly linked complex of government, drug companies, medical supply and equipment companies, health insurance companies, hospital networks and the like – and the shift to a narrow treatment-focused conceptualisation of health care'. This definition would appear to leave out the medical profession, but it is included as one of the providers along with all the other health professions and therapists. We might be tempted to consider that the problems associated with the medi-cal–industrial complex are peculiar to the US, the product of their free mar-ket ecology of healthcare organisations and industries. This contrasts with Western European NHS healthcare systems where the state is recognised as playing a key role in ensuring healthcare is delivered to the citizenry equita-bly – a responsibility taken on with the setting up of the welfare state after 1945. However, with the shift to neo-liberal policies of 'marketisation' and, later, 'privatisation', we must consider whether the medical–industrial com-plex has also come to dominate European healthcare. The medical–industrial complex implies the corporatisation of healthcare (Light, 2004, 2010). At the time Ehrenreich and Ehrenreich (1970) introduced the concept, 'corporatisa-tion' was part of the wider discourse on the fate of the medical profession, along with the other alternatives of de-professionalisation and de-skilling (Ehrenreich and Ehrenreich, 1977; Light and Levine, 1988). While corporati-sation implies a loss or lessening of autonomy and control, it is a situation to which professions would appear to be able to accommodate, for they would still retain control over the work processes (the means), even though they may no longer have control over the ends (Derber, 1982).

Relman (1980), the editor of the *New England Journal of Medicine*, while less radical than Ehrenreich and Ehrenreich (1970) on the subject of the medical–industrial complex, drew on the concept to highlight his concern that doctors should not have any direct financial interests in private health-care organisations and/or were on the boards of healthcare corporations. From his perspective, any pursuit of profit in this area would be against the patients' best interests and could in effect lead to iatrogenic medicine (Light, 2010) as, for example, in the tragic example of thalidomide (Illich,

1977) or, more recently, oxycontin that played such a devasting role in the opioid crisis in the US (Raddon Keefe, 2022). These awful stories concerning 'Big Pharma' have also impacted on Western European NHS systems (Abrahams, 2009; Green et al., 2019). This particularly worrying aspect of doctors' prescribing habits also reflects concerns over the lack of effective pharmaceutical industry regulation, including drugs promotion and marketing. These latter routinely involve senior members of the medical profession promoting the drugs in the role of 'opinion leaders'. Perhaps even more worryingly, is the capacity of pharmaceutical companies to convince regulatory bodies of the benefits of their drugs, despite their high cost (Abrahams, 2009). This includes where patients and patient groups have campaigned for earlier access to new drugs. Abraham (2009) cites the cases of recent breast cancer and dementia. The effect of these campaigns appear to depend on whether they coincide with the interests of the pharmaceutical companies concerned more than that of the patients. The pharmaceutical industry is but one aspect of the medical–industrial complex, which also includes medical devices, healthcare computing systems, health insurance companies, as well as private health providers of NHS care, which will be discussed later in this chapter.

Before going further, it is necessary to say something about the 'countervailing powers' theory of Light (1995) and its relevance for analysing the workings of the medical–industrial complex. For Light (2010), the theory resonates with and expands on the historical and comparative study of the professions by Krause (1996) in interaction with states and capitalist markets. According to Light (2010:271), these three contest with one other in the ongoing construction and reconstruction of 'the structure of markets, the culture of professional work and its organization, status, and power'. These countervailing forces give rise to various forms of professional work organisation, including academic research with strong links to the medical–industrial complex, private medicine operating within highly competitive markets and systems of managed care. This description relates primarily to the US but, with adjustments, parallels are also to be found within the Western European NHSs. The theory of countervailing power starts with the assumption that the medical profession is in a symbiotic relation with the state, in which both sides know it needs to accommodate to the concerns of the other to ensure the benefits of the relationship for both to continue to work. It is encapsulated in what Klein (1990) famously depicted as 'the politics of the double bed'. With the introduction of neo-liberalism and NPM, this assumption began to be questioned and there has been a move from 'protected' to 'contracted' professionalism for doctors (Light, 1995). This has marked a shift in the balance of countervailing powers between the profession and the state that led to greater managerial control and external regulation. This reflected significant changes between networks (professions), hierarchy (the state) and the market (medical–industrial complex).

Light (1995) does extend this scope to include patients (although he seemingly forgets nursing and the other healthcare professions). More recently, Light (2010) suggests that, to deal with the complexity of these relationships, we can draw on the 'linked ecologies' framework of Abbott (2005). This could include other health professions in the intertwining of events in adjacent ecologies and provide a detailed vocabulary for analysing them in terms of the dynamics of professions, markets and state. Particularly pertinent here are Abbott's use of the concepts 'jurisdictions' and 'settlements' (which will be returned to later, but not quite in the manner Abbott intended). For Light (2010), the main concern appears to be the medical profession's relationship with the market. Here he generally concludes, like Relman (2007), that medical practice should be de-commercialised with doctors being salaried and working within an NHS. Certainly, he does feel that Freidson (2001) was incorrect in assuming that codes of professionalism could be relied on to govern the behaviour of medical practitioners, as the healthcare professions do not embody a higher moral order and need to be rescued from market forces and their own self-interests. What, then, has been the effect of neo-liberalism on the European NHS systems and medical profession?

Western European NHS systems in the wake of neo-liberalism

The NHS systems across Europe fall broadly into two categories, according to the typology of Moran (2000):

- Entrenched command and control (United Kingdom (UK) and Scandinavia).
- Insecure command and control (Portugal, Spain, Italy, and Greece).

This distinction is premised on institutional embeddedness and governance. There are two preliminary points to be made here: first, the categories underplay the role of markets (being governance focused), which limit their usefulness for analysing the impact of neo-liberal policies, and, second, the 'insecure' variety is, apparently, defined either as an inferior or as an unfinished version of the first category. It is true that the Mediterranean health systems have largely adopted the UK NHS model, but the historical route these countries followed were different to that which gave rise to the UK – or even the Scandinavian – versions. The differences relate to their 'path dependencies' which not only emphasise the importance and inertia of history but also recognises that it is only as the result of crises or conjunctures (Wilsford, 1994) that radical change can come about. Consequently, on closer examination, we find Portugal, Spain, Italy and Greece as versions of the NHS all carry elements of their pre-existing healthcare arrangements, whether in relation to pre-existing social health insurance (SHI) systems, and private practice or, more subtly, in the form of clientelism and familialism. These dynamics have implications for the medical–industrial complex across Europe.

While this path dependency argument broadly explains the differences between UK and Scandinavia on the one hand and the Mediterranean NHS systems on the other, it remains that in the latter case these countries' states have to varying degrees lacked the institutional wherewithal to exert the controls to ensure their NHS systems work fully and effectively. One of the key differences is the matter of state formation. Unlike the UK or Scandinavia, the states of Italy and Greece are of relatively recent construction, and, like Portugal and Spain, suffered from authoritarian regimes in the twentieth century something that their northern European counterparts have not experienced for several centuries (Ferrera, 2005). These Mediterranean countries have also experienced military dictatorships in their relatively recent past, which, as Andreotti and colleagues (2001) and Mouzelis (1986) note, has had an important impact on their subsequent democracies. All to varying degrees have continuing challenges in establishing effective central state mechanisms for delivering health and social services across their territories. Italy, for example, only moved to a formally federal structure in the current century (Ferré et al., 2014), and continues to be challenged by great variations across the country in the quality and effectiveness of healthcare delivery, particularly between the north and south of the country. Here Italy has long been seen as being almost two countries (Andreotti et al., 2001) with the differences in healthcare performance being particularly marked (Ferré et al., 2014). These countries are now all members of the European Union (EU), which influences their health policies – including, for instance, the training and employment of health professionals such as doctors' maximum hours and the professional education and training of nurses (Dent, 2003).

Having established that the command and control typology of Moran (2000) is modestly useful but with limitations, we need to look at the impact of neo-liberal health policies on these NHS systems and assess what the implications might be for the medical–industrial complex. First, it is important to say something about managed care as this was the vehicle initially employed to carry the neo-liberal credo into Europe via the language of the internal market or quasi-market (Saltman and Figueras, 1998). In the US, it opened new opportunities for the private interests of the medical–industrial complex to make substantial profits (Ehrenreich, 2016; Waitzkin and the Working Group on Health Beyond Capitalism, 2018). This reflects the character of US capitalism where government is reluctant to intervene in the market. This includes healthcare and contrasts with European healthcare, especially the NHS variety, where governments do intervene.

The person credited with the introduction of managed care into European NHS systems, as Light (2004) notes, is Enthoven (1988). The idea is that an NHS system could be regarded as approximately the same as a Health Maintenance Organisation (HMO), and was, putatively, the innovative ingredient needed to shift an NHS system from a 'top-down' state-run organisation to a 'bottom-up' patient-responsive system premised on the 'market' (and not 'hierarchy'). Within an NHS system 'market' meant nothing like a free market, but a proxy called the 'internal' (or 'quasi') market in the UK (Enthoven, 1985; Dent, 2003). Patients were recast as 'consumers' – although in this they were unlike consumers in commercial or retail markets. The internal market never did fully materialise within Western European NHS systems for two main reasons. First, the 'internal/quasi market' lacked the flexibility and information flows necessary for an effective market to become established, and second, an NHS system is by its very nature political in that it is subject to government interventions. Nevertheless, the reforms did have a significant influence on the organisation and delivery of healthcare. This, however, was due more to the forces of managerialism than the logic of the market and gave rise to the phenomenon of the NPM (Dent, 2003; Dent and Barry, 2004). Hood (1995) famously summed up the principles of NPM, as: disaggregation/decentralisation, competition, parsimony, managerialism and (professional) performativity. These became virtual watchwords across the Western European NHS systems. One early adopter was Sweden, where the county councils (and municipalities) had a central part to play in overseeing the introduction of NPM. The decentralised approach was quite marked, giving rise at one stage to three different variants (Dent, 2003). This contrasted with the UK where the NHS introduced the instruments of NPM by central *fiat*. Interestingly, later, southern European adopters tended to follow the UK model.

Earlier I presented reasons for the broad differences between the northern and southern European NHS systems, which related to path dependency. The adoption of NPM by these Mediterranean countries had an impact in challenging strong regional autonomies, particularly evident in Spain and Italy and/or competing subsystems in Portugal. Moreover, it also challenged the embedded forces of clientelism (Dent, 2003), including the Italian version of *Partitocrazia* (Krause, 1996). Nevertheless, evidence suggests that these local practices have survived to some degree, as in the case of Italy. The particularisation of the configuration of these centrifugal forces (regionalisation, clientelism, as well as that of familialism) (Dent, 2003) means there are distinct variations between these southern European NHSs as well as their northern counterparts. These southern NHS systems, nevertheless, followed a similar path in as much as they were explicitly inspired by the UK NHS. One characteristic of this group is that they co-exist alongside other, longer established, providers. The Greek NHS is a notable example. It was established in 1983 but still operates alongside an SHI system, most notably IKA, the dominant SHI established in 1934 which still provides most of the primary healthcare in urban areas. The system is an NHS/SHI hybrid for economic and political reasons, which has also been plagued by a widespread system of unofficial co-payments in so far as patients and their families often pay *fakelakia* to ensure good medical treatment (Dent, 2003). More recently, since 2011, much of Greece's private health sector has contracted to the NHS through the National Organization for the

Provision of Health Services (Economou et al., 2017), with a particularly pragmatic approach to public–private partnership (PPP). PPPs are a variant of the Private Finance Initiative model (PFI) that go beyond simply constructing a hospital and delivering the service and maintenance function for around 30 years (Acerete, Stafford and Stapleton, 2011). PPPs contract to provide the clinical services too. The question for this chapter is whether and, to what extent, do PPPs expand the European medical–industrial complex?

Prior to the neo-liberal reforms in southern Europe in Italy, for example, the private sector would largely be hospitals and clinics provided by the Catholic church on a not-for-profit basis. In the 1990s a policy of privatisation in the form of PPP, including for-profit hospitals and clinics, was adopted by Italy although not taken up across much of the country. It has largely been concentrated in four regions, and there only accounting for about 30% of hospital stays (Ferré et al., 2014). Spain, by contrast, has been a real PPP innovator, at least in Valencia, with the introduction of the 'Alzira' model, which has strongly influenced other countries and provides an interesting and relevant comparator to the Independent Sector Treatment Centres (ISTCs) in England in 1990s (Acerete, Stafford and Stapleton, 2011, 2012). The Alzira innovation was a capitation-based PPP, that is, the health authorities agree to pay the provider an annual per patient fee. The advantage hoped for was the shift of risk from the public purse to the private sector, coupled with an assumption that the provider would be able to deliver services more efficiently (Bernal-Delgado et al., 2018). This latter assumption has been difficult to substantiate (Acerete, Stafford and Stapleton, 2011). Portugal has adopted a similar approach, inspired by the UK's approach (Simðes et al., 2017), but they too could find no clear evidence that PPP hospitals delivered greater efficiency or effectiveness. Interestingly, the process of PPP contracting has stalled in Portugal, while in Valencia in Spain, the hospitals and clinics contracted out under the Alzira PPP arrangements, which have now been taken back into the public sector (Comendeiro-Maaløe et al., 2019).

Unlike the current trend within southern European countries, England (but not Wales, Scotland, or Northern Ireland) (Anderson et al., 2022) continues to encourage publicly funded private sector health provision. This expansion is no longer limited to the ISTCs because since 2006 any private hospital is allowed to compete for NHS-funded elective care work. By 2012/13, these private hospitals were treating the majority (72.5%) of NHS-funded cases in the independent sector. However, it is important to note that, for 2018/19, the whole of the NHS-funded independent sector provision accounted for only 6% of NHS-funded elective surgery (Anderson et al., 2022). The Scandinavian countries similarly expanded their public–private ventures between 1990 and 2020s, with some rethinking during the early 2000s. In Sweden, for example, there were hospitals in the 1990s being completely franchised to private providers (Sveman and Essinger, 2001), whereas, in contrast, Swedish hospitals predominantly operate out of the public sector. The situation within Swedish primary care is somewhat different. Historically this sector was underdeveloped, and most people attended hospital outpatient clinics including those who would have been more appropriately treated within primary care. The expansion of primary care more recently has provided a sizeable opportunity for privatisation and today 40% of publicly funded primary care is now purchased from the private sector. The other area of growth in private provision of any significance has been private health insurance. In Sweden, this has grown substantially since the 1990s. Even so, the market only amounts to about 10% of the adult population. In Denmark, by contrast, the figure is much greater, at nearer 40% or 2.3 million persons. For comparison, the figure for the UK is much lower at a little over 4.5% of a population of around 65 million (Anderson et al., 2022) but this does deliver a higher number of policy holders, about three million people. These comparative figures in the cases of the UK and Sweden are most likely to reflect a concern to avoid waiting for treatment. Presumably something similar is at work in Denmark but it is unclear what the multiplier effect might be that has led to a quadrupling of the proportion of citizens taking out private health insurance.

Having reviewed the European NHS systems, albeit in summary form, it would seem that there are real, but limited, opportunities to expand the medical–industrial complex. This would be through the growth of the private sector services available within the neo-liberal NHS systems across Europe. However, the policies have been driven more by governments' attempts to reduce the cost to public finances for NHS healthcare, than wishing to create opportunities for the private sector to exploit patients and the NHS services. The central concern is the exponentially rising costs of healthcare – a consequence of the ageing population, citizen expectations and, relatedly, the cost of technology and drugs. That is not to say, however, that would not leave 'rich pickings' for the medical–industrial complex. But it is unlikely ever to equate to the US version of the medical–industrial complex with its concomitant price of making it impossible to 'provide integrated, cost-effective care [nor to] manage the major sources of inefficiency, fragmentation, and escalating costs' (Light, 2004:2).

The medical–industrial complex and the changing relations within Western European national health systems

What is becoming clear from reviewing the NHS systems across Western Europe is that the countervailing forces that make up the medical–industrial complex are rather different to those found in the US. The state plays a bigger role, exercising its monopolist power to ensure, for instance, the regulation and control of its relations with the pharmaceutical industry and the widespread adoption of cheaper generic, over trademarked, drugs. This also limits doctors' scope to prescribe compared to their colleagues working within SHI systems. For example, UK doctors' prescriptions are 85.3% generic medicines as compared to 30.2% in France and 29.2% in Germany

(Anderson et al., 2022). These controls also limit the extent of the doctors' clinical autonomy. Even so, Goldacre (2012) is still able to cite examples where patented drugs are being extensively prescribed unnecessarily in the UK. Similar points can be made in relation to healthcare information and communications technology. Here it is not primarily the doctors making the decisions, it is the state and/or senior NHS management, but that has not always meant success in terms of efficiency or effectiveness. The National Programme for Information Technology (NPfIT) for the English NHS was a highly sophisticated and expensive (£12.8 billion) system, which ultimately failed for being far too centralised and inflexible (Eason et al., 2011; Justinia, 2016). The experience has left the UK very wary of massive top-down health information technology initiatives (Anderson et al., 2022). Nevertheless, the Covid-19 pandemic did bring about something of a rethink. It led to a rapid deployment of health information technology aimed at improving patients' access to electronic health records and enabling effective teleconsultations. All this was achieved without the autocratic approach of NPfIT. Moreover, it has motivated the NHS across all four countries of the UK to again focus on developing and implementing strategies to enable access to integrated electronic health records across NHS health organisations and their patients (Anderson et al., 2022). No other Western European NHS system attempted anything as grand as NPfIT, but they have in varying degrees designed and implemented health information technology along similar lines but generally in a fairly decentralised way, with Norway (Saunes, Karanikolos and Sagan, 2020) being something of a centralised exception.

A similar story can be told in regard to medical technology more generally, such as medical devices, including diagnostic tools, prostheses, as well as larger and more expensive pieces of kit, the MRI scanners and similar machinery now used extensively within X-ray and imaging departments of virtually all hospitals. Here the NHSs within most Western European countries have introduced systems of Health Technology Assessment (HTA), which grew from the work of the National Institute for Clinical Excellence in the UK (later the National Institute for Health and Care Excellence – NICE) established in 1999. Almost all Western European NHS systems have their own HTA arrangements to help ensure cost-effective, good quality healthcare – Denmark, for example, adopted HTA fairly early on (Olejaz et al., 2012), whereas Portugal was a late adopter, set up in 2015 (Simões et al., 2017). Greece has still to make such arrangements, although work is progressing on its National Evaluation Centre of Quality and Technology in Health (Economou et al., 2017; Mentis, 2022). HTAs are designed to ensure the procurement of appropriate technology cost effectively, including medicines. Physicians are likely to have some influence on this process, particularly when they are the principal end-user, but this is within a complex of regulatory and financial parameters and alongside other actors, including managers and patients. HTA is a broad concept and varies between countries, depending, for example, on the level of decentralisation and role played by industry (Banta, 2003). In the context of this discussion of the medical–industrial complex, what HTA is meant to do to ensure efficiency and effectiveness in the procurement of medical devices is to harness the physicians' expertise within cost constraints and ensure no conflicts of interests.

While doctors are salaried employees, they have also been powerful, particularly at the local level. However, within the current neo-liberal policy world it would seem that this marks a weakening of medical power, and the ending of clinical autonomy (for example, in prescribing) along with any remnants of medical dominance (Freidson, 1970). Certainly, the medical profession no longer exercises the autonomous power it once did, but collectively it still has a lot of influence in the organisation and delivery of healthcare. It does this through its involvement in developing clinical protocols and guidelines, and engagement or otherwise with care pathways (Allen, 2009). While individual doctors find their clinical work constrained by these various protocols and practices, the designers of them are fellow members of the medical profession. This reflects an extension of the stratification within the profession that Freidson (1984) identified some years ago. These changes look somewhat like 'settlements' – even if Abbott (2005:250) would not recognise them as such (being professionally agreed arrangements) as he conceptualises these as different from the 'well defined and relatively stable jurisdictions of professions'. The changes that the medical profession has undergone in recent decades have the hallmarks of a new and ongoing 'settlement', in which they are having to renegotiate their work situation and professional jurisdiction, as, for instance, where nursing has taken on responsibilities previously the monopoly of doctors, including prescribing (Dent, 2003). These changes have, even so, not always meant the NHS purchasing drugs for the lowest prices as there have been cases of generic manufacturers in the medical–industrial complex, gaming prices. One case in the UK in 2019, for example, resulted in a 'refund' payment of £8 million to the NHS (Anderson et al., 2022). Nevertheless, overall, the system has been able to contain the cost of drugs within NHS systems, for example, the Kings Fund estimate that the UK NHS saved £7.1 billion in 2013/14 as compared to 1976 (Alderwick, 2015).

We must also mention the patients (and their families/carers), more particularly patient groups, for they too are one of the countervailing powers identified by Light (1995). Their influence has changed over recent decades as the policy orientation has shifted from the patient as consumer to that of co-producer (Dent, 2018). In the more managed healthcare system of NPM, user involvement in the organisation and delivery of healthcare has become integral to the system and co-production of services has become, formally at least, an integral part within at least some of the Western European NHS systems (Dent, 2018; Dent and Pahor, 2015; Kjellström, 2019; Voorberg, Bekkers and Tummers, 2015), possibly as an additional curb on professional autonomy and power (Dent, 2018). Another aspect to user involvement in healthcare, more connected to the 'voice' variety than that of 'co-production'

(Dent and Pahor, 2015) relates to the funding by pharmaceutical companies of health consumer and patients' organisations (HCPOs) (Baggott and Forster, 2008). Patient organisations include disease specific groups such as those for multiple sclerosis and breast cancer. These groups differ from the geographically based organisations, such as Healthwatch (Carter and Martin, 2016) in that the patient organisations are likely to have been co-created with health professionals (Pavolini and Spina, 2015) and funded in part, at least, by the pharmaceutical industry (Baggott and Forster, 2008). These cases are illustrative examples of the dynamics of the countervailing power of the medical profession and pharmaceutical industry and the kind of strategies used to try to ensure user involvement favours their interests.

In the case of the European states, however, their principal concern in recent years has been to contain healthcare costs, and this has been the key reason they have experimented with privatisation. Even so, we cannot ignore the political possibility that PPPs may have also been promoted to valorise healthcare services and provide opportunities for profit, couched in terms of a neo-liberal political philosophy. Even so, PPP schemes across Europe can hardly be interpreted as opportunities for profiteering 'carpetbaggers' given that the contract arrangements have tended to be subject to tight regulation and scrutiny, while profits appear to be modest (Barlow, Roehrich and Wright, 2013). One key development started in England with the setting up of NICE in 1999. NICE was set up 'to promote clinical excellence and the effective use of resources in England and Wales' (Davies, Wetherell and Barnett, 2006:269). The organisation is intended to 'square the circle', ensuring quality improvement across the NHS in cost-effective ways. The rationale that underpins this is evidence-based, originally focused on medicine (Sackett and Rosenberg, 1995) but soon extended to the other health professions and management (Rycroft-Malone et al., 2004). NICE inspired similar institutes across Europe, as it was one of the first national HTA bodies on the continent.

This has meant that these NHS systems have been reasonably effective at controlling their costs of medicines and medical devices, in the case of medicines, largely by promoting and enforcing generic substitution (Duerdon and Hughes, 2010). Within the EU, it is the European Medicines Agency (n.d.) that 'assesses applications from companies to market generic medicines'. This approach to cost-effective quality improvement has been further extended with the adoption of integrated care pathways designed to coordinate all the actors to play their prescribed part in the process (Allen, 2009). But, against these developments designed to ensure the delivery of efficient and effective healthcare, are set the concerns that arise around other policies that seem to open the NHS systems up to profiteering from the private sector. For instance, in the UK, the 2012 Health and Social Care Act included 'any qualified provider' who would be entitled to be contracted to provide NHS services. This appeared to open up the NHS to the danger of becoming little more than an agglomeration of private providers 'badged' as the NHS.

The new 2022 Health and Care Act has again given rise to these concerns, although the British Medical Association (2022) in its briefing to members point out that private providers are ruled out of wielding influence over commissioning decisions as members of NHS decision-making bodies. These concerns are not limited to NHS England; however, they affect all the other Western European NHSs too. Nonetheless, the regulatory arrangements that the Western European NHS systems variously operate, including the UK, should mean that the worst excesses of profit-seeking are avoided.

Unlike the US, Western European governments are very ready to intervene to regulate their NHS systems. In terms of countervailing powers, the West European state is an active and integral part of the multi-dimensional field of the medical–industrial complex. This is the case even when such governments pursue neo-liberal policies. One of the flagship neo-liberal policies, with England leading the way, was the PPP. Initially it took the form of the PFI, but over time this mutated into a version of PPP as in the case of ISTC clinics in the UK and the Alzira capitation model in Spain. But they never signified the absence of the state, only a modified role within reconfigured relations in this field.

Conclusion: future directions

In terms of the future direction of the Western European medical–industrial complex, the question is one of whether it will become more, or less, like its US counterpart. Gaffney and Muntaner (2018), cited right at the beginning of the chapter, usefully suggest a list four axes of health system neo-liberalism:

- Health system austerity.
- A retreat from universalism.
- A rise in cost-sharing.
- Health system privatisation.

They apply to their case studies of Greece, Spain and England and provide a reasonable analysis of each case, but it is important to make the point that they are primarily concerned to see how far European NHS systems provide a template for a 'single-payer national health program' in the US like an NHS system. Their conclusion is that the impact of neo-liberalism on the European NHS systems has meant that they themselves are under serious threat of being dismantled. While we can see the reasons for this conclusion, simply with reference to the four axes listed earlier, what they do not consider is the path dependencies that underpin each of the Western European NHS systems. In short, they overlook the inciteful nuances that a Weberian informed analysis can offer, as here with neo-institutionalism (Saks, 2016)

Even when neo-liberalism has been in the ascendance, for example, at the time of the 2012 Health and Social Care Act in England, Langley, the minister of health at the time, had to pause, take another round of public consultation, and moderate his attempts to open the NHS to widespread privatisation. What has happened since is that, while privatisation in the form of PPP has continued, as have concerns over the danger that inefficiently designed contractual arrangement remains high (Barlow, Roehrich and Wright, 2013), private provision within the NHS has remained fairly modest. Within other Western European NHS systems there are signs of a rowing back from their commitment to PPPs. In Portugal and Spain, for example, there has been a negative reaction to the Spanish Alzira model, mainly on political rather than technical grounds. But the evidence is not all one-way and PPPs are likely to remain part of the UK's and EU's armoury, at least, for the near to mid-future. On the other hand, these arrangements are likely to remain under scrutiny both from those with a technical interest in the comparative efficiencies of PPP as against public hospitals and from those politically opposed to private sector profiting from NHS healthcare activity. Whichever side of the debate taken, it is important to note that PPPs have never taken up more than a relatively small percentage of hospital activity within any NHS system. In 2019, for instance, the health expenditure as a percentage of Gross National Product (GDP) for the US was 17.6% (Statista, 2022), whereas the World Health Organization (WHO) European average was 8.5% (Anderson et al., 2022:54). This figure includes more than just the European NHS systems, which vary from Sweden at 10.9% at the highest expenditure to Greece at the lowest at 7.8%. The northern European countries discussed here spent 10% or more, while the Southern European countries all spent less, although that does not take account of what the Greeks call *fakelaki* – that is, illicit co-payments. The European NHS expenditures are all less than 11% of GDP and the average is nearer 9.5% which is just over half that for the US, which indicates a substantially smaller 'pot' for the medical–industrial complex to profit from within these NHS systems than that of the US.

A report by Saltman and Figueras (1998:108) in a WHO study some years ago concluded their comparison of the US and European healthcare systems with the statement that 'a central distinction is the importance of *collective* responsibility and political accountability in western European healthcare systems, as compared with the emphasis upon *individual* responsibility and financial accountability in US health policy' (*emphasis added*). The conclusion applies almost as much today as it did over 30 years ago when neoliberal health policies were first beginning to be adopted. It also applies to the distinction, *mutatis mutandus*, between the medical–industrial complex in Western European NHS systems and US healthcare. This reality will shape the future directions of both policy and relations between the healthcare systems and the complex of private industries that service them. Unlike the US healthcare system, European NHS systems are more given to 'stickiness' (Pierson, 2000) within the structures of policymaking, political cultures and powerful interest groups.

Gaffney and Muntaner (2018) argue that because the US experience is one where reforms are always vulnerable to 'reversal' or 'roll back', the European NHS systems are likewise vulnerable. But, in terms of countervailing powers, the dynamics within the different Western European NHS systems is markedly different, for the state – despite variations – plays a greater ongoing key role here in the configuration of forces than in the US. Certainly, there are real possibilities and evidence of 'rollbacks' to universal public health partially caused by a reaction to the 2008 financial crisis, as well as the appeal of neo-liberal policies to some Western European governments, including the UK, because they appear to shift financial cost and risk on to the private sector. But even in this neo-liberal context, it is government that sets the agenda, and seeks to control the outcomes – and costs. This contrasts with the US which, as Moran (2000:150) typified it, is a supply state. The implications for the medical–industrial complex are clear; the 'defining feature of the "supply state" is that both the providers and creators of medical technology are rampant' in contrast to the Western European command and control states. Gaffney and Muntaner (2018) observe that, even in the insecure variety, the government of provision and technology is on 'a pretty tight rein'. This applies, even when a government might wish to privatise healthcare along US lines, for they too are constrained by their own path dependencies, which barring major systems collapse, make it difficult to reform healthcare systems in a big way (Wilsford, 1994).

In conclusion, healthcare within the NHS systems has remained a public and not a private good, even where privatisation has been part of health policy. This has primarily shaped the medical–industrial complex within Western Europe. Whether this will remain the case in the future will depend on these countries' economic resilience, and the influence of ideologically committed neo-liberals within their respective governments.

References

Abbott, A. (2005) 'Linked ecologies: States and universities as environments for professions', *Sociological Theory* 23: 245–74.

Abrahams, J. (2009) 'The pharmaceutical industry, the state and the NHS', in Gabe, J. and Calnan, M. (eds) *The New Sociology of the Health Service*, London: Routledge.

Acerete, B., Stafford, A. and Stapleton, P. (2011) 'The Spanish healthcare public private partnerships: The "Alzira model"', *Critical Perspectives in Accounting* 22: 533–49.

Acerete, B., Stafford, A. and Stapleton, P. (2012) 'New developments: New global health care PPP development – A critique of a success story', *Public Money and Management* 32(4): 311–14.

Alderwick, H., Robertson, R., Appleby, J., Dunn, P. and Maguire, D. (2015) *Better Value in the NHS: The Role of Changes in Clinical Practice*, London: The Kings Fund.

Allen, D. (2009) 'From boundary concept to boundary object: The practice and politics of care pathway development', *Social Science and Medicine* 69(3): 354–61.

Anderson, M., Pitchforth, E., Edwards, N., Alderwick, H., McGuire, A. and Mossialos, E. (2022) 'The United Kingdom: Health systems review', *Health Systems in Transition* 24(1): i–192.

Andreotti, A., Garcia, S. M., Gomez, A., Hespanha, P., Kazepov, Y. and Mingione, E. (2001) 'Does a Southern European model exist?', *Journal of European Area Studies* 9(1): 43–62.

Baggott, R. and Forster, R. (2008) 'Health consumer and patients' organizations in Europe: Towards a comparative analysis', *Health Expectations* 11: 85–94.

Banta, D. (2003) 'The development of health technology assessment', *Health Policy* 63: 121–32.

Barlow, J., Roehrich, J. and Wright, S. (2013) 'Europe sees mixed results from public-private partnerships for building and managing health care facilities and services', *Health Affairs* 32(1): 146–54.

Bernal-Delgado, E., Garcia-Armesto, S., Oliva, J., Martinez, F. I. S., Repulla, J. R., Peña-Longobardo, L. M., Ridao-López, M. and Hernández-Quevedo, C. (2018) 'Spain: Health systems review', *Health Systems in Transition* 20(2): 1–179.

British Medical Association (2022) *The Health Care Act*. Available at: bma.org

Carter, P. and Martin, G. (2016) 'Challenges facing Healthwatch, a new consumer champion in England', *International Journal of Health Policy Management* 5(x): 1–5.

Comendeiro-Maaløe, M., Ridao-López, M., Gorgemans, S. and Bernal-Delgado, E. (2019) 'Public-private partnerships in the Spanish national health system: The reversion of the Alzira model', *Health Policy* 123: 408–11.

Davies, C., Wetherell, M. and Barnett, E. (2006) *Citizens at the Centre: Deliberative Participation in Healthcare Decisions*, Bristol: Policy Press.

Dent, M. (2003) *Remodelling Hospitals and Health Professions in Europe: Medicine, Nursing and the State*, Basingstoke: Palgrave Macmillan.

Dent, M. (2018) 'Health care governance, user involvement and medical regulation in Europe', in Chamberlain, J. M., Dent, M. and Saks, M. (eds) *Professional Health Regulation in the Public Interest: International Perspectives*, Bristol: Policy Press.

Dent, M. and Barry, J. (2004) 'New public management and the professions in the UK: Reconfiguring control?', in Dent, M., Chandler, J. and Barry, J. (eds) *Questioning the New Public Management*, Aldershot: Ashgate.

Dent, M. and Pahor, M. (2015) 'Patient involvement in Europe – A comparative framework', *Journal of Health Organization and Management* 29(5): 546–55.

Derber, C. (1982) *Professionals as Workers: Mental Labor in Advanced Capitalism*, Boston, MA: G. K. Hall.

Duerdon, M. G. and Hughes, D. A. (2010) 'Generic and therapeutic substitution in the UK: Are they a good thing?', *British Journal of Clinical Pharmacology* 70(3): 335–41.

Eason, K., Dent, M., Waterson, P., Tutt, D., Hurd, P. and Thornett, A. (2011) *Getting the Benefit From Electronic Patient Information That Crosses Organizational Boundaries*, Final Report: NIHR Service Delivery and Organisational Programme. Available at: https://fundingawards.nihr.ac.uk/award/08/1803/226

Economou, C., Kaitelidou, D., Karanikolos, M. and Maresso, A. (2017) 'Greece: Health system review', *Health Systems in Transition* 19(5). Available at: https://apps.who.int

Ehrenreich, B. and Ehrenreich, J. (1970) *The American Health Empire: Power, Profits and Politics*, New York: Vintage Books.

Ehrenreich, B. and Ehrenreich, J. (1977) 'The professional-managerial class', *Radical America* 11(2): 7–32.

Ehrenreich, J. (2016) *The Third Wave Capitalism: How Money, Power, and the Pursuit of Self-interest Have Imperiled the American Dream*, Ithaca, NY and London: ILR Press/Cornell University Press.

Enthoven, A. C. (1985) *Reflections on the Management of the National Health Service*, London: Nuffield Provincial Hospitals Trust.

Enthoven, A. C. (1988) *Theory and Practice of Managed Competition in Health Care Finance*, Amsterdam: North-Holland.

European Medicines Agency (n.d.) *Generic and Hybrid Applications Page*. Available at: EMA.europa.eu

Ferré, F., de Belvis, A. G., Valerio, L., Longhi, S., Lazzari, A., Fattore, G., Ricciardi, W. and Maresso, A. (2014) 'Italy: Health system review', *Health Systems in Transition* 16(4): i–168.

Ferrera, M. (2005) 'Democratisation and social policy: From expansion to "recalibration"', *Prepared for the UNRISD Project on Social Policy and Democratization*, Geneva: UNRISD: 3. Available at: www.researchgate.net/publication/238621676

Freidson, E. (1970) *Medical Dominance: The Social Structure of Medical Care*. Piscataway, NJ: Transaction Books.

Freidson, E. (1984) *Professionalism Reborn: Theory, Prophecy and Policy*, Chicago, IL: University of Chicago Press.

Freidson, E. (2001) *Professionalism: The Third Logic*, Cambridge: Polity Press.

Gaffney, A. and Muntaner, C. (2018) 'Austerity and health care', in Waitzkin, H. and the Working Group on Health Beyond Capitalism (eds) *Health Care Under the Knife: Moving Beyond Capitalism for Our Health*, New York: Monthly Review Press.

Goldacre, B. (2012) *Bad Pharma: How Medicine Is Broken, and How We Can Fix It*, London: Fourth Estate.

Green, K., O'Dowd, N. C., Watt, H., Majeed, A. and Pinder, R. J. (2019) 'Prescribing trends of gabapentin, pregabalin, and oxycodone: A secondary analysis of primary care prescribing patterns in England', *British Journal of General Practice Open*. Available at: http://doi.org/10.3399/bjgpopen19X101662

Hood, C. (1995) 'The "new public management" in the 1980s: Variations on a theme.' *Accounting, Organizations and Society* 20(2/3): 93–109.

Illich, I. (1977) *Limits to Medicine: Medical Nemesis: The Expropriation of Health*, Harmondsworth: Penguin.

Justinia, T. (2016) 'The UK's national programme for IT: Why was it dismantled?', *Health Services Management Research* 30(1): 2–9; 73: 1–23.

Kjellström, S., Areskoug-Josefsson, K., Gäre, B. A., Andersson, A.-C., Ockander, M., Käll, J., McGrath, J., Donetto, S. and Robert, G. (2019) 'Exploring, measuring and enhancing the coproduction of health and well-being at the national, regional and local levels through comparative case studies in Sweden and England: The "Samskapa" research programme protocol', *BMJ Open* 9: e029723. Available at: http://doi.org/10.1136/bmjopen-2019-029723

Klein, K. (1990) 'The state and the profession: The politics of the double bed', *British Medical Journal* 301: 700–2.

Krause, E. (1996) *Death of the Guilds: Professions, States and the Advance of Capitalism, 1930 to the Present*, New Haven, CT: Yale University Press.

Light, D. (1995) 'Countervailing powers: A framework for professions in transition', in Johnson, T., Larkin, G. and Saks, M. (eds) *Health Professions and the State in Europe*, London: Routledge.

Light, D. (2003) 'Universal health care: Lessons from the British experience', *American Journal of Public Health* 93(1): 25–30.

Light, D. (2004) 'Introduction – ironies of success: A new history of the American health care "system"', *Journal of Health and Social Behaviour* 45(Extra Issue): 1–24.

Light, D. (2010) 'Health care professions, markets and countervailing powers', in Bird, C., Conrad, P., Fremont, A. and Timmermans, S. (eds) *Handbook of Medical Sociology*, 6th edition, Nashville: Vanderbilt University Press.

Light, D. and Levine, S. (1988) 'The changing character of the medical profession', *The Milbank Quarterly* 66(2): 10–32.

Mentis, I. (2022) 'The introduction of Health Technology Assessment (HTA) in Greece and comparison with the European experience', *Archives of Hellenic Medicine* 39(3): 313–21.

Moran, M. (2000) 'Understanding the welfare state: The case of health care', *British Journal of Politics and International Relations* 2(2): 135–60.

Mouzelis, N. P. (1986) *Politics in the Semi-Periphery: Early Parliamentarism in the Balkans and Latin America*, Basingstoke: Macmillan.

Olejaz, M., Juul Nielson, A., Rudkjøbing, A., Birk, H., Krasnik, A. and Hernández-Quevedo, C. (2012) 'Denmark: Health system review', *Health Systems in Transition* 14(2): 1–192.

Pavolini, E. and Spina, E. (2015) 'Users' involvement in the Italian NHS: The role of associations and self-help groups', *Journal of Health Organization and Management* 29(5): 570–81.

Pierson, P. (2000) 'The limits of design: Explaining institutional origins and change', *Governance* 13(4): 475–99.

Raddon Keefe, P. (2022) *Empire of Pain*, Basingstoke: Picador.

Relman, A. S. (1980) 'The new medical-industrial complex', *New England Journal of Medicine* 303(17): 963–70.

Riska, E. (2001) 'Health professions and occupations', in Cockerham, W. C. (ed) *The Blackwell Companion to Medical Sociology*, Oxford: Blackwell.

Rycroft-Malone, J., Seers, K., Titchen, A., Harvey, G., Kitson, A. and McCormack, B. (2004) 'What counts as evidence in evidence-based practice?', *Journal of Advanced Nursing* 47(1): 81–90.

Sackett, D. L. and Rosenberg, W. M. C. (1995) 'The need for evidence-based medicine', *Journal of the Royal Society of Medicine* 88: 620–4.

Saks, M. (2016) 'A review of theories of professions, organizations and society: The case for neo-Weberianism, neo-institutionalism and eclecticism', *Journal of Professions and Organization* 3: 170–87.

Saltman, R. B. and Figueras, J. (1998) 'Analyzing the evidence on European health care reforms', *Health Affairs* 17(2): 85–108.

Saunes, I. S., Karanikolos, M. and Sagan, A. (2020) 'Norway: Health systems review', *Health Systems in Transition* 22(1): v–163.

Simões, J., Augusto, G. F., Fronteira, I. and Hernández-Quevedo, C. (2017) 'Portugal: Health systems review', *Health Systems in Transition* 19(2): 1–184.

Statista (2022) 'US national health expenditure as percent of GDP from 1960 to 2020', *Source CMS (Office of the Actuary)*. Available at: www.statista.com

Sveman, E. and Essinger, K. (2001) 'Procurement of health care services in Sweden in general, and the example of procurement of acute care in the Stockholm Region', in *European Integration and Health Care Systems: A Challenge for Social Policy*, Stockholm: Swedish Federation of County Councils. Available at: www.yumpu.com/en/document/view/30880148/procurement-of-health-care-services-in-sweden-in-general-the-

Voorberg, W. H., Bekkers, V. J. J. M. and Tummers, L. G. (2015) 'A systematic review of co-creation and co-production: Embarking on the social innovation journey', *Public Management Review* 17(9): 1333–57.

Waitzkin, H. and the Working Group on Health Beyond Capitalism (2018) *Health Care Under the Knife: Moving Beyond Capitalism for Our Health*, New York: Monthly Review Press.

Wilsford, D. (1994) 'Path dependency, or why history makes it difficult but not impossible to reform health care systems in a big way', *Journal of Public Policy* 14(3): 251–83.

Conclusion

Challenges, reforms and future perspectives

Guido Giarelli and Mike Saks

Introduction

At the end of our collective undertaking, it is worth trying to synthesise the main results that emerged from the various chapters of the book within a neo-Weberian and neo-institutionalist frame of reference (Saks, 2016). Here we shall briefly summarise the answers to the questions posed to contributors in this part of the book, as set out in the Introduction, by drawing on the comparative perspective provided by the British, Scandinavian and Mediterranean macro-regions with National Health Services (NHSs) in Western Europe. In doing so, we shall also consider the specific analyses that we have asked the authors to undertake in Part II of the book – about the role played by the actors involved in the NHSs in comparison with different healthcare systems, namely, the state, the medical and health professions, patients and the public, and the medical–industrial complex. A key question here is that of how this role, has or has not, has changed in facing the challenges of the last four decades as a consequence of neo-liberal reform policies in the societies concerned. This in turn provides an important pointer to the future development of such healthcare systems as distinct from others – such as those based on social insurance and private insurance – in Western Europe.

The timing of the origins of the National Health Services

If we start with a short historical reconstruction of the origins of NHSs in the three European health macro-regions, we are immediately faced with chronological differences in terms of their historical periods of origin. The first was the British NHS in 1948. This was followed by the transformation of the previous Scandinavian social insurance systems into universal public schemes from the 1950s to the early 1970s – Sweden in 1955, Norway in 1967 and Denmark in 1971. Finally, in the Mediterranean countries, NHSs were established between the end of the 1970s and the 1980s – in 1978 in Italy, in 1979 in Portugal, in 1983 in Greece and in 1986 in Spain. This means that, in terms of timing, there is a gap of almost 40 years between the first (UK) and the last (Spain) in setting up the NHSs.

DOI: 10.4324/9781003139799-20

This is a long time during which many things have changed, including the transition from the 'golden age' of the welfare state of the post-war era (Pierson, 1998), the economic crisis of the 1970s, and the neo-liberal reforms from the 1980s. This has not been without consequences in terms of the political, economic and cultural contexts of the NHS. The British NHS enjoyed a long period of stability until the first reform of 1974, despite the problems of scarcity of allocated resources and a lack of strategic planning and weak upward accountability. Nordic social insurance systems could also develop during this period through a gradual expansion of their coverage and organisation for the delivery of healthcare services guided by the ideals of public planning and public health promotion of a consolidated social democratic political tradition.

On the other hand, the Mediterranean NHSs were set up at the end of the period as part of a more general democratisation process of political and social institutions, after the overthrow of previous authoritarian regimes in Spain, Portugal and Greece, and the demand for a more universalistic model of healthcare supported by left-wing parties and social and political movements of the 1960s and 1970s in Italy. However, the change in the general international political and cultural climate during the 1980s, with the emergence of neo-liberal policies and New Public Management (NPM) strategies in healthcare, has made the time for the implementation of these NHS systems much shorter and more problematic than in the British and Nordic cases. The questioning of the welfare state and universalistic healthcare systems in the new climate has stirred up social forces and actors such as private insurances, private hospitals and most doctors who were ideologically averse to the new universalistic systems in these countries. This has made the implementation of the new NHSs in these countries extremely complex and difficult, which in each country were answered by governments with different results.

In Italy, the implementation of the *Servizio Sanitario Nazionale* (SSN) was severely hampered during the 1980s by scarce funding and delays in enacting regulations. This has made the process of its institutionalisation extremely hard, due to the difficulties in transforming the structures of the previous scattered and unequal social insurance system into the new unified national system. Moreover, this process has been poorly governed at both national and local levels of government: at national level, the minister of health was a member of the Liberal Party, the only party that had voted against the institution of the SSN; at local level, the newly instituted management boards of the SSN, the *Comitati di Gestione* were divided up among the political parties and, consequently, they gave a very bad account of themselves in terms of incompetence and corruption.

In Spain, the existence of one single fund instituted in 1943 by the Franco government as a compulsory health insurance scheme (*Seguro Obligatorio de Enfermidad*) has made the transition to the new *Sistema Nacional de Salud* (SNS) easier, although this process needed to be carried out gradually as a result of the progressive inclusion of all pre-existent health-care services into a single institution. This did not mean that there were no obstacles, especially by public employees and armed forces funds and anti-reformist social actors such as doctors. However, the new democratic regime was able to overcome these problems thanks to the general political and cul-tural climate and the democratisation of decision-making, in particular with the devolution of central power to the regions (*Comunidades Autónomas*) and the progressively regionally decentralised character of the SNS.

If Italy and Spain were substantially able to introduce their own NHSs even if there were significant problems, it was different in the other two Med-iterranean countries. In Portugal, the establishment of the *Serviço Nacional de Saúde* (SNS) did not lead to the abolition of the previous social insurance schemes, which continued to cover almost a quarter of the population. This had the consequence of creating a three-tier system, with the SNS supple-mented by social funds and private voluntary insurances. This only partial implementation of radical reforms and strategic plans has also typically char-acterised subsequent attempts at reform the SNS.

In Greece, things got worse when, with the restoration of democracy in 1974 after seven years of dictatorship, in 1980 the first attempt to estab-lish an NHS by a right-wing government was rejected. In 1983, the subse-quent socialist government was able to approve its constitution, but it largely remained as a paper exercise as it was never or only partially implemented in practice – neither through urban primary healthcare centres nor through the unification of health insurance funds. Consequently, a three-tier system was created here too, given the impossibility of undermining the power of the sickness funds and the strong and persistent role of the private health sector incorporating clinics, laboratories and doctors.

Recent healthcare reforms: are they neo-liberal?

What qualifies a healthcare reform as 'neo-liberal'? If we follow the three general principles of neo-liberalism outlined by McGregor (2001) of free markets, individualism and decentralisation, we can consider the first as implying in healthcare a policy oriented towards controlling costs and public health expenditures, economic efficiency, privatisation and competition/mar-ketisation of service delivery. This has materialised over the past four decades in two main strategies: austerity and the NPM. The former has represented the dominant response at international level to the financial crisis that has spread across the world since 2007, mainly based on the retrenchment of public services and employees, and on the privatisation of public services (Basu, Carney and Kenworths, 2017). The latter is a style of governance of public services and administration centred on the principles of private enter-prise and managerialism aimed at improving their efficiency (Lane, 2000).

But if the first characteristic of a neo-liberal policy is 'marketisation' (Van der Hoeven and Sziráczki, 1997), the second feature is individualism, which assumes that people act independent of each other, rationally pursuing their own self-interest. This is based on an idea of the individual who rationally chooses in the market; when applied to healthcare, the ideal patient is considered to be a responsible and informed consumer, able to choose among different service options which are viewed as commodities. Freedom of choice is therefore strictly linked to marketisation, as choice is believed to fuel competition between healthcare providers, thereby promoting quality and maximising efficiency (Gabe, Harley and Calnan, 2015). The third interlinked feature of a neo-liberal policy is decentralisation, which – although it can have other ideological origins – implies a rescaling of services and their management to the territorial levels closest to the user to improve quality and efficiency. It is argued that this promotes greater accountability of services for citizens and their needs, and greater responsiveness to them at local and regional levels of governance.

If we apply these three neo-liberal tenets to a comparative analysis of the healthcare reforms implemented during the last four decades in the three health macro-regions, we can see that is not possible to designate all of them as 'neo-liberal'. While in the British health macro-region, we can certainly define as such all the reforms adopted by the English governments from Thatcher to date, it is problematic to apply the same label to the Scottish and Welsh health policies carried out after devolution. Their objectives and content are more oriented towards greater equity in access to public healthcare services, instead of freedom of choice between public and private services, and improvement in the quality of healthcare services through citizen involvement and co-production instead of marketisation. Even the decentralisation adopted has not meant, as in England, the delegation of contracts and delivery of services to local private purchasers and agencies, but rather a greater involvement of local communities in their NHSs.

The picture in the Scandinavian health macro-region is also diverse: in each country, different types of health policies have been adopted in different periods. In Sweden, most of the reforms introduced since the 1990s can be considered neo-liberal, since they were mainly oriented towards marketisation by experimenting with market-oriented organisational models like the purchaser–provider split and performance-based payment. They also allowed freedom of choice for patients between public and private providers, in particular specialist physicians and general practitioners (GPs). However, some of these reforms were later modified or reversed by subsequent governments of a different political orientation, making their implementation quite discontinuous and intermittent. Decentralisation was instead a fundamental characteristic of the previous system in the post-war period, but it meant a complex division of labour and responsibility between the national, regional and local levels. Various attempts were made to re-scale the system of multi-level governance from the 1990s – which led to a re-centralisation of governing power by merging county councils into larger regions and strengthening national authorities, but they either failed or were only partially applied.

In Denmark, no significant neo-liberal reforms have been introduced, since GPs and specialist physicians were already private, albeit tightly integrated into public planning and regulation, whereas the ownership of hospitals has remained public. However, here the 2007 structural reform created larger municipalities and regions by merging former counties, thus moving a previously decentralised multi-level governance system towards centralisation and increasing the power of national government. Overall, the Danish case has shifted towards a form of New Public Governance (NPG) based on a multi-level network collaboration of democratic public institutions, including the state, regions and municipalities. However, this has been combined with limited elements of neo-liberal governance such as the use of performance-based incentives for regions and hospitals, the growth of voluntary health insurance and the inclusion of private hospitals and clinics into treatment guarantee policies to assert patient rights and create pressure on public hospitals.

In Norway, the situation is different again, since a major reform was introduced by the Labour government in 2002 transferring hospital ownership from county councils to the central government following the principles of the NPM and a private enterprise model. The adoption of activity-based funding in hospitals in 1997, the Family Doctor Reform in 2001 by which GPs were essentially privatised, and the free choice of all public and private hospitals in 2014 were also part of the general trend of implementing neo-liberal reforms, albeit based on centralisation.

Even in Mediterranean countries, the situation is rather disparate. In Italy, neo-liberal reform was concentrated in the early 1990s period, with the corporatisation of Local Health Authorities transforming them into public enterprises governed by managers and replacing previous management committees. Moreover, during the 2010s, after the economic crisis, severe austerity health policies were adopted which significantly reduced both public hospitals and personnel. However, between the first reform introducing the NHS in 1978 and the third reforms of 1999 and 2000 promoting primary healthcare, the more integrated social and healthcare services in the districts and regionally decentralised management of services were more oriented towards equity in access to services and a form of managed cooperation different to neo-liberal managed competition.

In Spain, the most serious attempt at implementing a neo-liberal reform of the NHS with some success was the austerity policy adopted by the Coalition government in 2012 because of the severe economic crisis. This led to an increasing role of central government in a strongly decentralised system on regional basis, budgetary cuts and retrenchment measures, and a restriction of universal access to healthcare through a return to a corporatist entitlement excluding unauthorised immigrants. While the Spanish NHS has shown a low degree of permeability to neo-liberal measures, in Portugal, the implementation of neo-liberal health policies in a three-tier system has been much easier since the 1990s, with the adoption of NPM strategies and public–private partnerships in the hospital sector. These were further strengthened by the austerity policy enacted after the 2008 financial crisis and the Memorandum of Understanding signed by the Portuguese government with the Troika (the European Union Commission, European Central Bank and International Monetary Fund), which imposed a readjustment programme with punitive austerity measures to increase cost containment and public debt reduction up to middle of 2015.

The austerity policy was even worse in Greece. After the neo-liberal strategies adopted by the conservative government in 1992 in favour of an already strong private sector containing clinics, hospitals and diagnostic centres, the three Economic Adjustment Programmes implemented during the period 2010 to 2018 as consequence of the Memorandum of Understanding (MoU) signed by the Greek government with the Troika resulted in the loss of social health insurance rights of over 2.5 million people – as well as the imposition of public health spending restrictions, increased user charges and co-payments, and salary cuts and layoffs of healthcare personnel.

Overall, we can say that only the case of England shows real continuity in the adoption of neo-liberal policies during the last four decades, while in the case of Scotland and Wales and the other two health macro-regions there was an evident discontinuity of health policies in the same period. In the latter countries and regions, not all the policies introduced were of a neo-liberal orientation, so we can more correctly speak of a plurality of reforms based on different policy orientations.

The impact of the health reform policies

As regards the impact of the health reform policies, these will be considered on the architecture of the NHSs, and on the related issue of population health. We shall first examine to what extent these policies have or not significantly altered the three fundamental components of an NHS: financing, service organisation, and governance of the system. Starting with funding, in none of the NHSs in the three health macro-regions considered has public financing based on taxation been modified or cancelled. Indeed, this is probably the only point in common between neo-liberal and non-neo-liberal policies, although there has been a significant increase in private health insurance in certain of the countries, such as in England and societies in Scandinavia, where they were traditionally more marginal.

The picture changes significantly when we look at the organisation of services: here practically in all the NHSs, the impact of neo-liberal policies altered the ratio between public and private healthcare services in favour of the latter. This is not true for the hospital sector, which has remained mostly public, apart from some not very encouraging experimentation with public–private partnerships in England, Spain and Portugal. However, especially in Scandinavian and Mediterranean NHSs such as Italy, there was a radical rationalisation of public hospitals, with a marked decrease of hospital beds, reduction of staff, shortening of hospital stays, and increased specialisation among hospitals. Unlike the position with funding, in terms of service organisation, this has inevitably impacted on population health in terms of access to care.

GPs and medical specialists, on the other hand, have increasingly become self-employed professionals, as in Sweden, together with their clinics, diagnostic and health centres in most counties. Here there has been a significant difference between those purely in private practice who operate in the free market on a fee-for-service basis, such as in Portugal and Greece, and those who are paid on capitation basis by the government like in England, or by the municipalities as in Norway. In general, this has corresponded to a strengthening of primary care services, in terms of both freedom of choice and chance of access to services, especially in those NHSs where the primary sector was considerably weaker than the secondary one, such as in Sweden with its Primary Care Choice Reform in 2010.

In other countries like Spain, where the primary healthcare sector was already stronger, GPs and medical specialists have remained public employees working in public health centres. What has continued to be problematic, though, in almost all cases, is long-term care for the chronically ill and elderly, where considerable problems of funding and integration between public and private, hospital and municipal, health and social services persist. Neo-liberal reforms have therefore left these issues substantially unchanged to the detriment of users. Some improvements have only been made in England, Scotland, Wales, Sweden, Denmark and Norway with reforms that attempted to create unified pathways for patients to overcome the fragmentation and silo organisation of services, even if their implementation has proved problematic.

However, neo-liberal reforms have undoubtedly left the greatest imprint on the governance of NHS systems. The 'internal market' or the 'quasi-market', as it has been called since it has only been partially implemented in experiments (Le Grand and Bartlett, 1993), probably represents the hallmark of neo-liberal governance. However, apart from England where the split between purchasers and providers was tested for the first time and is still in place, it was only loosely adopted in Sweden by some counties, in Norway with the hospital reform, very partially in the Italian NHS with the reform of 1992 and in Denmark with the 'free choice of hospitals' from 1993 and treatment guarantees with a choice of private hospitals if waiting times exceed 30 days for diagnosis in public hospitals. In such cases, cracks have appeared in market-based health provision for consumers. In this light, it is not surprising that Scotland and Wales dismantled the internal market after devolution, returning to a unified governance system defined as 'state stewardship'.

As has been seen, a distinctive trait of neo-liberal policies in terms of population health has been the NPM, which has found widespread application especially in England and the Scandinavian countries, and less fully in Italy and Spain, changing the style of traditional hierarchical government of public administration to a private enterprise style of governance. It was introduced especially for hospital management to improve medical quality and the efficiency of services. However, even though it has made professionals more productive and responsive to patient demands, in most cases it has resulted in high levels of stress for practitioners, and a shift in the traditional relationship of trust between doctor and patient. Although there is widespread empathy from the public, this has been challenged in Britain by the recent wave of strikes over pay and conditions by health personnel from paramedics to nurses – the latter of whom have never before taken such action, not least in the history of the NHS (Ford, 2023).

Another effect of neo-liberal governance has sometimes been re-centralisation, even though it appears to have gone against one of the fundamental neo-liberal principles of decentralisation. Nonetheless, if we look at the Scandinavian countries where it has been mostly implemented, its rationale was the same as that of decentralisation – to improve the quality and efficiency of the services while containing their cost. Therefore, the actual rationale behind it is not specifically decentralisation, but a re-scaling process that could enable these objectives to be pursued. In other words, re-scaling in Scandinavian countries has taken the form of re-centralisation because their traditional multi-level decentralised structure of governance was believed to hinder the effective and coordinated pursuit of neo-liberal policies to the benefit of users.

Although patterns of re-centralisation – and indeed, in some circumstances, decentralisation – may have had positive effects for patients, austerity, which is a further feature that neo-liberal governance has assumed in the NHSs considered, definitively has not. This is especially true of Mediterranean countries like Portugal and Greece, the governments of which signed the MoU with the Troika during the 2010s due to their sovereign debts. This meant that most of the governance powers of their national governments shifted to international actors. As a result, the harsh punitive measures imposed by the Troika's package negatively impacted on population health by leading to increased social inequalities in healthcare and the reduction of healthcare expenditure and services in their NHSs.

In terms of gauging the overall impact of neo-liberal reforms on population health, though, one problem is that it is difficult to separate the net effect of health policy reforms from other causal factors, such as other policies, economic situations, and medical technology innovations. However, what it is possible to do is to consider major upward trends in life expectancy at birth, healthy life years at birth and infant mortality rates, all of which were positive except in the two countries of Portugal and Greece. Here, as noted, they were subjected to the austerity measures imposed by the Troika, where the prevalence of non-communicable diseases and psychological distress were among the highest in Europe – even before the arrival of Covid-19. After the pandemic, epidemiological indicators significantly deteriorated in several other Western European countries. Nonetheless, even the positive trends before Covid-19 could be reversed in the coming years if the public health sector is not adequately strengthened in face of possible future pandemics.

Are the National Health Services sustainable in the near future?

As is well known, the issue of sustainability cannot be reduced simply to the financial viability of healthcare systems, since the political issue of public legitimacy by citizens who pay for them and the socio-epidemiological issue of their ability to meet the needs and demands of the population are equally relevant. Adopting this comprehensive perspective, it appears that European NHSs should be able to survive according to the LSE-Lancet Commission (Anderson et al., 2021), despite demographic and epidemiological trends that pose serious challenges for the foreseeable future in terms of population ageing and the prevalence of chronic diseases. Among these challenges, the rising demand for more and higher quality social and healthcare services requires a radical transformation focused on prevention and early intervention, and a reconfiguration of services to develop primary and community care and relieve the hospital sector. Of course, this will require not only more funding and efficiency savings but also doing 'only what is needed' as a key mechanism for increasing value for money under the 'prudent healthcare principles' proposed by countries such as Wales.

In terms of political sustainability and public legitimacy, a number of complementary issues should be addressed. First is growing inequalities in health in relation to social class, territorial divides and ethnicity (particularly linked to immigrants and refugees), where there is a problem of trust regarding professionals in public health authorities, which requires a dialogue respectful of cultural differences about life-style changes. There is also a problem of fragmentation especially in primary care services; privatisation and competition among providers has destroyed the previous system of locally based responsibility for population health in countries like Sweden, reducing prevention and promotion of health to individualised issues. In addition, the strong growth of private health insurance in all countries with NHSs increases the risk of gradually creating a two-tiered system with the emergence of a parallel private market – a risk that will grow if the NHSs are not be able to satisfy the needs and demands of users.

This brings us to a final dimension of sustainability based on socio-epidemiology, which relates to issues such as waiting lists, the digital divide, social and healthcare integration, preparedness for future pandemics and availability of human resources – including the tendency for doctors and nurses to seek employment outside the public sector and, indeed, to leave the profession altogether. Maintaining a satisfactory service and quality standard in the NHS is a critical challenge for its future, which requires consideration of expectations and health needs on one side and organisational, professional and technological possibilities on the other. Market-based reforms have not shown evidence of real benefits to date in this respect (Anderson et al., 2021);

the continuation of a 'publicly funded NHS for all' remains the baseline from which to move to imagine and implement new creative solutions, which are less doctor-centric and hospital-oriented, and capable of addressing both communicable and non-communicable diseases – in light of known social determinants of health and environmental and behavioural risk factors.

Conclusion

How far, then, have the neo-liberal health reforms of the last four decades significantly changed the NHSs of Western Europe? And to what extent have they remained national health systems? All the authors of this volume agree here that – despite the more or less strong impact that the neo-liberal reforms have had and the significant changes they have produced – the NHSs have proved to be resilient institutions. They continue to be based on solid and still valid principles of equality, universalism, comprehensiveness and solidarity (Allsop, 1995), capable of responding to old and new challenges such as scarce resources, rising costs, increasing demands and rising expectations by adapting their structures and processes of functioning.

Certainly, the analysis of the historical construction of the NHS in the three health macro-regions has shown that the implementation of the Mediterranean NHSs has been particularly troubled. Moreover, the architecture of all the NHSs has more or less radically changed as a consequence of neo-liberal reforms. If public funding of them has remained largely untouched, the organisation and management of services have been changed due to their increased marketisation and privatisation, and the introduction of NPM business management principles – not least in the English and Scandinavian NHSs. However, the lack of evidence that the stated objectives of these neo-liberal reforms have been achieved has generated general political resistance. It has also underlined the need to experiment with new and alternative forms of service organisation which are less market-oriented, like co-production in Scotland and the NPG in Denmark, with stronger democratic participation in the governance of healthcare. Furthermore, most of the NHSs considered have shown a high degree of continuity based on path dependence in terms of their overall structures and processes, pointing to the important role of historical, political, economic and cultural contexts in shaping reform (Wilsford, 1994).

According to the supporters of 'hybridisation' theory (Schmid et al., 2010), we should perhaps speak of the emergence of hybrid systems as a soft form of convergence among different types of national health systems instead of solid state NHSs. As the same scholars admit, the growing relevance of marketisation and privatisation does not imply a structural change in the state-led systems because the implementation of neo-liberal reforms has entailed further state interventions to guarantee the functioning of the quasi-market. What has actually happened is that the NHSs have integrated state hierarchy with market-style modes of regulation. However, as we have seen, this has not been generalised on a contiguous timescale. In practice the various cases considered have, to a greater or lesser degree, had different orientations, so that we should speak more correctly of a plurality of reforms. Therefore, following the suggestion by Hassenteufel and Palier (2007) about 'neo-Bismarckian' healthcare systems with regard to social health insurance in France and Germany, we could similarly define as 'neo-Beveridgian' the NHS-type systems after the last four decades of pluralistic reforms in Western Europe, which have both preserved and renewed their identity. In summary, then, the original Beveridgian principles of the NHS still remain, but must be updated and regenerated to address ever-occurring challenges if their sustainability is to be ensured in the future.

References

Allsop, J. (1995) *Health Policy and the NHS*, 2nd edition, London: Longman.

Anderson, M., Pitchforth, E., Asaria, M., et al. (2021) 'LSE-Lancet Commission on the future of the NHS: Re-laying the foundations for an equitable and efficient health and care service after COVID-19', *Lancet Commissions* 397(10288): 1915–78.

Basu, S., Carney, M. A. and Kenworths, N. J. (2017) 'Ten years after the financial crisis: The long reach of austerity and its global impact on health', *Social Science and Medicine* 187: 203–7.

Ford, M. (2023) 'Nurses fighting for fair pay head to Downing Street', *Nursing Times*, 2 February. Available at: www.nursingtimes.net/news/workforce/nurses-fighting-for-fair-pay-head-to-downing-street-02-02-2023/

Gabe, J., Harley, K. and Calnan, M. (2015) 'Healthcare choice: Discourses, perceptions, experiences and practice', *Current Sociology* 63(5): 623–35.

Hassenteufel, P. and Palier, B. (2007) 'Towards neo-Bismarckian health care states? Comparing health insurance reforms in Bismarckian welfare systems', *Social Policy and Administration* 41(6): 574–96.

Lane, J.-E. (2000) *New Public Management. An Introduction*, London: Routledge.

Le Grand, J. and Bartlett, W. (1993) *Quasi-markets and Social Policy*, London: Palgrave Macmillan.

McGregor, S. (2001) 'Neoliberalism and health care', *International Journal of Consumer Studies* 25(2): 82–9.

Pierson, C. (1998) 'Contemporary challenges to welfare state development', *Political Studies* 66(4): 777–94.

Saks, M. (2016) 'Review of theories of professions, organizations and society: Neo-Weberianism, neo-institutionalism and eclecticism', *Journal of Professions and Organization* 3(2): 170–87.

Schmid, A., Cacace, M., Götze, R., Rothgang, H. (2010) 'Explaining health care system change: Problem pressure and the emergence of "hybrid" health care systems', *Journal of Health Politics, Policy and Law* 35(4): 455–86.

Van der Hoeven, R. and Sziráczki, G. (1997) *Lessons From Privatization*, Geneva: International Labour Organization.

Wilsford, D. (1994) 'Path dependency, or why history makes it difficult but not impossible to reform health care systems in a big way', *Journal of Public Policy* 14: 251–83.

Index

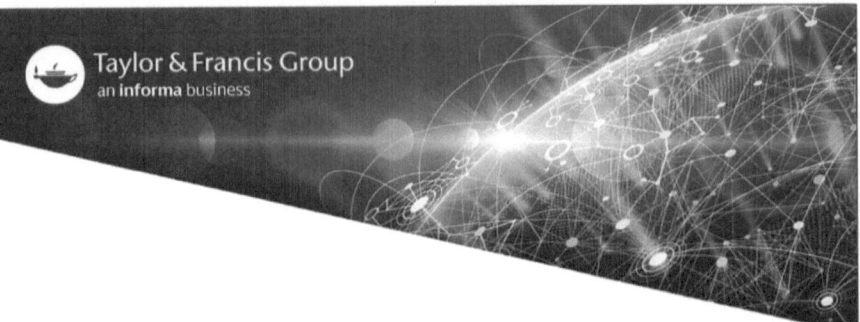
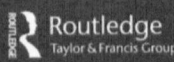
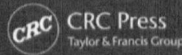